Novel Advances in Glucocorticoids

Novel Advances in Glucocorticoids

Edited by **Reginald Thornburg**

hayle
medical

New York

Published by Hayle Medical,
30 West, 37th Street, Suite 612,
New York, NY 10018, USA
www.haylemedical.com

Novel Advances in Glucocorticoids
Edited by Reginald Thornburg

International Standard Book Number: 978-1-63241-301-7 (Hardback)

Contents

Preface

Glucocorticoids have been acknowledged as one of the most essential steroid hormones, for its therapeutic benefits have been used in clinical treatments, particularly in anti-inflammation cases. Glucocorticoids controls several processes in the body also with the mobilization of energy stores, immune system, gene expression, and upholding of the homeostasis as well as the stress response, this is not unexpected that the theory of "glucocorticoids" is talked about in almost all medical books that aims on definite organs or systems such as the cardiovascular system, the immune system, and the neuroendocrine system. This book aims to reveal the newest researches linked to glucocorticoids, from the laboratory or from clinical case studies, and targets to create a scope of balancing the therapeutic benefits and problems caused by glucocorticoids.

All of the data presented henceforth was collaborated in the wake of recent advancements in the field. The aim of this book is to present the diversified developments from across the globe in a comprehensible manner. The opinions expressed in each chapter belong solely to the contributing authors. Their interpretations of the topics are the integral part of this book, which I have carefully compiled for a better understanding of the readers.

At the end, I would like to thank all those who dedicated their time and efforts for the successful completion of this book. I also wish to convey my gratitude towards my friends and family who supported me at every step.

Editor

Behind the Curtain: The Mechanisms of the Impacts of Glucocorticoids

Mechanisms of Glucocorticoid Receptor (GR) Mediated Corticotropin Releasing Hormone Gene Expression

Rosalie M. Uht

Additional information is available at the end of the chapter

1. Introduction

Normal physiologic functioning is dependent on the maintenance of homeostasis in the face of numerous stressors. Responses to stress include the fight or flight reaction and activation of the sympathetic nervous and endocrine systems. The central component of the endocrine response is the hypothalamic-pituitary-adrenal (HPA) axis, which when activated leads to increased levels of circulating glucocorticoids. Indeed, an increase in glucocorticoids has been used as an operational definition of stress.

The HPA axis is activated by a wide range of stimuli which includes perception of danger, pain, sepsis, and others. These stimuli are integrated at points throughout the central nervous system and ultimately impinge on the HPA axis motor neurons in the paraventricular nucleus of the hypothalamus (PVH). HPA neurons synthesize and secrete corticotropin releasing factors (crfs), the best known of which is the 41 amino acid peptide corticotropin releasing hormone (CRH);(Vale et al 1981)). CRH travels through the hypothalamic portal circulation to the anterior pituitary where it binds CRH receptors. This in turn leads to adrenocorticotrophic hormone (ACTH) secretion into the systemic circulation which stimulates the adrenal cortex to secrete glucocorticoids.

Glucocorticoids elicit gluconeogenesis, which increases circulating levels of glucose. Although this mechanism is adaptive in the face of a homeostatic challenge, glucocorticoids can also have deleterious effects. Dysregulation of the HPA axis underlies classic endocrine disorders, such as Cushing's disease. and is highly correlated with a number of psychiatric disorders, including post-traumatic stress disorder, anorexia nervosa, and depression. In addition, high circulating levels of glucocorticoids lead to osteopenia and immunosuppression. Thus, regulation of the HPA axis must be exquisitely controlled.

There are numerous components to HPA axis down-regulation; one of the most significant of these is the end product of HPA axis regulation itself – glucocorticoids. Glucocorticoids down-regulate axis activity by acting at numerous loci in the HPA axis and in extra-hypothalamic regions of the brain, such as the hippocampus(de Kloet et al 2005, (Sapolsky et al 1984). Glucocorticoid regulation in the hippocampus, extra-hypothalamic sites and pituitary are reviewed below.

1.1. Glucocorticoidregulation of the hippocampal-hypothalamic pathway

Glucocorticoid receptors (GRs) are most densely concentrated in the hippocampus of the central nervous system (CNS), and in fact it is in the hippocampus where glucocorticoid binding sites were first detected(McEwen et al 1979). GRs were first classified by their binding characteristics. Two types were identified, distinguished in part by their binding characteristics to corticosterone and the synthetic glucocorticoid dexamethasone (Dex) (de Kloet et al 1975). After steroid receptor cloning it became apparent that the two receptors correlate to the mineralocorticoid receptor (MR) and the GR. The GR is recruited in the presence of high levels of circulating glucocorticoids elicited in the face of stress (de Kloet et al 2005).

Down-regulatory signals from the hippocampus are processed through a multisynaptic pathway. Hippocampal projections to the subiculum elicit excititory signals in the form of glutamatergic synapses in the basal nucleus of the stria terminalis (BNST). These stimulate inhibitory output from the BNST, which in turn down regulates the HPA axis. Thus, damage to the hippocampus leads to loss of HPA axis inhibition (Choi et al 2007, Herman et al 2003).

1.2. Glucocorticoid regulation at the level of the pituitary

One of the best studied components of glucocorticoid down-regulation of the HPA axis is ligand-bound GR-mediated down-regulation of the gene that codes for the ACTH precursor, pre-pro-opiomenlanocortin (POMC)(Bicknell 2008). As is the case   in other cells, glucocorticoids gain entry to the cyptoplasm and bind the cytoplasmic GR. Ligand binding activates the receptor, a process that includes dissociation from the heat shock protein 90 (hsp90) as reviewed by Pratt and Dittmar(Pratt & Dittmar 1998). The ligand-bound receptor is transported into the nucleus where it interacts with numerous nuclear proteins and chromatin to regulate transcription. Prototypically, the GR binds to glucocorticoid response elements that are inverted palindromes; however, the regulatory region of *pomc* does not have such elements. Rather, it has a negative glucocorticoid response elements (nGREs) – hybrid elements also called composite elements. GRs bind these sites as monomers and interact with monomers of other transcription factors to down-regulate *pomc* transcription. GRs also repress transcription in the absence of direct DNA binding by modulating the activity of other transcription factors. In these aspects *pomc* regulation is similar to regulation of *crh*.

A significant difference between the synthesis of CRH and ACTH is the relative contribution of post-translational enzymatic processing. In the case of CRH synthesis, one peptide is produced, thus, the majority of regulatory steps are pre-translational. Conversely, numerous peptides are generated from *pomc* These include ACTH, beta-endorphin, and alpha-melanocyte stimulating hormone. Thus, pre-pro-POMC enzymatic processing plays a major role in determining levels of functional ACTH.

1.3. Hypothalamic crfs

CRH-expressing parvocellular neurons are the final common integrators of humeral and synaptic input. Located in the mpPVH, they receive inputs from numerous sites in the CNS: the hippocampus, brainstem, amygdala, intrahypothalamic sites, and PVH interneurons. (Swanson & Sawchenko 1980).

Although CRH is the most potent and best known crf, it is only one of several. Prior to the biochemical characterization of CRH(Vale et al 1981), arginine vasopressin (AVP) and oxytocin were also known to have crf properties(Gibbs 1986). Perhaps the most studied of these is AVP, best known for its activity as an anti-diuretic hormone. AVP arises from PVH magnocellular neurons whose terminals secrete AVP directly into the systemic circulation.The AVP that acts as a crf is synthesized in parvocellular neurons of the PVH. Interestingly, all parvocellular neurons that express AVP also express CRH. Furthermore, all of these express GRs(Cintra et al 1987, Uht et al 1988), and their function is measured by the ability to translocate into the nucleus in the presence of Dex(Uht et al 1988).

2. Glucocorticoid receptors

Many biochemical and pharmacologic properties of GRs were characterized prior to cloning (Gustafsson et al 1987). The existence of the MR and the GR was determined pharmacologically. In the absence of ligand the GR was present in a cytoplasmic complex. In the presence of ligand, the GR was present in the nucleus. Furthermore, ligand bound GR had been shown to bind specific sites in DNA, which came to be known as glucocorticoid response elements (GREs). Thus, before cloning the fundamental differences between a steroid receptor and receptors for other hormones had been determined. The GR was an intracellular receptor rather than a plasma membrane bound receptor and its mechanism of action involved binding DNA. Hence the term that evolved -- Ligand activated nuclear receptors.

2.1. Glucocorticoid receptor cloning and identification of functional domain

The initial cloning of the GR revealed two GRs: alpha and beta. Oakley *et al* discovered that GR beta did not bind ligand(Oakley et al. 1996) -- biological functions of GR-beta are still in the early stages of discovery(Yudt & Cidlowski 2002). This review focuses on GR-alpha, which will be referred to as GR.

2.2. GR as a founding member of the nuclear receptor (NR) superfamily

The GR and the estrogen receptor (ER) are founding members of the NR superfamily, and were cloned within the same time period(Green et al 1986, Greene et al 1986). They are highly homologous and are composed of domains that retain much of their function when dissociated from each other. Both GR and ER have three major domains, the NTD, DBD and LBD, as do all steroid receptors (Fig 1). The domains are dissociable and for certain functions are also interchangeable. For example, an ER chimera, which contains a GR binding domain, activates transcription in the presence of estradiol but does so by binding a GRE(Green & Chambon 1987).

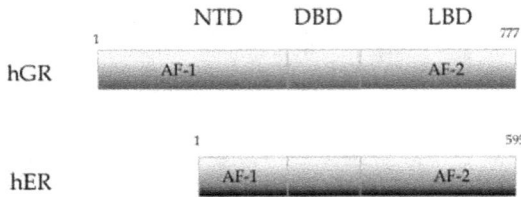

Figure 1. Domains of the GR and ER. (hGR) human glucocorticoid receptor, (hER) human estrogen receptor, (AF-1 and AF-2) activation functions 1 and 2, respectively

3. GR-regulated gene repression: response elements

Prior to the late 1980s, a prevailing view of GR-mediated repression was that it would require a palindromic DNA binding site. This assumption could not explain the fact that glucocorticoids repress a number of genes in the absence of a prototypic GRE. The discovery of composite elements and the discovery that elements for other transcription factors could sustain GR-mediated inhibition of gene activation were major advances in the understanding of GR-mediated repression.

3.1. Repression mediated by composite elements

Composite elements are hybrids (Lefstin & Yamamoto 1998). In the case of GR regulation they consist of half sites, one for a GR monomer and one for a monomer of a distinct transcription factor -- *e.g.* a monomer of an activator protein-1 (AP-1) family member. They are found in numerous genes, including those directly involved in regulating the HPA-axis - - *crh* and *pomc*.

Much of the initial molecular analysis of composite elements was performed using the proliferin gene (*proliferin*).The *proliferin* composite element consists of half sites for GRE and AP-1 binding and confers both activation and repression, dictated by the specific AP-1 family member bound (Diamond et al 1990, Pearce et al 1998). AP-1 family members include c-Jun, cFos and similar proteins. A GR monomer bound in the presence of a c-Jun monomer will stimulate activation from the *proliferin* element, whereas high levels of c-Fos inhibit activation(Diamond et al 1990). Like the *proliferin* element, the *crh* nGRE is composed of GRE and AP-1 half sites. In addition, the extent to which the nGRE directs repression is dependent on the AP-1 family member bound to the composite element (Malkoski & Dorin 1999).

3.2. Repression mediated through other transcription factors and components of the basal transcriptional activity

Three papers published simultaneously in 1990 reported that glucocorticoid-bound GR could down-regulate AP-1 stimulated gene expression (Jonat et al 1990, Schule et al 1990, Yang-Yen et al 1990). Mechanisms by which the GR down-regulates AP-1 activity and activity of other transcription factors are still being elucidated -- some interact with coregulators and others interact directly with components of the general transcription machinery. An example of the latter is GR down-regulation of nuclear factor-kappa B (NF-kB) activity. In the context of the interleukin-8 gene(il-8), GR is a physical and functional intermediary between the RelA (p65) component of NF-kB and the C'-terminal domain of polymerase II (pol II). GR alters the phosphorylation state of the C'-terminal domain of pol II and thus regulates its activity(Nissen & Yamamoto 2000). The GR also down-regulates il-8 expression by interfering with the activity of the transcription elongation factor-b (Luecke & Yamamoto 2005). Thus, GR targets both initiation and elongation steps in the context of the il-8 promoter. It is unknown whether or not GR works through either of these mechanisms in the context of crh.

4. Identification of NR coregulators

By the 1990s it was clear that NRs required additional factors to regulate gene expression. The discovery of NR co-regulators — coactivators and corepressors — permitted a quantum leap in the elucidation of NR mechanisms of gene regulation.

4.1. NR coactivators

Although there are numerous coactivators, this review focuses on the three members of the p160 family commonly referred to as SRCs-1, -2, and -3. In addition, a nomenclature group has codified the names of these coactivators as NCoA 1-3. Here they will be referred to collectively as the p160 family and individually the names first reported will be used with the agreed upon nomenclature indicated, e.g. SRC-1 (NCoA 1).

The first p160 was discovered by O'Malley as a coactivator for a progesterone receptor -- the steroid receptor co-activator-1, SRC-1 (NCoA 1)(Onate et al 1995). Subsequently, Stallcup reported a p160 coactivator for the mouse GR, Glucocorticoid Receptor Interacting Protein 1 GRIP1(Hong et al 1997, Hong et al 1996), also designated NCoA 2. The third p160, reported by several investigators, bears many names, including AIB1(Anzick et al 1997) and RAC3(Li et al 1997) but it is often referred to as SRC-3 (NCoA 3).

Each p160 contains two highly conserved regions. In the center of the protein is a cluster of three Leucine-X-X-Leucine-Leucine (LXXLL) motifs, in which X denotes any amino acid(Ding et al 1998, Heery et al 1997). These are also referred to as NR-boxes. The motifs are a requisite site of interaction with nuclear receptors; mutations of these sites abrogate NR activation functions (Feng et al 1998). p160s also contain a domain that binds to histone acetylases, e.g. the cAMP regulatory element binding protein (CREB)-binding protein (CBP), which remodel chromatin by acetylating specific lysines in histones(Marmorstein 2001).

Mechanisms by which p160s regulate *crh* expression are not well understood. The best studied of these is SRC-1. The SRC-1a isoform mRNA has been mapped to the PVH, and CRH mRNA levels have been evaluated in SRC-1 knockout mice (Lachize et al 2009). Paradoxically, SRC-1 is associated with *crh* repression(van der Laan et al 2008). There is precedent for this -- Rogatsky and colleagues reported that GRIP1 has a repressive function(Rogatsky et al 2001). The GRIP1 domain that supports this function, however, is unique to the GRIP1 p160. Thus, the mechanisms of SRC-1a down-regulation have yet to be identified.

4.1.1. Coactivator interaction with histone acetyl transferases (HATs)

The discovery of the p160s and the discovery of a coactivator for the cAMP regulatory element binding protein (CREB) - binding protein (CBP) and its homologue p300 occurred contemporaneously. In addition to a p160 binding domain the two coactivators contain a histone acetylase domain. CBP is a coactivator for numerous transcription factors that include a number of nuclear receptors and factors involved in inflammation, *e.g.* STAT1 (Horvai et al 1997). In addition to CBP and p300, other acetylases such as the p300/CBP-associated factor (p/CAF;(Yang et al 1996)play a role in nuclear receptor regulation; however, their role in GR regulated *crh* expression is poorly understood.

4.2. Nuclear receptor co-repressors

Some members of the NR family, such as the thyroid hormone receptor (TR), maintain a constitutively silent state of gene expression. The search for a co-repressor for TR led to the discovery of the Nuclear Receptor Corepressor (NCoR), whose homologue is known as the silencing mediator of retinoic acid receptor and the thyroid receptor (SMRT). The NR interaction site in NCoR is remarkably similar to the NR-boxes in the p160 coactivator family. The corepressor motif is L/I XXI/V-I, compared to the p160 coactivator motif, LXXLL. The corepressor motif is referred to as a CoRNR box. These features of coactivator and corepressor regulated gene expression are summarized in Table 1.

Coregulator	Interaction Site	Associated Enzyme	Enzymatic Action	Effect on Chromatin	Effect on Transcription
Coactivator	NR box LXXLL	HAT	Histone Acetylation	Decondensation	Activation
Corepressor	CoRNR box L/I XXI/V-I	HDAC	Histone Deacetylation	Condensation	Deactivation or Repression

Table 1. The chain of events for activation parallels that for repression.

The mechanisms by which co-repressors interact with GR to down-regulate *crh* expression are largely uncharacterized. Using transient transfection/reporter assays, van der Laan *et al.* reported that cotransfection of NCoR and SMRT did not accentuate glucocorticoid mediated *crh* repression. Instead, these repressors accentuated corticosterone inhibition of forskolin-stimulated expression(van der Laan et al 2008).

The corepressors NCoR and SMRT bind to histone deacetylases (HDACs). The specificity of an HDAC for a given receptor has been elucidated in some studies. An early report revealed that HDAC3 but not HDAC1 is involved in TR repression (Guenther et al 2001). Given the conserved nature of many functions across nuclear receptors one might predict that like the TR, GR- repressed transcription of *crh* expression would involve HDAC3 but not HDAC1. In the context of the *crh* promoter, however, the reverse is true(Miller et al 2011).

5. Structural analysis of GR

Structural analysis of GR permits identification not only of a single protein structure but also of protein interfaces involved in specific inter-molecular interactions.

5.1. The DNA binding domain

Crystallographic analysis of a GR dimer bound to its DNA recognition site revealed that GR zinc fingers intercalate with DNA (Freedman et al 1988, Luisi et al 1991). Subsequent NMR analysis of the DBD structure revealed inherent stability in the absence of DNA (Berglund et al 1992). The DBD is now known to have several functions in addition to binding DNA, and it may be that the inherent structure supports these functions.

5.2. The ligand binding domain

A characteristic of all NRs is that the LBD is longer and less structured than the DBD. This partially explains why the crystal structure of two smaller nuclear receptors, RXR-alpha and TR were the first to be solved (Bourguet et al 1995, Wagner et al 1995). The TR was the first ligand-bound NR to be crystallized; even so, it took years to optimize LBD purification in sufficient quantities to permit crystallization (Apriletti et al 1995, Apriletti et al 1988) (McGrath et al 1994). This process was facilitated by use of a radioactively labeled ligand (Apriletti et al 1995, Apriletti et al 1988), which allowed LBD to be tracked throughout purification. The discovery of NR boxes was taking place simultaneously with efforts to crystalize the TR LBD. Thus, crystallization of the ligand-bound TR bound to a GRIP1NR box followed shortly thereafter (Darimont et al 1998, Wagner et al 1995).

The next LBD structure to be solved was ER-alpha, again bound to ligand and an NR box. As a member of the steroid receptor branch of the NR superfamily it has a longer, more complex LBD than the TR. Thus, the protein is inherently more difficult to crystalize, and its crystal structure more difficult to solve. Coordinates used to solve the TR structure permitted ER modeling (Shiau et al 1998). Indeed, in the absence of TR crystal structure coordinates, solution of the ER crystal structure may have been intractable at the time.

The GR LBD is even less structured than either TR or ER-alpha. In fact, a mutation in the GR LBD was required to generate crystals. Co-crystallization of GR LBD bound to Dex and to an NR box revealed that the overall structure of the receptor LBD is the same as the TR and ER-alpha with three key differences: an additional dimerization function, a second set of charge clamps, and an additional pocket (Bledsoe et al 2002, Bledsoe et al 2004). These distinctive features underscore the complexity of GR (Bledsoe et al 2004).

6. Epigenetics and chromatin modification

Strictly defined, the term epigenetics refers to an inheritable factor composed of something other than unmodified genomic DNA— this is distinct from chromatin modifications that regulate processes that are not inherited. Thus, most of the processes referred to here are not truly epigenetic, but rather consist of chromatin modifications that modulate gene expression.

6.1. Histone acetylation

Although typically associated with transcriptional activation, histone acetylation is also associated with repressed states of gene expression (Shahbazian & Grunstein 2007). The initial focus of study in this field was on chromatin acetylation via recruitment of histone acetyl transferases (HATs). The addition of an acetyl to a lysine (Lys) neutralizes the acid-base interaction with DNA. This neutralization, as well as the steric hindrance conferred by Lys acetylation, destabilizes histone:DNA interactions, and allows proteins such as transcription factors, transcription initiators, and elongation factors access to DNA binding sites.

6.2. Histone Deacetylation

Deacetylation is the counterpart to acetylation. Histone Deacetylases (HDACs) are comprised of a family of enzymes with three subdivisions. The nomenclature of mammalian HDACs is somewhat confounding, having arisen from sequential numbering as the enzymes were discovered. Class I includes HDAC 1-3, 8 and 11. They have one catalytic domain and for the most part are nuclear. Class II HDACs are larger than Class I and are divided into two subclasses, IIa and IIb. Class IIa HDACs include HDAC 4, 5, 7and have an N'-terminal domain unique to this class. In addition, Class IIa HDACs shuttle between the nucleus and cytoplasm. Class IIb HDACs, 6 and 10, have two HDAC domains instead of a unique N'-terminus, and are predominantly found in the cytoplasm (Verdin et al 2003). Class III HDACs are distinguished by their requirement for NAD^+. They are named sirtuins due to similarity to the yeast Sir2. Like Sir2, they are targets of intense study given their association with aging and neurodegenerative processes. Because HDACs are tightly correlated with repression they have been examined in the context of GR-repressed *crh* expression (Miller et al 2011).

7. Corticotropin Releasing Hormone (CRH)

Although CRH is widely expressed in the mammalian CNS, the focus here is on regulation of *crh* in the medial parvocellular region of the PVH (mpPVH).

7.1. CRH cloning

In 1983, a fragment of the human *crh* was cloned that contained the proximal promoter and coding region. The predicted amino acid sequence differs from the ovine by seven residues (Shibahara et al 1983). Cloning the rat cDNA and a portion of the promoter were reported in 1987(Thompson et al 1987). The rat cDNA has high sequence homology to human cDNA, and in fact the peptide sequences are identical. Rat and human proximal promoter sequences are also highly conserved (Thompson et al 1987).

7.2. *crh* regulation

A cAMP regulatory element (CRE) at approximately -200 in the proximal promoter plays a pivotal role in activating *crh* expression by recruitment of (CREB)(Seasholtz et al 1988, Thompson et al 1987). Interestingly this site not only mediates activation but also mediates repression by recruiting the inducible cAMP early repressor(Aguilera & Liu 2012). In addition, a negative GRE in the 200 base span contributes to *crh* down-regulation (Malkoski & Dorin 1999,(Malkoski et al 1997). Indeed the entire first 200 bases of the proximal promoter are highly conserved, underscoring the importance of this region to regulation of the stress response(Yao et al 2007).

Specific mechanisms of GR-mediated *crh* down-regulation have been difficult to parse, as is case for most glucocorticoid down-regulated genes. At the most basic level it is unclear whether glucocorticoids suppress *crh*-activated expression only, or if they also suppress basal levels of expression. This distinction is important in that recruitment of signal-specific co-activators would be required prior to GR inhibition. Repression of basal activity, however, would entail recruiting a corepressor.

Most studies of inhibited *crh* regulation have used transient transfection assays or isolated DNA. In neither case is DNA in its natural state of chromatinization. More recent studies of *crh* expression underscore the importance of considering the chromatin environment.

8. Impact of chromatin modifications on analysis of GR-mediated *crh* down-regulation

A number of factors regulate the *crh* chromatin environment. Inhibition of activated *crh* expression involves both the CRE and the nGRE, and maintenance of basal activity involves histone acetylation and DNA methylation. Numerous steps in mechanisms of inhibition and repression have yet to be elucidated.

8.1.1. Repression of cAMP activated crh expression

CRE is required for regulation of *crh* expression through signal transduction. Phosphorylated CREB (pCREB) can interact with an inhibitory member of the CREB family, the inducible cAMP early repressor (ICER). ICER is a dominant negative of pCREB and decreases cAMP activated expression. Further details on the role of pCREB and its family members in regulating *crh* expression can be found in the Aguilera and Liu review(Aguilera & Liu 2012).

8.1.2. Regulation through the nGRE

Repression mediated through the nGRE in the proximal *crh* promoter is similar to repression mediated through the *proliferin* nGRE. A monomer of GR and a monomer of the AP-1 family bind the composite element. The prototypic coactivator for pCREB is CBP, which is also a coactivator for AP-1(Bannister & Kouzarides 1995, Bannister et al 1995). Thus, in the context of *crh*, CBP might permit a functional interaction between the GR:AP-1 dimer and a dimer of CREB family members bound to the CRE.

8.2. Maintenance of basal levels of activation

Basal levels of activation involve a balance of activation and repression. There are numerous ways in which this balance may be maintained -- one is to maintain a constant state of chromatin modification. Two modification types that play a role in *crh* regulation are histone acetylation and methylation of CpG islands.

8.2.1. Histone acetylation

Activated *crh* expression involves CBP recruitment to the proximal promoter. CBP is a HAT coactivator for both pCREB and c-Jun, so activation of either the pKA pathway or the pKC pathway could be involved in CBP recruitment.

Analysis of global histone 3 and 4 (H3 and H4) acetylation in the context of estradiol-regulated *crh* expression has been reported(Lalmansingh & Uht 2008). As is the case in estradiol regulation, Dex regulates H3 and H4 acetylation differentially, as measured by chromatin immunoprecipitation followed by PCR amplification(Miller et al 2011). Dex increases H4 acetylation, a finding that underscores the fact that acetylation may be associated a state of repression as well as activation.

The level of histone acetylation is a function of the presence of enzymatically active HATs and HDACs. In the case of Dex-regulated *crh* expression, the amount of ligand bound GR is increased in the region of the promoter(Miller et al 2011). When measured at the same time, HDAC levels are also increased. Furthermore, GR binds HDAC1 in a Dex-dependent manner, suggesting the possibility that GR recruits HDAC1 to the *crh* promoter (Figure 2).

Like the differential acetylation of H3 and H4, the Dex associated increase in HDACs displays a degree of specificity — although HDAC1 is increased at the promoter, HDAC3 is not (Miller et al 2011). The mechanisms by which these enzymes leave and are recruited to chromatin are poorly understood and merit further study.

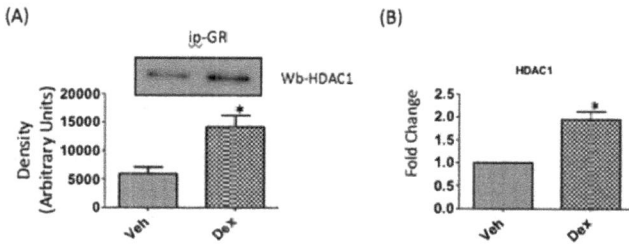

Figure 2. Dex treatment leads to increased HDAC1:GR complexes and increased HDAC1 at the *crh* promoter. (A) Co-immunoprecipitation analysis; nuclear extract was immunoprecipitated with a polyclonal antibody against GR. Western blot analysis of the immune-precipitate revealed an increase in the co-immunoprecipitation of HDAC1. n=3; Bars represent the mean ± SEM and are represented as the fold difference of the Veh *, P < 0.05. (B) ChIP analysis of the CRH promoter; cells were treated with Dex and chromatin was immune-precipitated with an anti HDAC1 antibody. Quantitative RT-PCR analysis of the immune-precipitated DNA indicates enrichment of HDAC1 at the promoter. n=3; Bars represent the mean ± SEM and are represented as the fold difference of the Veh *, P < 0.05.

8.2.2. DNA methylation

Methylation of CpG islands of the GR promoter was one of the earliest reported true epigenetic phenomena in that it was associated with inheritance -- in this case a behavioral phenotype(Weaver et al 2004). More recently, CpG island methylated *crh* has been described in the context of social defeat(Elliott et al 2010).

The first report of CpG island methylation in the context of *crh* regulation was an offshoot from a study of a mouse model of Rett Syndrome. This syndrome occurs in girls and manifests as diminished intelligence, repetitive motor movements, and anxiety — all of which have variable penetrance. The genetic lesion in Rett Syndrome is a mutation in the methyl CpG (meCpG) binding protein 2 (MeCP2). This protein binds to meCpG islands and represses the expression of bound genes. McGill and colleagues found that one of these genes is *crh*. Remarkably, mice bearing the MeCP2 mutation have a hyperactive HPA axis associated with elevated levels of CRH mRNA in the PVH, central amygdala, and BNST— all regions that express GRs and which are associated with HPA axis regulation. In addition, meCpG sites have been mapped in the *crh* proximal promoter region and were found to be present in the same region as the CRE and nGRE(McGill et al 2006). These findings underscore the importance of this region in *crh* regulation.

9. A role for bioinformatics in GR-regulated *crh* expression

Dalwadi and Uht recently investigated expression patterns of two neuronal cell lines, which were derived from embryonic PVH and amygdala. Paradoxically, even though neurons in these populations express CRH and contain GRs, they differ in the response to glucocorticoid treatment. In the mpPVH, glucocorticoids down-regulate *crh* expression whereas in the amygdala they up-regulate it. Expression microarrays are currently being analyzed using the expression pattern of two neuronal cell lines, amygdalar AR-5 and hypothalamic IVB - both differentially express *crh* in response to Dex treatment. The number of genes associated with development of projections is similar between the two cell lines, whereas the number of genes involved in steroid hormone responsiveness is two-fold greater in the hypothalamic line compared to the amygdalar line. Given the importance of the hypothalamus relative to amygdala in regulation of steroid hormone physiology, these results are not unexpected. However, the two lines also differ in the relative expression of genes associated with response to oxidative stress and to DNA binding, as categorized in the Gene Ontology database (GO; Figure 3). These differences are intriguing and have spurred further investigation.

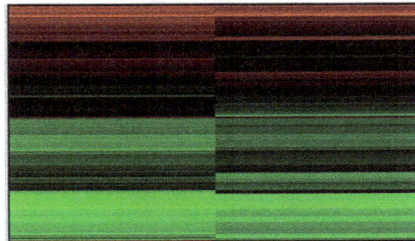

GO Term	AR-5	IVB
DNA Binding	36	21
Neuron Projection Development	9	8
Response to Oxidative Stress	10	6
Response to Steroid Hormone Stimulus	6	12

Figure 3. Hierarchal cluster showing relative abundance of genes between the AR-5 and IVB cell lines (red - abundant, green - less abundant). (GO) Gene Ontology as defined by the DAVID analysis program. (AR-5) Amygdalar cell line, (IVB) Hypothalamic cell line.

More refined techniques are now available for bioinformatics analysis of gene expression. One of those is the combination of chromatin immunoprecipitation and microarray assays (ChIP-chip). In this approach, DNA isolated from ChIPs is used to probe a genomic microarray. ChIP-chip has been used to analyze GR binding sites. So and colleagues used a combination of conventional expression array analysis followed by ChIP-chip. When glucocorticoid-induced genes were compared to glucocorticoid-repressed genes, analysis revealed that the GR-holoreceptor induced all genes that were regulated via a conventional palindrome. In distinction, none of the genes repressed contained such an element (So et al 2007). Such a clear-cut distinction is rare in biology.

A second example of a bioinformatics approach useful in the analysis of NR mediated gene regulation is global run-on and sequencing (GRO-seq)(Core et al 2008). This technique permits unbiased analysis of all RNA transcripts, which allows detection of both mRNA and non-coding RNAs. It has been used in a number of biological systems, including use of this technique to determine the nature of transcripts induced by 17estradiol treatment of MCF-7 cells, a prototypic breast cancer cell line. To date, however, there are no reports of GRO-seq analysis of glucocorticoid regulated genes.

10. Summary

In the last fifteen years an explosion of new information has facilitated novel ways of looking at GR mediated gene expression. The seminal findings by Yamamoto in the early 1980s — that GRs bind to specific palindromic glucocorticoid response elements(Payvar et al 1983)— is now frequently referred to as the classic mechanism of gene regulation. At present, numerous alternate mechanisms of gene regulation are being elucidated. Many of these involve interactions with coregulatory factors. Such interactions have helped bridge the gap between transcription and chromatin remodeling, which in turn has resulted in the intersection of the NR field with the field of epigenetics.

This review has focused on glucocorticoid regulation of genomic effects via the GR. Other areas currently being investigated include the actions of GR splice variants, and the role of glucocorticoid regulation of heat shock proteins. Lastly, the effects of glucocorticoids at the cell membrane (non-genomic events), mechanisms of cell membrane transport of glucocorticoids, and nuclear import of the GR holoreceptors are all steps in regulation that merit further analysis.

Author details

Rosalie M. Uht

Institute for Aging and Alzheimer's Disease Research and Department of Pharmacology and Neuroscience University of North Texas Health Science Center, USA

Acknowledgement

Dedicated to the Memory of Wylie Vale 1941 - 2012.

The data for figures were generated by Dharmendra Sharma (Fig 2) and Dhwanil Dalwadi (Fig 3).

The author thanks Teresa Olsen for editing the manuscript.

Funding obtained from UNTHSC startup funds and NIHR01 RMH082900A (RMU).

11. References

Aguilera G, Liu Y. 2012. The molecular physiology of CRH neurons. *Frontiers in neuroendocrinology* 33: 67-84

Anzick SL, Kononen J, Walker RL, Azorsa DO, Tanner MM, et al. 1997. AIB1, a steroid receptor coactivator amplified in breast and ovarian cancer. *Science* 277: 965-8

Apriletti JW, Baxter JD, Lau KH, West BL. 1995. Expression of the rat alpha 1 thyroid hormone receptor ligand binding domain in Escherichia coli and the use of a ligand-induced conformation change as a method for its purification to homogeneity. *Protein expression and purification* 6: 363-70

Apriletti JW, Baxter JD, Lavin TN. 1988. Large scale purification of the nuclear thyroid hormone receptor from rat liver and sequence-specific binding of the receptor to DNA. *The Journal of biological chemistry* 263: 9409-17

Bannister AJ, Kouzarides T. 1995. CBP-induced stimulation of c-Fos activity is abrogated by E1A. *The EMBO journal* 14: 4758-62

Bannister AJ, Oehler T, Wilhelm D, Angel P, Kouzarides T. 1995. Stimulation of c-Jun activity by CBP: c-Jun residues Ser63/73 are required for CBP induced stimulation in vivo and CBP binding in vitro. *Oncogene* 11: 2509-14

Berglund H, Kovacs H, Dahlman-Wright K, Gustafsson JA, Hard T. 1992. Backbone dynamics of the glucocorticoid receptor DNA-binding domain. *Biochemistry* 31: 12001-11

Bicknell AB. 2008. The tissue-specific processing of pro-opiomelanocortin. *Journal of neuroendocrinology* 20: 692-9

Bledsoe RK, Montana VG, Stanley TB, Delves CJ, Apolito CJ, et al. 2002. Crystal structure of the glucocorticoid receptor ligand binding domain reveals a novel mode of receptor dimerization and coactivator recognition. *Cell* 110: 93-105

Bledsoe RK, Stewart EL, Pearce KH. 2004. Structure and function of the glucocorticoid receptor ligand binding domain. *Vitamins and hormones* 68: 49-91

Bourguet W, Ruff M, Chambon P, Gronemeyer H, Moras D. 1995. Crystal structure of the ligand-binding domain of the human nuclear receptor RXR-alpha. *Nature* 375: 377-82

Choi DC, Furay AR, Evanson NK, Ostrander MM, Ulrich-Lai YM, Herman JP. 2007. Bed nucleus of the stria terminalis subregions differentially regulate hypothalamic-pituitary-adrenal axis activity: implications for the integration of limbic inputs. *The Journal of neuroscience : the official journal of the Society for Neuroscience* 27: 2025-34

Cintra A, Fuxe K, Harfstrand A, Agnati LF, Wikstrom AC, et al. 1987. Presence of glucocorticoid receptor immunoreactivity in corticotrophin releasing factor and in growth hormone releasing factor immunoreactive neurons of the rat di- and telencephalon. *Neuroscience letters* 77: 25-30

Core LJ, Waterfall JJ, Lis JT. 2008. Nascent RNA sequencing reveals widespread pausing and divergent initiation at human promoters. *Science* 322: 1845-8

Darimont BD, Wagner RL, Apriletti JW, Stallcup MR, Kushner PJ, et al. 1998. Structure and specificity of nuclear receptor-coactivator interactions. *Genes & development* 12: 3343-56

de Kloet ER, Joels M, Holsboer F. 2005. Stress and the brain: from adaptation to disease. *Nature reviews. Neuroscience* 6: 463-75

de Kloet R, Wallach G, Mc EBS. 1975. Differences in Corticosterone and Dexamethasone Binding to Rat Brain and Pituitary. *Endocrinology* 96: 598-609

Diamond MI, Miner JN, Yoshinaga SK, Yamamoto KR. 1990. Transcription factor interactions: selectors of positive or negative regulation from a single DNA element. *Science* 249: 1266-72

Ding XF, Anderson CM, Ma H, Hong H, Uht RM, et al. 1998. Nuclear receptor-binding sites of coactivators glucocorticoid receptor interacting protein 1 (GRIP1) and steroid receptor coactivator 1 (SRC-1): multiple motifs with different binding specificities. *Mol Endocrinol* 12: 302-13

Elliott E, Ezra-Nevo G, Regev L, Neufeld-Cohen A, Chen A. 2010. Resilience to social stress coincides with functional DNA methylation of the Crf gene in adult mice. *Nature neuroscience* 13: 1351-3

Feng W, Ribeiro RC, Wagner RL, Nguyen H, Apriletti JW, et al. 1998. Hormone-dependent coactivator binding to a hydrophobic cleft on nuclear receptors. *Science* 280: 1747-9

Freedman LP, Luisi BF, Korszun ZR, Basavappa R, Sigler PB, Yamamoto KR. 1988. The function and structure of the metal coordination sites within the glucocorticoid receptor DNA binding domain. *Nature* 334: 543-6

Gibbs DM. 1986. Vasopressin and oxytocin: hypothalamic modulators of the stress response: a review. *Psychoneuroendocrinology* 11: 131-9

Green S, Chambon P. 1987. Oestradiol induction of a glucocorticoid-responsive gene by a chimaeric receptor. *Nature* 325: 75-8

Green S, Walter P, Kumar V, Krust A, Bornert J-M, et al. 1986. Human oestrogen receptor cDNA: sequence, expression and homology to v-*erb*-A. *Nature* 320: 134-39

Greene GL, Gilna P, Waterfield M, Baker A, Hort Y, Shine J. 1986. Sequence and expression of human estrogen receptor complementary DNA. *Science* 231: 1150-4

Guenther MG, Barak O, Lazar MA. 2001. The SMRT and N-CoR corepressors are activating cofactors for histone deacetylase 3. *Molecular and cellular biology* 21: 6091-101

Gustafsson JA, Carlstedt-Duke J, Poellinger L, Okret S, Wikstrom AC, et al. 1987. Biochemistry, molecular biology, and physiology of the glucocorticoid receptor. *Endocrine reviews* 8: 185-234

Heery DM, Kalkhoven E, Hoare S, Parker MG. 1997. A signature motif in transcriptional co-activators mediates binding to nuclear receptors. *Nature* 387: 733-6

Herman JP, Figueiredo H, Mueller NK, Ulrich-Lai Y, Ostrander MM, et al. 2003. Central mechanisms of stress integration: hierarchical circuitry controlling hypothalamo-pituitary-adrenocortical responsiveness. *Frontiers in neuroendocrinology* 24: 151-80

Hong H, Kohli K, Garabedian MJ, Stallcup MR. 1997. GRIP1, a transcriptional coactivator for the AF-2 transactivation domain of steroid, thyroid, retinoid, and vitamin D receptors. *Molecular and cellular biology* 17: 2735-44

Hong H, Kohli K, Trivedi A, Johnson DL, Stallcup MR. 1996. GRIP1, a novel mouse protein that serves as a transcriptional coactivator in yeast for the hormone binding domains of steroid receptors. *Proceedings of the National Academy of Sciences of the United States of America* 93: 4948-52

Horvai AE, Xu L, Korzus E, Brard G, Kalafus D, et al. 1997. Nuclear integration of JAK/STAT and Ras/AP-1 signaling by CBP and p300. *Proceedings of the National Academy of Sciences of the United States of America* 94: 1074-9

Jonat C, Rahmsdorf HJ, Park K-K, Cato ACB, Gebel S, et al. 1990. Antitumor promotion and antiinflammation: down-modulation of AP-1 (fos/jun) activity by glucocorticoid hormone. *Cell* 62: 1189-204

Lachize S, Apostolakis EM, van der Laan S, Tijssen AM, Xu J, et al. 2009. Steroid receptor coactivator-1 is necessary for regulation of corticotropin-releasing hormone by chronic stress and glucocorticoids. *Proceedings of the National Academy of Sciences of the United States of America* 106: 8038-42

Lalmansingh AS, Uht RM. 2008. Estradiol regulates corticotropin-releasing hormone gene (crh) expression in a rapid and phasic manner that parallels estrogen receptor-alpha and -beta recruitment to a 3',5'-cyclic adenosine 5'-monophosphate regulatory region of the proximal crh promoter. *Endocrinology* 149: 346-57

Lefstin JA, Yamamoto KR. 1998. Allosteric effects of DNA on transcriptional regulators. *Nature* 392: 885-8

Li H, Gomes PJ, Chen JD. 1997. RAC3, a steroid/nuclear receptor-associated coactivator that is related to SRC-1 and TIF2. *Proceedings of the National Academy of Sciences of the United States of America* 94: 8479-84

Luecke HF, Yamamoto KR. 2005. The glucocorticoid receptor blocks P-TEFb recruitment by NFkappaB to effect promoter-specific transcriptional repression. *Genes & development* 19: 1116-27

Luisi BF, Xu WX, Otwinowski Z, Freedman LP, Yamamoto KR, Sigler PB. 1991. Crystallographic analysis of the interaction of the glucocorticoid receptor with DNA. *Nature* 352: 497-505

Malkoski SP, Dorin RI. 1999. Composite glucocorticoid regulation at a functionally defined negative glucocorticoid response element of the human corticotropin-releasing hormone gene. *Mol Endocrinol* 13: 1629-44

Malkoski SP, Handanos CM, Dorin RI. 1997. Localization of a negative glucocorticoid response element of the human corticotropin releasing hormone gene. *Molecular and cellular endocrinology* 127: 189-99

Marmorstein R. 2001. Structure and function of histone acetyltransferases. *Cellular and molecular life sciences : CMLS* 58: 693-703

McEwen BS, Davis PG, Parsons B, Pfaff DW. 1979. The brain as a target for steroid hormone action. *Annual review of neuroscience* 2: 65-112

McGill BE, Bundle SF, Yaylaoglu MB, Carson JP, Thaller C, Zoghbi HY. 2006. Enhanced anxiety and stress-induced corticosterone release are associated with increased Crh expression in a mouse model of Rett syndrome. *Proceedings of the National Academy of Sciences of the United States of America* 103: 18267-72

McGrath ME, Wagner RL, Apriletti JW, West BL, Ramalingam V, et al. 1994. Preliminary crystallographic studies of the ligand-binding domain of the thyroid hormone receptor complexed with triiodothyronine. *Journal of molecular biology* 237: 236-9

Miller L, Foradori CD, Lalmansingh AS, Sharma D, Handa RJ, Uht RM. 2011. Histone deacetylase 1 (HDAC1) participates in the down-regulation of corticotropin releasing hormone gene (crh) expression. *Physiology & behavior* 104: 312-20

Nissen RM, Yamamoto KR. 2000. The glucocorticoid receptor inhibits NFkappaB by interfering with serine-2 phosphorylation of the RNA polymerase II carboxy-terminal domain. *Genes & development* 14: 2314-29

Oakley RH, Sar M, Cidlowski JA. 1996. The human glucocorticoid receptor beta isoform. Expression, biochemical properties, and putative function. *The Journal of biological chemistry* 271: 9550-9

Onate SA, Tsai SY, Tsai MJ, O'Malley BW. 1995. Sequence and characterization of a coactivator for the steroid hormone receptor superfamily. *Science* 270: 1354-7

Payvar F, DeFranco D, Firestone GL, Edgar B, Wrange O, et al. 1983. Sequence-specific binding of glucocorticoid receptor to MTV DNA at sites within and upstream of the transcribed region. *Cell* 35: 381-92

Pearce D, Matsui W, Miner JN, Yamamoto KR. 1998. Glucocorticoid receptor transcriptional activity determined by spacing of receptor and nonreceptor DNA sites. *The Journal of biological chemistry* 273: 30081-5

Pratt WB, Dittmar KD. 1998. Studies with Purified Chaperones Advance the Understanding of the Mechanism of Glucocorticoid Receptor-hsp90 Heterocomplex Assembly. *Trends in endocrinology and metabolism: TEM* 9: 244-52

Rogatsky I, Zarember KA, Yamamoto KR. 2001. Factor recruitment and TIF2/GRIP1 corepressor activity at a collagenase-3 response element that mediates regulation by phorbol esters and hormones. *The EMBO journal* 20: 6071-83

Sapolsky RM, Krey LC, McEwen BS. 1984. Stress down-regulates corticosterone receptors in a site-specific manner in the brain. *Endocrinology* 114: 287-92

Schule R, Rangarajan P, Kliewer S, Ransone LJ, Bolado J, et al. 1990. Functional antagonism between oncoprotein c-jun and the glucocorticoid receptor. *Cell* 62: 1217-26

Seasholtz AF, Thompson RC, Douglass JO. 1988. Identification of a cyclic adenosine monophosphate-responsive element in the rat corticotropin-releasing hormone gene. *Molec Endocrinol* 2: 1311-19

Shahbazian MD, Grunstein M. 2007. Functions of site-specific histone acetylation and deacetylation. *Annual review of biochemistry* 76: 75-100

Shiau AK, Barstad D, Loria PM, Cheng L, Kushner PJ, et al. 1998. The structural basis of estrogen receptor/coactivator recognition and the antagonism of this interaction by tamoxifen. *Cell* 95: 927-37

Shibahara S, Morimoto Y, Furutani Y, Notake M, Takahashi H, et al. 1983. Isolation and sequence analysis of the human corticotropin-releasing factor precursor gene. *The EMBO journal* 2: 775-9

So AY, Chaivorapol C, Bolton EC, Li H, Yamamoto KR. 2007. Determinants of cell- and gene-specific transcriptional regulation by the glucocorticoid receptor. *PLoS genetics* 3: e94

Swanson L, Sawchenko P. 1980. Paraventricular nucleus: a site for the integration of neuroendocrine and autonomic mechanisms. *Neuroendocrinol* 31: 410-17

Swanson LW, Sawchenko PE, Lind RW, Rho JH. 1987. The CRH motor euron: differential peptide regulation in neurons with possible synaptic, paracrine, and endocrine outputs. *Annals of the New York Academy of Sciences* 512: 12-23

Thompson RC, Seasholtz AF, Douglass JO, Herbert E. 1987. *The rat corticotropin releasing hormone gene*. New York: New York Academy of Sciences. 1-11 pp.

Uht RM, McKelvy JF, Harrison RW, Bohn MC. 1988. Demonstration of glucocorticoid receptor-like immunoreactivity in glucocorticoid-sensitive vasopressin and corticotropin-releasing factor neurons in the hypothalamic paraventricular nucleus. *Journal of neuroscience research* 19: 405-11, 68-9

Vale W, Spiess J, Rivier C, Rivier J. 1981. Characterization of a 41-residue ovine hypothalamic peptide that stimulates secretion of corticotropin and beta-endorphin. *Science* 213: 1394-7

van der Laan S, Lachize SB, Vreugdenhil E, de Kloet ER, Meijer OC. 2008. Nuclear receptor coregulators differentially modulate induction and glucocorticoid receptor-mediated repression of the corticotropin-releasing hormone gene. *Endocrinology* 149: 725-32

Verdin E, Dequiedt F, Kasler HG. 2003. Class II histone deacetylases: versatile regulators. *Trends in genetics : TIG* 19: 286-93

Wagner RL, Apriletti JW, McGrath ME, West BL, Baxter JD, Fletterick RJ. 1995. A structural role for hormone in the thyroid hormone receptor. *Nature* 378: 690-7

Weaver IC, Cervoni N, Champagne FA, D'Alessio AC, Sharma S, et al. 2004. Epigenetic programming by maternal behavior. *Nature neuroscience* 7: 847-54

Yang XJ, Ogryzko VV, Nishikawa J, Howard BH, Nakatani Y. 1996. A p300/CBP-associated factor that competes with the adenoviral oncoprotein E1A. *Nature* 382: 319-24

Yang-Yen H-F, Chambard J-C, Sun Y-L, Smeal T, Schmidt TJ, et al. 1990. Transcriptional interference between c-Jun and the glucocorticoid receptor: mutual inhibition of DNA binding due to direct protein-protein interaction. *Cell* 62: 1205-15

Yao M, Stenzel-Poore M, Denver RJ. 2007. Structural and functional conservation of vertebrate corticotropin-releasing factor genes: evidence for a critical role for a conserved cyclic AMP response element. *Endocrinology* 148: 2518-31

Yudt MR, Cidlowski JA. 2002. The glucocorticoid receptor: coding a diversity of proteins and responses through a single gene. *Mol Endocrinol* 16: 1719-26

Chapter 2

Mechanism of Glucocorticoid-Induced Osteoporosis: An Update

Xing-Ming Shi, Norman Chutkan, Mark W. Hamrick and Carlos M. Isales

Additional nformation is available at the end of the chapter

1. Introduction

Synthetic oral steroids were initially developed in the 1940-1950's. Although their use was initially limited by their high cost, as they became more affordable and began to be used for treatment of a wide variety of conditions, side effects associated with their use became much more prevalent. In fact, glucocorticoid-induced osteoporosis is now the most common secondary cause of osteoporosis. Until relatively recently, the mechanism of action of these drugs and the mechanisms involved in the development of side effects such as osteoporosis and the higher incidence of bone fractures was not known. Although steroids are widely viewed as mainly catabolic for bone a distinction needs to be made between physiologic and pharmacologic doses of steroids. Recent evidence demonstrates that steroids can clearly be anabolic for bone. In this chapter we review recent findings and mechanisms of glucocorticoid action on bone and some of the clinical consequences of pharmacologic doses of these compounds on bone.

2. Glucocorticoids and osteoporosis

Glucocorticoids are among the most potent anti-inflammatory and immunosuppressive agents and are key therapeutic agents for the management of chronic inflammatory diseases, including rheumatic diseases [1-4], pulmonary disease [5;6], asthma [7-11] and post transplantation immunotherapy [12]. However, long-term glucocorticoid therapy (>3 months) causes bone loss resulting in osteoporosis (glucocorticoid-induced osteoporosis or GIOP) [3;4;13-15], a severe-side effect that occurs in 30 – 50% of patients [16-18]. The incidence of GIOP is indiscriminate of race, age and gender [19;20]. Children, as young as 4 years of age, and adolescents who are on glucocorticoid therapy for various pediatric disorders, including asthma [20-22], juvenile rheumatoid arthritis [23;24], Crohn's disease [25], systemic lupus erythematosus [26;27], and inflammatory bowel disease [28;29] have been reported to endure significant bone density decrease. There is no clearly defined threshold for safe use of glucocorticoids. In practice, a dose equal to or greater than 5mg/day of prednisone is considered as low, and 10mg/day or more is high. The severity of bone loss in GIOP is both time- and dose-dependent. GIOP occurs in two phases: a rapid, early phase in which bone mineral density is reduced, within the first 5 to 7 months of therapy, possibly as a result of excessive bone resorption, and a slower, progressive phase in which bone mineral density declines because of impaired bone formation [30]. Bone loss continues as long as treatment is maintained.

3. Glucocorticoid mechanism of action as anti-inflammatory and immunosuppressant drugs

Glucocorticoids exert their actions via intracellular glucocorticoid receptors (GRs) [31;32]. The GR belongs to the ligand-regulated nuclear receptor superfamily [33]. Like other members in this superfamily, GR contains three major functional domains: a N-terminal activation domain required for transcriptional activation and association with basal transcription factors; a central DNA-binding domain (DBD) consisting of two highly conserved zinc finger regions that are critical for dimerization, DNA binding, transcriptional activation and repression; and a C-terminal ligand-binding domain (LBD) that serves as the binding site for glucocorticoids, chaperone proteins, and coactivators [34;35]. In the absence of ligand, GR is predominantly retained in the cytoplasm as an inactive multi-protein complex consisting of heat shock protein (hsp90) and a number of other proteins, including the immunophilins. The binding of glucocorticoid triggers a conformational change in the GR and leads to dissociation of the multi-protein complex and exposure of a nuclear localization sequence resulting in its nuclear translocation. Once in the nucleus, GR, in the form of a homodimer, binds to a palindromic glucocorticoid-response element (GRE) in the target gene promoter and activates transcription (e.g., of the tyrosine amino transferase gene), or it can bind to a negative GRE (nGRE) to repress transcription (e.g., of the osteocalcin gene) [36].

Glucocorticoids suppress the expression of a panel of inflammatory-relevant genes including cytokines [interleukins (IL) and tumor necrosis factors (TNF-α,β], chemokines (Regulated upon Activation Normal T-cell Expressed and Secreted or RANTES, Macrophage Inflammatory Protein-1-alpha or MIP-1α, Monocyte Chemotactic Protein or MCP-1, -3, and -4], inflammatory enzymes (COX-2, iNOS), and adhesion molecules (Intercellular Adhesion Molecule 1 or ICAM-1, E-selectin) that play a key role in the recruitment of inflammatory cells to the inflammation sites [37-39]. However, most of these genes do not have negative GREs in their promoter regions, and therefore, they are not directly regulated by the binding of GRs to such regulatory elements. These genes do contain NF-κB- and/or AP-1-binding sites and are activated through these sites by NF-κB and/or AP-1 in response to stimuli (cytokines). Thus, one mechanism by which glucocorticoids could regulate transcription would be modulation of NF-κB or AP-1 DNA-binding activity. In 1990, three independent groups found cross-talk between GR and AP-1 [40-42]. In these studies, it was found that activated GR can interact with c-Jun/AP-1 and that the formation of a GR-c-Jun complex prevents c-Jun/AP-1 DNA-binding, resulting in the inhibition of gene expression. Later, it was found that the activated GR can associate with the p65 subunit of NF-κB and inhibit gene activation mediated by NF-κB [43;44]. These findings led to the establishment of the **protein-protein interaction model**.

In 1995, it was found that glucocorticoids induce the expression of a cytoplasmic inhibitor of NF-κB, the IκB-α [45;46]. These studies led to the establishment of a second model, **the IκB-α upregulation model**. This model proposes that glucocorticoids induce the expression of IκB-α and that the newly synthesized IκB-α sequesters the p65 subunit of the NF-κB in the cytoplasm and thereby inhibits NF-κB nuclear functions. However, this mechanism has been challenged by a number of studies. It has now been established that the effect of glucocorticoids on IκB-α expression, and subsequently NF-κB nuclear translocation, is cell-type specific. In some cell types glucocorticoid inhibition of proinflammatory stimuli-induced p65 nuclear translocation is coupled with the induction of IκB-α [45-48]. In other cell types, however, these two events are uncoupled [49;50]. Moreover, a GR mutant that does not enhance IκB-α expression, is still able to repress NF-κB activity [51].

4. Glucocorticoid effects on bone cells

Glucocorticoids have both anabolic and catabolic effects on bone. However, the outcome of glucocorticoid therapy is a net loss of bone [4;52;53]. Corticosteroid 11-β-hydroxysteroid dehydrogenase 2 [11β-HSD2] is an enzyme that oxidizes the active form of glucocorticoid cortisol to the inactive metabolite cortisone, thus the levels of expression and activity of this enzyme is critical for glucocorticoid signaling. *In vivo* studies show that bone-specific transgenic overexpression of 11β-HSD2, under the control of type I collagen promoter, impairs osteoblast differentiation and bone acquisition [54-56]. These studies demonstrate that the endogenous glucocorticoid signaling is essential for normal skeletal development. However, glucocorticoid in excess such as patients with Cushing's syndrome [22] or the patients on glucocorticoid therapy rapidly lose bone mass resulting in osteoporosis. The direct effects of glucocorticoids on bone cells are illustrated in Figure 1.

5. Glucocorticoid effects on bone marrow Mesenchymal Stem Cells (MSCs)

Bone marrow MSCs are multipotent cells that can give rise to several distinct cell lineages, including osteoblasts, adipocytes, and chondrocytes [57-60]. Patients on glucocorticoid therapy not only lose bone but also accumulate large amounts of marrow fat (fatty marrow), indicating that glucocorticoid has altered lineage commitment of MSC to adipocytes at the expense of osteoblasts because these two pathways have a reciprocal relationship [61-64]. Thus, one possible mechanism by which glucocorticoids alter MSC fate determination is through the induction of the master adipogenic regulator peroxisome proliferator-activated receptor gamma (PPARγ) [65;66], which is transcriptionally activated by the CCAAT/enhancer binding protein (C/EBP) family transcription factors in response to glucocorticoid [67-70] (Figure 2). Indeed, Weinstein and colleagues showed that administration of glucocorticoids to mice reduces the numbers of osteoprogenitor cells [71].

This could be achieved through induction of PPARγ since under the same condition bone marrow adipogenesis is enhanced [72], and that a reduction in PPARγ dosage (haploinsufficiency) in mice results in reduced adipogenesis and enhanced osteogenesis from bone marrow progenitors [73].

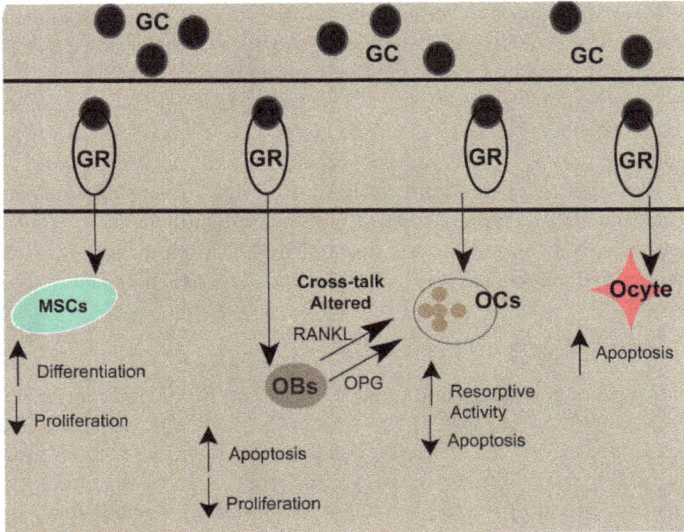

Figure 1. Glucocorticoids bind to the glucocorticoid receptor (GR) and affect mesenchymal stem cell (MSC), osteoblast (OB), osteoclast (OC) and osteocyte (Ocyte) function. The net result is decreased bone formation and increased bone resorption. ↑increase; ↓decrease.

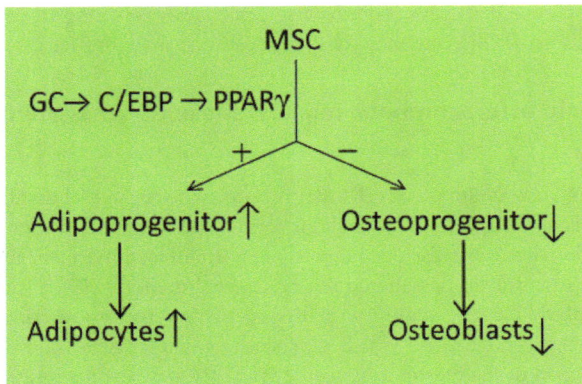

Figure 2. Glucocorticoid reduces the number of osteoprogenitors from MSC by promoting adipogenic differentiation pathway. Glucocorticoid induces the expression of C/EBP family transcription factors that directly activate the transcription of PPARγ, the master regulator of adipogenesis, and shifts the lineage commitment of MSCs to adipocyte pathway, thus reducing the number of osteoprogenitor cells.

6. Glucocorticoid effects on osteoblasts and osteocytes

It has been known for decades that glucocorticoid inhibits bone formation [52;74], but only recently have we realized that glucocorticoids directly target bone cells. By administering a high dose of prednisolone to mice, Weinstein and colleagues found that glucocorticoid induces the death of mature osteoblasts and osteocytes [71;75]. In the same study, the authors also showed that the same is true in bone biopsy samples obtained from patients with glucocorticoid-induced osteoporosis. These results were further strengthened in a transgenic mouse model, in which the glucocorticoid signaling is disrupted by overexpression of 11β-HSD2 specifically in osteoblasts. The study showed that the 11β-HSD2 transgenic mice are protected from glucocorticoid-induced osteoblasts and osteocytes apoptosis and suppression of bone formation [76]. These studies demonstrate that glucocorticoids cause bone loss by restricting the supply of bone building cells, the osteoblasts, and by interfering with the communication network within bone environment via osteocyte death. The osteocytes are the mechanosensory cells that detect and send signals for bone formation in response to damages caused by mechanical loading and unloading [77;78].

7. Glucocorticoid effects on osteoclasts

Osteoclasts are bone resorbing cells and play a key role in the maintenance of bone homeostasis through bone remodeling. In patients, glucocorticoid-induced osteoporosis features a rapid early phase increase in bone resorption, followed by a slow progressive decrease in bone formation [52]. Earlier studies showed that glucocorticoids stimulate osteoclast differentiation and increase their activity [72;79;80]. It is now recognized that glucocorticoids increase the longevity of osteoclasts but may inhibit their bone resorptive activity [81;82]. Moreover, a recent study suggests that glucocorticoids do not inhibit, but modify osteoclast resorptive behavior, making osteoclasts erode bone surfaces over long distances without interruption [83].

8. Glucocorticoid-induced Leucine Zipper (GILZ): A new glucocorticoid anti-inflammatory effect mediator

The protein-protein interaction and the IκB-α upregulation models described earlier in this chapter were established prior to the discovery of a glucocorticoid-inducible protein named glucocorticoid-induced leucine zipper (GILZ), which was identified in 1997 [84]. GILZ is a member of the leucine zipper protein family [84;85] and belongs to the transforming growth factor-beta (TGF-β)-stimulated clone-22 (TSC-22d3) family of transcription factors [86;87]. Members of this family of proteins contain three distinct domains; an N-terminal domain containing a TSC box (N-Ter), a middle leucine zipper domain (LZ), and a C-terminal poly-proline rich domain (PRR).

Unlike IκB-α, which is induced by glucocorticoids in certain cell types [49;50;88], GILZ is induced by glucocorticoids virtually in all cell types examined so far, including bone marrow mesenchymal stem cells, osteoblasts, adipocytes, macrophages and epithelial cells [89]. *In vitro* studies show that overexpression of GILZ protects T-cells from apoptosis induced by anti-CD3 monoclonal antibody, but not other apoptosis-inducing agents such as dexamethasone, ultraviolet irradiation, starvation, or triggered by cross-linked anti-Fas mAb [84]. T-cell-specific transgenic overexpression of GILZ results in thymocyte apoptosis *ex vivo*, possibly through down-regulation of Bcl-xL [90]. The *in vitro* actions of GILZ have been shown to be mediated through direct protein-protein interactions between GILZ and NF-κB, and between GILZ and AP-1 [86;91;92]. The interaction between GILZ and NF-κB blocks NF-κB nuclear translocation and DNA-binding, and the interaction with AP-1 inhibits the binding of AP-1 to its DNA elements [91;92]. GILZ also interacts directly with the mitogen-activated protein kinase (MAPK) family members, Ras and Raf-1, resulting in inhibition of Raf-1 phosphorylation and subsequently, inhibition of MEK/ERK-1/2 phosphorylation and AP-1-dependent transcription [86;93]. Moreover, GILZ can deactivate macrophages [94], inhibit proinflammatory cytokine-induced inflammatory enzymes such as cyclooxygenase-2 [95], inhibit IL-2/IL-2 receptor and IL-5 expression [91;96], and stimulate the production of anti-inflammatory IL-10 by immature dendritic cells, thereby, preventing the production of inflammatory chemokines by CD40L-activated dendritic cells [97]. These studies demonstrate that GILZ is a glucocorticoid anti-inflammatory effect mediator and utilizes very similar mechanisms, to those GR uses [98].

9. GILZ mediates the anabolic effect of glucocorticoids

GILZ is a direct GR target gene with several GREs present in its promoter region [99]. In the absence of glucocorticoid stimulation GILZ is expressed at a very low basal level. However, in the presence of glucocorticoid, GILZ expression is rapidly induced (Figure 3] but GR is also activated, and the activated GR negatively impacts bone, both directly (i.e., inhibits osteocalcin gene transcription) and indirectly through other pathways as illustrated (Figure 4]. Because of that, it is impossible to determine the role of GILZ in osteoblast differentiation and bone formation without the influence of GR, which plays a negative role and may override GILZ actions. To further study this problem, a retrovirus-mediated GILZ overexpression system was established in bone marrow MSCs/osteoprogenitor cells. Studies carried out in this system showed that GILZ has potent pro-osteogenic activity as demonstrated by significantly increased alkaline phosphatase activity, enhanced mineralized bone nodule formation, and the expression of osteoblast-associated genes such as Runx2, type I collagen, alkaline phosphatase, and osteocalcin [100]. Furthermore, our recent studies have shown that overexpression of GILZ can antagonize the inhibitory effect of TNF-α on MSC osteogenic differentiation [101]. Possible mechanisms underlying this antagonism may include GILZ inhibition of TNF-α-induced ERK/MAP kinase activation, which has been shown to be responsible for TNF-α down-regulation of a key osteogenic factor Osx [102;103], and inhibition of TNF-α-induced expression of E3 ubiquitin ligase Smurf proteins, which have been shown to accelerate the degradation of Runx2 protein [104-106].

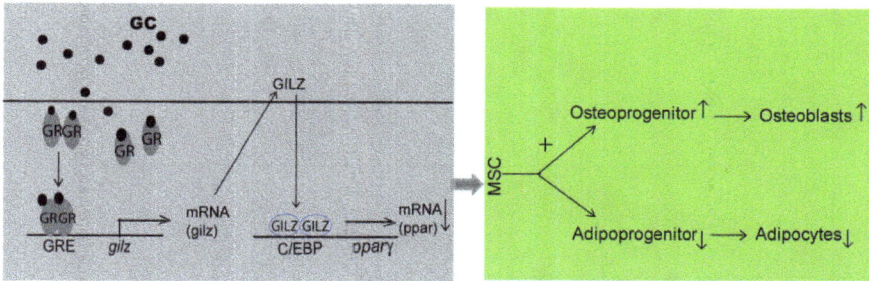

Figure 3. GILZ enhances MSC osteogenic differentiation by shifting MSC lineage preference to osteogenic pathway.

10. GR mediates the catabolic effects of glucocorticoids

There are many glucocorticoid effectors involved in the regulation of bone development or metabolism through different pathways. However, it was only recently demonstrated that the GR was directly responsible for glucocorticoid-induced bone loss *in vivo*. Using a bone-specific GR knockout mouse model, Rauch et al showed that glucocorticoids are unable to induce bone loss or to inhibit bone formation in these mice because the GR-deficient osteoblasts become refractory to glucocorticoid-induced apoptosis, inhibition of proliferation, and differentiation [107]. Interestingly, data from this study also demonstrated that GR-deficiency results in a low bone mass phenotype, confirming the previous studies that the endogenous glucocorticoid signaling is critical for normal bone acquisition [54-56]. Other evidence supporting the role of GR in glucocorticoid-induced bone loss includes: 1] the glucocorticoid-activated GR binds directly to the negative glucocorticoid response elements (nGREs) in the promoter region of the osteocalcin (*Ocn*) gene, an osteoblast-specific gene that plays an important role in bone mineralization and inhibit its transcription [36;108]; 2] GR transcriptionally activates the expression of MAP kinase phosphatase-1 (MKP-1) [109], which inactivates MAP kinase and thus inhibits osteogenic differentiation [64;110;111]; and 3] GR can physically interact with and inhibit the transcriptional functions of Smad3, an intracellular signaling mediator of transforming growth factor-beta (TGF-β) [112] (Figure 4]. Glucocorticoids have been known to antagonize TGF-β action in bone [113-115] and TGF-β stimulates osteoprogenitor cell proliferation [116-119] and attract osteoprogenitor cells to the remodeling sites during bone remodeling [120]. It is important to note that while the catabolic effects of glucocorticoids are often associated with long-term glucocorticoid excess [1-4;7], a short term exposure to glucocorticoid seems beneficial; for example, treatment of bone marrow stromal cells or osteoblasts with dexamethasone enhances, rather than inhibits, alkaline phosphatase (ALP) activity. The ALP is expressed at the early stage of osteoblast differentiation program and the increase of ALP expression or activity marks the entry of cells into the osteoblast lineage.

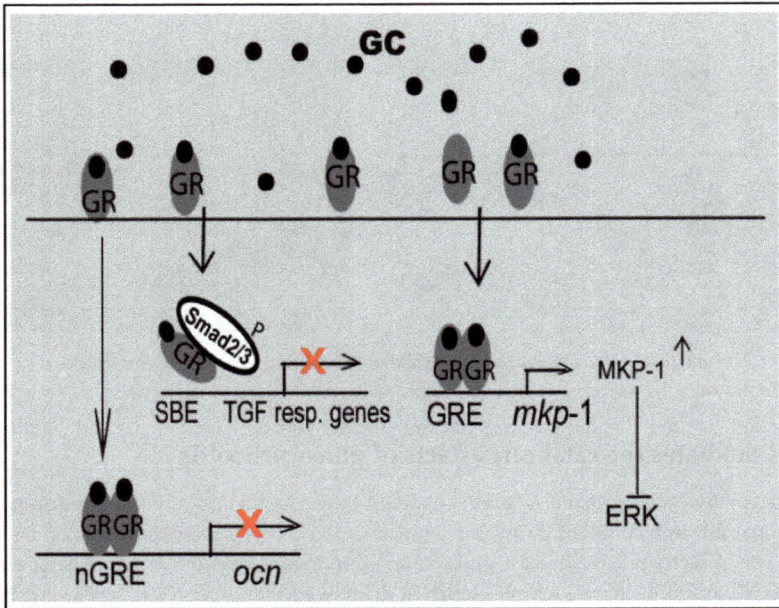

Figure 4. GR inhibits MSC proliferation, ERK activation and Ocn expression. Ligand-bound GR physically interacts with: 1] TGF-β signaling mediator Smad3 and disrupts its transcriptional activity; 2] Activates mkp-1 transcription, by binding to GRE in the mkp-1 promoter region, resulting inhibition of ERK activation; and 3] Suppresses Ocn expression by binding to nGRE in the Ocn promoter region.

11. Glucocorticoid-Induced Osteoporosis (GIOP)

Although glucocorticoids are an essential hormone for survival and normal function, when present in excess (pharmacologic doses) lead to a number of serious side effects including bone loss and fractures. In fact, it is estimated that 30-50% of patients chronically exposed to high levels of glucocorticoids will develop a bone fracture [121]. Glucocorticoid excess can result from either endogenous (Cushing's) or exogenous (iatrogenic) sources. Glucocorticoids are widely used for the treatment of a variety of inflammatory and autoimmune conditions. It is estimated that 0.5% of the population receives steroid therapy and exogenous steroids are thus the most common cause of secondary osteoporosis [122]. There has been a lot of discussion on the dose, duration and mode of administration of steroids and the impact on the development of osteoporosis. There has been a lot of debate on a "safe" dose for glucocorticoid replacement. Doses as low as 2.5 mg of prednisolone have been reported to result in osteoporosis [122]. Even patients on "physiologic" glucocorticoid replacement for Addison's disease have been reported to have lower bone density than controls, although clearly many of these patients were overreplaced with steroid therapy [123]. Further, steroids even when given in an intermittent, rather than continuous fashion, or in an inhaled rather than oral fashion, are still associated with an increased risk of fracture. In treatment guidelines by the American College of Rheumatology in 2010, it was recommended that for patients with low fracture risk receiving more than 7.5 mg of prednisolone equivalents for more than 3 months receive some form of therapy for fracture prevention. In contrast for patients at high fracture risk it was recommended that they receive some form of therapy even at glucocorticoid doses lower than 5 mg and even for periods for less than one month [124].

12. Mechanism

Glucocorticoids have multiple effects on bone and bone cells. In addition, in cases where the glucocorticoids are given to treat systemic inflammatory conditions (e.g. rheumatoid arthritis), the underlying condition also contributes to bone loss. Glucocorticoids also inhibit endogenous production of sex steroids (testosterone and estrogen) in addition to production of adrenal androgens, all of which may have protective effects against bone loss [125]. Further, prolonged high dose glucocorticoid use results in both muscle weakness thus predisposing to an increased number of falls and muscle wasting. Bone-muscle interactions may also contribute to maintaining bone health. Glucocorticoids also decrease intestinal calcium absorption thus further predisposing to osteoporosis. Recently, effects of glucocorticoids on decreasing bone vasculature, has also been implicated as a potential mechanism for glucocorticoid effects on bone [126]. There also seems to be an age-dependence of glucocorticoid effects on bone. The likelihood of fractures with glucocorticoids appears to increase with increasing patient age. Glucocorticoid-induced bone loss appears to be biphasic with an initial rapid phase of bone loss of 5-15% /year followed by a more sustained bone loss rate of 2% [121].

Glucocorticoids affect all bone cells, they result in osteocytic and osteoblastic apoptosis and decreased function of both osteoclasts and osteoblasts. However, they decrease osteoclastic apoptosis. Thus, the net effect is reduced bone formation and increased bone breakdown. Trabecular bone seems to be particularly sensitive to the detrimental effects of steroids resulting in a higher incidence of vertebral and femoral neck fractures [121]. Vertebral compression fractures are commonly missed since only about 30% of them are symptomatic. A study by Angeli et al [127] which examined the prevalence of vertebral fractures in patients receiving glucocorticoids for a variety of autoimmune conditions determined that over 37% of patients had at least one asymptomatic vertebral compression fracture and more than 14% had two or more asymptomatic fractures.

Glucocorticoid effects on bone appear to be generally reversible and once therapy is stopped bone repair occurs over the year following drug cessation. Thus, if feasible, steroid cessation may be the therapy of choice for GIOP.

13. Diagnosis

Determining fracture risk for patients on steroids is difficult since even patients with normal bone densitometry on steroids have a higher fracture risk. Current use of steroids is one of the risk factors used in the calculation of the FRAX (Fracture Risk Assessment) score.

However a recent joint position statement by the International Society for Clinical Densitometry and the International Osteoporosis Foundation concluded that when using the FRAX tool there probably was an underestimation of fracture risk with daily prednisone doses greater than 7.5 mg and an overestimation of fracture risk with daily prednisone doses of less than 2.5 mg. In addition, FRAX probably underestimated fracture risk when high dose inhaled steroids were used. Finally, it was concluded that for patients with adrenal insufficiency receiving appropriate replacement steroid doses this not be included in the FRAX calculation [128].

The American College of Rheumatology recommends that some form of therapy be considered for all patients receiving prolonged steroid therapy and that for those who have a bone densitometry test (Dual energy x-ray absorptiometry or DXA), a T-score of less than -1.0 be considered abnormal [125].

14. Therapy

Since glucocorticoids interfere with intestinal calcium absorption, all patients about to start glucocorticoid therapy should be placed on calcium and vitamin D replacement. Antiresorptive agents such as bisphosphonates (both oral and IV) have been used for the therapy of GIOP, are effective in decreasing the increased fracture risk associated with steroids and are approved for this indication. However, as discussed by Teitelbaum et al. [129], although initial use of steroids is associated with increased bone resorption (osteoclast mediated and related to decreased osteoclastic apoptosis and a situation in which antiresorptive use makes sense), more prolonged steroid use is associated with decreased bone formation and antiresorptive agents have the theoretical possibility of making things worse by further suppressing a low bone turnover state. Thus, use of an anabolic agent such as teriparatide (synthetic parathyroid hormone) for treatment of GIOP would appear more appropriate. In fact in a clinical trial, comparing alendronate vs. teriparatide for 18 months in 428 men/women with established osteoporosis and who had received at least 5mg of prednisone for at least 3 months, teriparatide was significantly more effective in both increasing bone mineral density at the spine [7.2 vs 3.4%) and in decreasing new vertebral fractures [0.6% vs 6.1%) [130]. Of note, this was a secondary instead of a primary osteoporosis prevention trial and there was a greater incidence of side effects associated with teriparatide use as compared to controls [131]. In addition, use of teriparatide by patients is currently limited to two years, thus alternative and better forms of therapy for GIOP need to be developed.

15. Conclusion

Although adverse side effects of glucocorticoids on bone have been long recognized, both from endogenous sources as described by Harvey Cushing in the 1930's or from exogenous sources after development of glucocorticoids in the 1950's the mechanisms involved in this process have only recently began to be understood. It is clear that although physiologic levels of glucocorticoids are important in normal bone development, pharmacologic doses result in a high level of fractures, particularly of vertebral bone. Thus, it would seem that glucocorticoids have both anabolic and catabolic actions on bone. Data from our labs and from others suggest that GILZ may be an important mediator of GR's anabolic actions and thus may be an attractive therapeutic target for drug development.

Author details

Xing-Ming Shi
Institute of Molecular Medicine and Genetics, Department of Pathology
Georgia Health Sciences University, Augusta, GA, USA

Norman Chutkan
Department of Orthopaedic Surgery, Georgia Health Sciences University, Augusta, GA, USA

Mark W. Hamrick
Departments of Cellular Biology & Anatomy and Orthopaedic Surgery, Georgia Health Sciences University, Augusta, GA, USA

Carlos M. Isales
Institute of Molecular Medicine and Genetics, Departments of Orthopaedic Surgery and Medicine, Georgia Health Sciences University, Augusta, GA, USA

Acknowledgement

This work was supported by grants from the National Institutes of Health (DK76045] and National Institute on Aging (P01AG036675].

16. References

[1] Harris, E.D., Jr., Emkey, R.D., Nichols, J.E., and Newberg, A. 1983. Low dose prednisone therapy in rheumatoid arthritis: a double blind study. *J.Rheumatol.* 10:713-721.

[2] Conn, D.L. 2001. Resolved: Low-dose prednisone is indicated as a standard treatment in patients with rheumatoid arthritis. *Arthritis Rheum.* 45:462-467.

[3] Locascio, V., Bonucci, E., Imbimbo, B., Ballanti, P., Adami, S., Milani, S., Tartarotti, D., and DellaRocca, C. 1990. Bone loss in response to long-term glucocorticoid therapy. *Bone Miner.* 8:39-51.

[4] Nishimura, J. and Ikuyama, S. 2000. Glucocorticoid-induced osteoporosis: pathogenesis and management. *J.Bone Miner.Metab* 18:350-352.

[5] The Lung Health Study Research Group. 2000. Effect of inhaled triamcinolone on the decline in pulmonary function in chronic obstructive pulmonary disease. *N.Engl.J.Med.* 343:1902-1909.

[6] Walsh, L.J., Wong, C.A., Oborne, J., Cooper, S., Lewis, S.A., Pringle, M., Hubbard, R., and Tattersfield, A.E. 2001. Adverse effects of oral corticosteroids in relation to dose in patients with lung disease. *Thorax* 56:279-284.

[7] Ruegsegger, P., Medici, T.C., and Anliker, M. 1983. Corticosteroid-induced bone loss. A longitudinal study of alternate day therapy in patients with bronchial asthma using quantitative computed tomography. *Eur.J.Clin.Pharmacol.* 25:615-620.

[8] Bazzy-Asaad, A. 2001. Safety of inhaled corticosteroids in children with asthma. *Curr.Opin.Pediatr.* 13:523-527.

[9] Corren, J., Nelson, H., Greos, L.S., Bensch, G., Goldstein, M., Wu, J., Wang, S., and Newman, K. 2001. Effective control of asthma with hydrofluoroalkane flunisolide delivered as an extrafine aerosol in asthma patients. *Ann.Allergy Asthma Immunol.* 87:405-411.

[10] Fernandes, A.L., Faresin, S.M., Amorim, M.M., Fritscher, C.C., Pereira, C.A., and Jardim, J.R. 2001. Inhaled budesonide for adults with mild-to-moderate asthma: a randomized placebo-controlled, double-blind clinical trial. *Sao Paulo Med.J.* 119:169-174.

[11] Adinoff, A.D. and Hollister, J.R. 1983. Steroid-induced fractures and bone loss in patients with asthma. *N.Engl.J.Med.* 309:265-268.

[12] Park, S.J., Nguyen, D.Q., Savik, K., Hertz, M.I., and Bolman, R.M., III. 2001. Pre-transplant corticosteroid use and outcome in lung transplantation. *J.Heart Lung Transplant.* 20:304-309.

[13] Dequeker, J. and Westhovens, R. 1995. Low dose corticosteroid associated osteoporosis in rheumatoid arthritis and its prophylaxis and treatment: bones of contention. *J.Rheumatol.* 22:1013-1019.

[14] Adachi, J.D., Olszynski, W.P., Hanley, D.A., Hodsman, A.B., Kendler, D.L., Siminoski, K.G., Brown, J., Cowden, E.A., Goltzman, D., Ioannidis, G. *et al.* 2000. Management of corticosteroid-induced osteoporosis. *Semin.Arthritis Rheum.* 29:228-251.

[15] Saag, K.G., Koehnke, R., Caldwell, J.R., Brasington, R., Burmeister, L.F., Zimmerman, B., Kohler, J.A., and Furst, D.E. 1994. Low dose long-term corticosteroid therapy in rheumatoid arthritis: an analysis of serious adverse events. *Am.J.Med.* 96:115-123.

[16] Braun, J. and Sieper, J. 2001. [Glucocorticoid-induced osteoporosis]. *Orthopade* 30:444-450.

[17] Clowes, J.A., Peel, N., and Eastell, R. 2001. Glucocorticoid-induced osteoporosis. *Curr.Opin.Rheumatol.* 13:326-332.

[18] Lukert, B.P. and Raisz, L.G. 1990. Glucocorticoid-induced osteoporosis: pathogenesis and management. *Ann.Intern.Med.* 112:352-364.

[19] Klein, G. 2004. Glucocorticoid-induced bone loss in children. *Clinical Reviews in Bone and Mineral Metabolism* 2:37-52.

[20] VAN STAA, T.P., COOPER, C., Leufkens, H., and Bishop, N. 2003. Children and the Risk of Fractures Caused by Oral Corticosteroids. *Journal of Bone and Mineral Research* 18:913-918.

[21] Boot, A.M., de Jongste, J.C., Verberne, A.A.P.H., Pols, H.A.P., and de Muinck Keizer-Schrama, S. 1997. Bone mineral density and bone metabolism of prepubertal children with asthma after long-term treatment with inhaled corticosteroids. *Pediatr.Pulmonol.* 24:379-384.

[22] Covar, R.A., Leung, D.Y., McCormick, D., Steelman, J., Zeitler, P., and Spahn, J.D. 2000. Risk factors associated with glucocorticoid-induced adverse effects in children with severe asthma. *J Allergy Clin Immunol* 106:651-659.

[23] Burnham, J.M. and Leonard, M.B. 2004. Bone disease in pediatric rheumatologic disorders. *Curr.Rheumatol.Rep.* 6 70-78.

[24] Viswanathan, A. and Sylvester, F. 2008. Chronic pediatric inflammatory diseases: Effects on bone. *Reviews in Endocrine & Metabolic Disorders* 9:107-122.

[25] Burnham, J.M., Shults, J., Semeao, E., Foster, B., Zemel, B.S., Stallings, V.A., and Leonard, M.B. 2004. Whole Body BMC in Pediatric Crohn Disease: Independent Effects of Altered Growth, Maturation, and Body Composition. *Journal of Bone and Mineral Research* 19:1961-1968.

[26] Lilleby, V., Lien, G., Frey Fr_Eslie, K., Haugen, M., Flat_È, B., and F_Èrre, ś. 2005. Frequency of osteopenia in children and young adults with childhood-onset systemic lupus erythematosus. *Arthritis & Rheumatism* 52:2051-2059.

[27] Compeyrot-Lacassagne, S., Tyrrell, P.N., Atenafu, E., Doria, A.S., Stephens, D., Gilday, D., and Silverman, E.D. 2007. Prevalence and etiology of low bone mineral density in juvenile systemic lupus erythematosus. *Arthritis & Rheumatism* 56:1966-1973.

[28] Walther, F., Fusch, C., Radke, M., Beckert, S., and Findeisen, A. 2006. Osteoporosis in pediatric patients suffering from chronic inflammatory bowel disease with and without steroid treatment. *J Pediatr.Gastroenterol.Nutr.* 43:42-51.

[29] Boot, A.M., Bouquet, J., Krenning, E.P., and Muinck Keizer-Schrama, S.M.P.F. 1998. Bone mineral density and nutritional status in children with chronic inflammatory bowel disease. *Gut* 42:188-194.

[30] Mazziotti, G., Angeli, A., Bilezikian, J.P., Canalis, E., and Giustina, A. 2006. Glucocorticoid-induced osteoporosis: an update. *Trends in Endocrinology & Metabolism* 17:144-149.

[31] Webster, J.C. and Cidlowski, J.A. 1999. Mechanisms of Glucocorticoid-receptor-mediated Repression of Gene Expression. *Trends in Endocrinology and Metabolism* 10:396-402.

[32] Kumar, R. and Thompson, E.B. 2005. Gene regulation by the glucocorticoid receptor: Structure:function relationship. *The Journal of Steroid Biochemistry and Molecular Biology* 94:383-394.

[33] Kallio, P.J., Palvimo, J., and Janne, O.A. 1994. [Nuclear hormone receptors]. *Duodecim* 110:383-394.

[34] Giguere, V., Hollenberg, S.M., Rosenfeld, M.G., and Evans, R.M. 1986. Functional domains of the human glucocorticoid receptor. *Cell* 46:645-652.

[35] Parker, M.G. 1990. Structure and function of nuclear hormone receptors. *Semin.Cancer Biol* 1:81-87.

[36] Morrison, N. and Eisman, J. 1993. Role of the negative glucocorticoid regulatory element in glucocorticoid repression of the human osteocalcin promoter. *J Bone Miner.Res.* 8:969-975.

[37] De Bosscher, K., Vanden Berghe, W., and Haegeman, G. 2003. The Interplay between the Glucocorticoid Receptor and Nuclear Factor-{kappa}B or Activator Protein-1: Molecular Mechanisms for Gene Repression. *Endocr Rev* 24:488-522.

[38] De Bosscher, K., Vanden Berghe, W., and Haegeman, G. 2000. Mechanisms of anti-inflammatory action and of immunosuppression by glucocorticoids: negative

interference of activated glucocorticoid receptor with transcription factors. *J Neuroimmunol.* 109:16-22.

[39] Zitnik, R.J., Whiting, N.L., and Elias, J.A. 1994. Glucocorticoid inhibition of interleukin-1-induced interleukin-6 production by human lung fibroblasts: evidence for transcriptional and post-transcriptional regulatory mechanisms. *Am J Respir.Cell Mol Biol* 10:643-650.

[40] Yang-Yen, H.F., Chambard, J.C., Sun, Y.L., Smeal, T., Schmidt, T.J., Drouin, J., and Karin, M. 1990. Transcriptional interference between c-Jun and the glucocorticoid receptor: mutual inhibition of DNA binding due to direct protein-protein interaction. *Cell* 62:1205-1215.

[41] Jonat, C., Rahmsdorf, H.J., Park, K.K., Cato, A.C., Gebel, S., Ponta, H., and Herrlich, P. 1990. Antitumor promotion and antiinflammation: down-modulation of AP-1 (Fos/Jun) activity by glucocorticoid hormone. *Cell* 62:1189-1204.

[42] Schule, R., Rangarajan, P., Kliewer, S., Ransone, L.J., Bolado, J., Yang, N., Verma, I.M., and Evans, R.M. 1990. Functional antagonism between oncoprotein c-Jun and the glucocorticoid receptor. *Cell* 62:1217-1226.

[43] Ray, A. and Prefontaine, K.E. 1994. Physical association and functional antagonism between the p65 subunit of transcription factor NF-kappa B and the glucocorticoid receptor. *Proc.Natl.Acad.Sci.U.S.A* 91:752-756.

[44] Scheinman, R.I., Gualberto, A., Jewell, C.M., Cidlowski, J.A., and Baldwin, A.S., Jr. 1995. Characterization of mechanisms involved in transrepression of NF-kappa B by activated glucocorticoid receptors. *Mol.Cell.Biol.* 15:943-953.

[45] Auphan, N., DiDonato, J.A., Rosette, C., Helmberg, A., and Karin, M. 1995. Immunosuppression by glucocorticoids: inhibition of NF-kappa B activity through induction of I kappa B synthesis. *Science* 270:286-290.

[46] Scheinman, R.I., Cogswell, P.C., Lofquist, A.K., and Baldwin, A.S., Jr. 1995. Role of transcriptional activation of I kappa B alpha in mediation of immunosuppression by glucocorticoids. *Science* 270:283-286.

[47] Crinelli, R., Antonelli, A., Bianchi, M., Gentilini, L., Scaramucci, S., and Magnani, M. 2000. Selective inhibition of NF-kB activation and TNF-alpha production in macrophages by red blood cell-mediated delivery of dexamethasone. *Blood Cells Mol Dis* 26:211-222.

[48] Thiele, K., Bierhaus, A., Autschbach, F., Hofmann, M., Stremmel, W., Thiele, H., Ziegler, R., and Nawroth, P.P. 1999. Cell specific effects of glucocorticoid treatment on the NF-kappaBp65/IkappaBalpha system in patients with Crohn's disease. *Gut* 45:693-704.

[49] De Bosscher, K., Schmitz, M.L., Vanden Berghe, W., Plaisance, S.p., Fiers, W., and Haegeman, G. 1997. Glucocorticoid-mediated repression of nuclear factor-_Bdependent transcription involves direct interference withΓĆётransactivation. *PNAS* 94:13504-13509.

[50] Brostjan, C., Anrather, J., Csizmadia, V., Stroka, D., Soares, M., Bach, F.H., and Winkler, H. 1996. Glucocorticoid-mediated Repression of NF__B Activity in Endothelial Cells Does Not Involve Induction of I__B__ Synthesis. *J.Biol.Chem.* 271:19612-19616.

[51] Heck, S., Bender, K., Kullmann, M., Gottlicher, M., Herrlich, P., and Cato, A.C. 1997. I kappaB alpha-independent downregulation of NF-kappaB activity by glucocorticoid receptor. *EMBO J* 16:4698-4707.

[52] Canalis, E., Mazziotti, G., Giustina, A., and Bilezikian, J.P. 2007. Glucocorticoid-induced osteoporosis: pathophysiology and therapy. *Osteoporos.Int* 18:1319-1328.

[53] Lukert, B.P. and Raisz, L.G. 1994. Glucocorticoid-induced osteoporosis. *Rheum. Dis. Clin. North Am.* 20:629-650.

[54] Sher, L.B., Woitge, H.W., Adams, D.J., Gronowicz, G.A., Krozowski, Z., Harrison, J.R., and Kream, B.E. 2004. Transgenic Expression of 11__-Hydroxysteroid Dehydrogenase Type 2 in Osteoblasts Reveals an Anabolic Role for Endogenous Glucocorticoids in Bone. *Endocrinology* 145:922-929.

[55] Sher, L.B., Harrison, J.R., Adams, D.J., and Kream, B.E. 2006. Impaired cortical bone acquisition and osteoblast differentiation in mice with osteoblast-targeted disruption of glucocorticoid signaling. *Calcif.Tissue Int* 79:118-125.

[56] Yang, M., Trettel, L.B., Adams, D.J., Harrison, J.R., Canalis, E., and Kream, B.E. 2010. Col3.6-HSD2 transgenic mice: A glucocorticoid loss-of-function model spanning early and late osteoblast differentiation. *Bone* 47:573-582.

[57] Bruder, S.P., Jaiswal, N., and Haynesworth, S.E. 1997. Growth kinetics, self-renewal, and the osteogenic potential of purified human mesenchymal stem cells during extensive subcultivation and following cryopreservation. *J.Cell Biochem.* 64:278-294.

[58] Engler, A.J., Sen, S., Sweeney, H.L., and Discher, D.E. 2006. Matrix Elasticity Directs Stem Cell Lineage Specification. *Cell* 126:677-689.

[59] Pittenger, M.F., Mackay, A.M., Beck, S.C., Jaiswal, R.K., Douglas, R., Mosca, J.D., Moorman, M.A., Simonetti, D.W., Craig, S., and Marshak, D.R. 1999. Multilineage Potential of Adult Human Mesenchymal Stem Cells. *Science* 284:143-147.

[60] Prockop, D.J. 1997. Marrow stromal cells as stem cells for nonhematopoietic tissues. *Science* 276:71-74.

[61] Ahdjoudj, S., Lasmoles, F., Oyajobi, B.O., Lomri, A., Delannoy, P., and Marie, P.J. 2001. Reciprocal control of osteoblast/chondroblast and osteoblast/adipocyte differentiation of multipotential clonal human marrow stromal F/STRO-1(+) cells. *J Cell Biochem.* 81:23-38.

[62] Beresford, J.N., Bennett, J.H., Devlin, C., Leboy, P.S., and Owen, M.E. 1992. Evidence for an inverse relationship between the differentiation of adipocytic and osteogenic cells in rat marrow stromal cell cultures. *J.Cell Sci.* 102 (Pt 2):341-351.

[63] Gori, F., Thomas, T., Hicok, K.C., Spelsberg, T.C., and Riggs, B.L. 1999. Differentiation of human marrow stromal precursor cells: bone morphogenetic protein-2 increases OSF2/CBFA1, enhances osteoblast commitment, and inhibits late adipocyte maturation. *J.Bone Miner.Res.* 14:1522-1535.

[64] Jaiswal, R.K., Jaiswal, N., Bruder, S.P., Mbalaviele, G., Marshak, D.R., and Pittenger, M.F. 2000. Adult human mesenchymal stem cell differentiation to the osteogenic or adipogenic lineage is regulated by mitogen-activated protein kinase. *J.Biol.Chem.* 275:9645-9652.

[65] Barak, Y., Nelson, M.C., Ong, E.S., Jones, Y.Z., Ruiz-Lozano, P., Chien, K.R., Koder, A., and Evans, R.M. 1999. PPAR gamma is required for placental, cardiac, and adipose tissue development. *Mol.Cell* 4:585-595.

[66] Rosen, E.D., Sarraf, P., Troy, A.E., Bradwin, G., Moore, K., Milstone, D.S., Spiegelman, B.M., and Mortensen, R.M. 1999. PPAR gamma is required for the differentiation of adipose tissue in vivo and in vitro. *Mol.Cell* 4:611-617.

[67] Shi, X.M., Blair, H.C., Yang, X., McDonald, J.M., and Cao, X. 2000. Tandem repeat of C/EBP binding sites mediates PPARgamma2 gene transcription in glucocorticoid-induced adipocyte differentiation. *J.Cell Biochem.* 76:518-527.

[68] Wu, Z., Bucher, N.L., and Farmer, S.R. 1996. Induction of peroxisome proliferator-activated receptor gamma during the conversion of 3T3 fibroblasts into adipocytes is mediated by C/EBPbeta, C/EBPdelta, and glucocorticoids. *Mol.Cell.Biol.* 16:4128-4136.

[69] Tang, Q.Q., Zhang, J.W., and Daniel Lane, M. 2004. Sequential gene promoter interactions by C/EBP[beta], C/EBP[alpha], and PPAR[gamma] during adipogenesis. *Biochemical and Biophysical Research Communications* 318:213-218.

[70] Clarke, S.L., Robinson, C.E., and Gimble, J.M. 1997. CAAT/Enhancer Binding Proteins Directly Modulate Transcription from the Peroxisome Proliferator- Activated Receptor [gamma]2 Promoter. *Biochemical and Biophysical Research Communications* 240:99-103.

[71] Weinstein, R.S., Jilka, R.L., Parfitt, A.M., and Manolagas, S.C. 1998. Inhibition of osteoblastogenesis and promotion of apoptosis of osteoblasts and osteocytes by glucocorticoids. Potential mechanisms of their deleterious effects on bone. *J Clin.Invest* 102:274-282.

[72] Yao, W., Cheng, Z., Busse, C., Pham, A., Nakamura, M.C., and Lane, N.E. 2008. Glucocorticoid excess in mice results in early activation of osteoclastogenesis and adipogenesis and prolonged suppression of osteogenesis: A longitudinal study of gene expression in bone tissue from glucocorticoid-treated mice. *Arthritis & Rheumatism* 58:1674-1686.

[73] Akune, T., Ohba, S., Kamekura, S., Yamaguchi, M., Chung, U.I., Kubota, N., Terauchi, Y., Harada, Y., Azuma, Y., Nakamura, K. *et al.* 2004. PPARgamma insufficiency enhances osteogenesis through osteoblast formation from bone marrow progenitors. *J.Clin.Invest* 113:846-855.

[74] Canalis, E. 2005. Mechanisms of glucocorticoid action in bone. *Curr.Osteoporos.Rep.* 3:98-102.

[75] Weinstein, R.S. 2001. Glucocorticoid-induced osteoporosis. *Rev.Endocr.Metab Disord.* 2:65-73.

[76] O'Brien, C.A., Jia, D., Plotkin, L.I., Bellido, T., Powers, C.C., Stewart, S.A., Manolagas, S.C., and Weinstein, R.S. 2004. Glucocorticoids Act Directly on Osteoblasts and Osteocytes to Induce Their Apoptosis and Reduce Bone Formation and Strength. *Endocrinology* 145:1835-1841.

[77] Robling, A.G., Niziolek, P.J., Baldridge, L.A., Condon, K.W., Allen, M.R., Alam, I., Mantila, S.M., Gluhak-Heinrich, J., Bellido, T.M., Harris, S.E. *et al.* 2008. Mechanical Stimulation of Bone in Vivo Reduces Osteocyte Expression of Sost/Sclerostin. *J.Biol.Chem.* 283:5866-5875.

[78] Gluhak-Heinrich, J., Ye, L., Bonewald, L.F., Feng, J.Q., MacDougall, M., Harris, S.E., and Pavlin, D. 2003. Mechanical Loading Stimulates Dentin Matrix Protein 1 (DMP1] Expression in Osteocytes In Vivo. *Journal of Bone and Mineral Research* 18:807-817.

[79] Hirayama, T., Sabokbar, A., and Athanasou, N.A. 2002. Effect of corticosteroids on human osteoclast formation and activity. *J Endocrinol* 175:155-163.

[80] Sivagurunathan, S., Muir, M.M., Brennan, T.C., Seale, J.P., and Mason, R.S. 2005. Influence of Glucocorticoids on Human Osteoclast Generation and Activity. *Journal of Bone and Mineral Research* 20:390-398.

[81] Jia, D., O'Brien, C.A., Stewart, S.A., Manolagas, S.C., and Weinstein, R.S. 2006. Glucocorticoids Act Directly on Osteoclasts to Increase Their Life Span and Reduce Bone Density. *Endocrinology* 147:5592-5599.

[82] Kim, H.J., Zhao, H., Kitaura, H., Bhattacharyya, S., Brewer, J.A., Muglia, L.J., Ross, F.P., and Teitelbaum, S.L. 2006. Glucocorticoids suppress bone formation via the osteoclast. *J Clin Invest* 116:2152-2160.

[83] S_Ée, K. and Delaiss_®, J.M. 2010. Glucocorticoids maintain human osteoclasts in the active mode of their resorption cycle. *Journal of Bone and Mineral Research* 25:2184-2192.

[84] D'Adamio, F., Zollo, O., Moraca, R., Ayroldi, E., Bruscoli, S., Bartoli, A., Cannarile, L., Migliorati, G., and Riccardi, C. 1997. A new dexamethasone-induced gene of the leucine zipper family protects T lymphocytes from TCR/CD3-activated cell death. *Immunity.* 7:803-812.

[85] Cannarile, L., Zollo, O., D'Adamio, F., Ayroldi, E., Marchetti, C., Tabilio, A., Bruscoli, S., and Riccardi, C. 2001. Cloning, chromosomal assignment and tissue distribution of human GILZ, a glucocorticoid hormone-induced gene. *Cell Death.Differ.* 8:201-203.

[86] Ayroldi, E., Zollo, O., Macchiarulo, A., Di Marco, B., Marchetti, C., and Riccardi, C. 2002. Glucocorticoid-induced leucine zipper inhibits the Raf-extracellular signal-regulated kinase pathway by binding to Raf-1. *Mol.Cell Biol.* 22:7929-7941.

[87] Shibanuma, M., Kuroki, T., and Nose, K. 1992. Isolation of a gene encoding a putative leucine zipper structure that is induced by transforming growth factor beta 1 and other growth factors. *J.Biol.Chem.* 267:10219-10224.

[88] Newton, R., Hart, L.A., Stevens, D.A., Bergmann, M., Donnelly, L.E., Adcock, I.M., and Barnes, P.J. 1998. Effect of dexamethasone on interleukin-1beta-(IL-1beta)-induced nuclear factor-kappaB (NF-kappaB) and kappaB-dependent transcription in epithelial cells. *Eur J Biochem* 254:81-89.

[89] Eddleston, J., Herschbach, J., Wagelie-Steffen, A.L., Christiansen, S.C., and Zuraw, B.L. 2007. The anti-inflammatory effect of glucocorticoids is mediated by glucocorticoid-induced leucine zipper in epithelial cells. *J Allergy Clin Immunol* 119:115-122.

[90] Delfino, D.V., Agostini, M., Spinicelli, S., Vito, P., and Riccardi, C. 2004. Decrease of Bcl-xL and augmentation of thymocyte apoptosis in GILZ overexpressing transgenic mice. *Blood.*

[91] Ayroldi, E., Migliorati, G., Bruscoli, S., Marchetti, C., Zollo, O., Cannarile, L., D'Adamio, F., and Riccardi, C. 2001. Modulation of T-cell activation by the glucocorticoid-induced leucine zipper factor via inhibition of nuclear factor kappaB. *Blood* 98:743-753.

[92] Mittelstadt, P.R. and Ashwell, J.D. 2001. Inhibition of AP-1 by the glucocorticoid-inducible protein GILZ. *J.Biol.Chem.* 276:29603-29610.

[93] Ayroldi, E., Zollo, O., Bastianelli, A., Marchetti, C., Agostini, M., Di Virgilio, R., and Riccardi, C. 2007. GILZ mediates the antiproliferative activity of glucocorticoids by negative regulation of Ras signaling. *J Clin Invest* 117:1605-1615.

[94] Berrebi, D., Bruscoli, S., Cohen, N., Foussat, A., Migliorati, G., Bouchet-Delbos, L., Maillot, M.C., Portier, A., Couderc, J., Galanaud, P. *et al.* 2003. Synthesis of glucocorticoid-induced leucine zipper (GILZ) by macrophages: an anti-inflammatory and immunosuppressive mechanism shared by glucocorticoids and IL-10. *Blood* 101:729-738.

[95] Yang, N., Zhang, W., and Shi, X.M. 2007. Glucocorticoid-induced leucine zipper (GILZ) mediates glucocorticoid action and inhibits inflammatory cytokine-induced COX-2 expression. *J Cell Biochem* 103:1760-1771.

[96] Arthaningtyas, E., Kok, C.C., Mordvinov, V.A., and Sanderson, C.J. 2005. The conserved lymphokine element 0 is a powerful activator and target for corticosteroid inhibition in human interleukin-5 transcription. *Growth Factors* 23:211-221.

[97] Cohen, N., Mouly, E., Hamdi, H., Maillot, M.C., Pallardy, M., Godot, V., Capel, F., Balian, A., Naveau, S., Galanaud, P. *et al.* 2005. GILZ expression in human dendritic cells redirects their maturation and prevents antigen-specific T lymphocyte response. *Blood*2005-2007.

[98] Ayroldi, E. and Riccardi, C. 2009. Glucocorticoid-induced leucine zipper (GILZ): a new important mediator of glucocorticoid action. *FASEB J.* 23:1-10.

[99] Asselin-Labat, M.L., Biola-Vidamment, A., Kerbrat, S., Lombes, M., Bertoglio, J., and Pallardy, M. 2005. FoxO3 Mediates Antagonistic Effects of Glucocorticoids and Interleukin-2 on Glucocorticoid-Induced Leucine Zipper Expression. *Mol Endocrinol* 19:1752-1764.

[100] Zhang, W., Yang, N., and Shi, X.M. 2008. Regulation of Mesenchymal Stem Cell Osteogenic Differentiation by Glucocorticoid-induced Leucine Zipper (GILZ). *J.Biol.Chem.* 283:4723-4729.

[101] He, L., Yang, N., Isales, C.M., and Shi, X.M. 2012. Glucocorticoid-Induced Leucine Zipper (GILZ) Antagonizes TNF-__ Inhibition of Mesenchymal Stem Cell Osteogenic Differentiation. *PLoS ONE* 7:e31717.

[102] Nakashima, K., Zhou, X., Kunkel, G., Zhang, Z.P., Deng, J.M., Behringer, R.R., and de Crombrugghe, B. 2002. The novel zinc finger-containing transcription factor Osterix is required for osteoblast differentiation and bone formation. *Cell* 108:17-29.

[103] Lu, X., Gilbert, L., He, X., Rubin, J., and Nanes, M.S. 2006. Transcriptional Regulation of the Osterix (Osx, Sp7) Promoter by Tumor Necrosis Factor Identifies Disparate Effects of Mitogen-activated Protein Kinase and NF+¦B Pathways. *J.Biol.Chem.* 281:6297-6306.

[104] Gilbert, L., He, X., Farmer, P., Rubin, J., Drissi, H., van Wijnen, A.J., Lian, J.B., Stein, G.S., and Nanes, M.S. 2002. Expression of the Osteoblast Differentiation Factor RUNX2 (Cbfa1/AML3/Pebp2alpha A) Is Inhibited by Tumor Necrosis Factor-alpha. *J.Biol.Chem.* 277:2695-2701.

[105] Kaneki, H., Guo, R., Chen, D., Yao, Z., Schwarz, E.M., Zhang, Y.E., Boyce, B.F., and Xing, L. 2006. Tumor Necrosis Factor Promotes Runx2 Degradation through Up-regulation of Smurf1 and Smurf2 in Osteoblasts. *J.Biol.Chem.* 281:4326-4333.

[106] Zhao, M., Qiao, M., Oyajobi, B.O., Mundy, G.R., and Chen, D. 2003. E3 ubiquitin ligase Smurf1 mediates core-binding factor alpha1/Runx2 degradation and plays a specific role in osteoblast differentiation. *J.Biol.Chem.* 278:27939-27944.

[107] Rauch, A., Seitz, S., Baschant, U., Schilling, A.F., Illing, A., Stride, B., Kirilov, M., Mandic, V., Takacz, A., Schmidt-Ullrich, R. *et al.* 2010. Glucocorticoids Suppress Bone Formation by Attenuating Osteoblast Differentiation via the Monomeric Glucocorticoid Receptor. *Cell Metabolism* 11:517-531.

[108] Yao, W., Cheng, Z., Busse, C., Pham, A., Nakamura, M.C., and Lane, N.E. 2008. Glucocorticoid excess in mice results in early activation of osteoclastogenesis and adipogenesis and prolonged suppression of osteogenesis: A longitudinal study of gene expression in bone tissue from glucocorticoid-treated mice. *Arthritis & Rheumatism* 58:1674-1686.

[109] Kassel, O., Sancono, A., Kratzschmar, J., Kreft, B., Stassen, M., and Cato, A.C.B. 2001. Glucocorticoids inhibit MAP kinase via increased expression and decreased degradation of MKP-1. *EMBO J* 20:7108-7116.

[110] Suzuki, A., Guicheux, J., Palmer, G., Miura, Y., Oiso, Y., Bonjour, J.P., and Caverzasio, J. 2002. Evidence for a role of p38 MAP kinase in expression of alkaline phosphatase during osteoblastic cell differentiation. *Bone* 30:91-98.

[111] Park, O.J., Kim, H.J., Woo, K.M., Baek, J.H., and Ryoo, H.M. 2010. FGF2-activated ERK Mitogen-activated Protein Kinase Enhances Runx2 Acetylation and Stabilization. *J.Biol.Chem.* 285:3568-3574.

[112] Song, C.Z., Tian, X., and Gelehrter, T.D. 1999. Glucocorticoid receptor inhibits transforming growth factor-beta signaling by directly targeting the transcriptional activation function of Smad3. *Proc Natl Acad Sci U.S.A* 96:11776-11781

[113] Iu, M.F., Kaji, H., Sowa, H., Naito, J., Sugimoto, T., and Chihara, K. 2005. Dexamethasone suppresses Smad3 pathway in osteoblastic cells. *J Endocrinol* 185:131-138.

[114] Periyasamy, S. and Sánchez, E.R. 2002. Antagonism of glucocorticoid receptor transactivity and cell growth inhibition by transforming growth factor-[beta] through AP-1-mediated transcriptional repression. *The International Journal of Biochemistry & Cell Biology* 34:1571-1585.

[115] Song, C.Z., Tian, X., and Gelehrter, T.D. 1999. Glucocorticoid receptor inhibits transforming growth factor-beta signaling by directly targeting the transcriptional activation function of Smad3. *Proc Natl Acad Sci U.S.A* 96:11776-11781.

[116] Locklin, R.M., Oreffo, R.O.C., and Triffitt, J.T. 1999. Effects of TGF[beta] and BFGF on the differentiation of human bone marrow stromal fibroblasts. *Cell Biology International* 23:185-194.

[117] Alliston, T., Choy, L., Ducy, P., Karsenty, G., and Derynck, R. 2001. TGF-[beta]-induced repression of CBFA1 by Smad3 decreases cbfa1 and osteocalcin expression and inhibits osteoblast differentiation. *EMBO J* 20:2254-2272.

[118] Kassem, Kveiborg, and Eriksen. 2000. Production and action of transforming growth factor-__ in human osteoblast cultures: dependence on cell differentiation and modulation by calcitriol. *European Journal of Clinical Investigation* 30:429-437.

[119] Edwards, J.R., Nyman, J.S., Lwin, S.T., Moore, M.M., Esparza, J., O'Quinn, E.C., Hart, A.J., Biswas, S., Patil, C.A., Lonning, S. *et al.* 2010. Inhibition of TGF-beta signaling by 1D11 antibody treatment increases bone mass and quality in vivo. *jbmrn-a*.

[120] Tang, Y., Wu, X., Lei, W., Pang, L., Wan, C., Shi, Z., Zhao, L., Nagy, T.R., Peng, X., Hu, J. *et al.* 2009. TGF-beta1-induced migration of bone mesenchymal stem cells couples bone resorption with formation. *Nat.Med.* 15:757-765.

[121] Bouvard, B., Audran, M., Legrand, E., and Chappard, D. 2009. Ultrastructural characteristics of glucocorticoid-induced osteoporosis. *Osteoporosis International* 20:1089-1092.

[122] Berris, K.K., Repp, A.L., and Kleerekoper, M. 2007. Glucocorticoid-induced osteoporosis. *Current Opinion in Endocrinology, Diabetes and Obesity* 14.

[123] L_Èv_źs, K., Gjesdal, C.G., Christensen, M., Wolff, A.B., Alm_źs, B.È., Svartberg, J., Fougner, K.J., Syversen, U., Bollerslev, J., Falch, J.A. *et al.* 2009. Glucocorticoid replacement therapy and pharmacogenetics in Addison's disease: effects on bone. *Eur J Endocrinol* 160:993-1002.

[124] Grossman, J.M., Gordon, R., Ranganath, V.K., Deal, C., Caplan, L., Chen, W., Curtis, J.R., Furst, D.E., McMahon, M., Patkar, N.M. *et al.* 2010. American College of Rheumatology 2010 recommendations for the prevention and treatment of glucocorticoid-induced osteoporosis. *Arthritis Care Res* 62:1515-1526.

[125] van Staa, T. 2006. The Pathogenesis, Epidemiology and Management of Glucocorticoid-Induced Osteoporosis. *Calcified Tissue International* 79:129-137.

[126] Weinstein, R.S. 2010. Glucocorticoids, osteocytes, and skeletal fragility: The role of bone vascularity. *Bone* 46:564-570.

[127] Angeli, A., Guglielmi, G., Dovio, A., Capelli, G., de Feo, D., Giannini, S., Giorgino, R., Moro, L., and Giustina, A. 2006. High prevalence of asymptomatic vertebral fractures in post-menopausal women receiving chronic glucocorticoid therapy: A cross-sectional outpatient study. *Bone* 39:253-259.

[128] Leib, E.S., Saag, K.G., Adachi, J.D., Geusens, P.P., Binkley, N., McCloskey, E.V., and Hans, D.B. 2011. Official Positions for FRAX_« Clinical Regarding Glucocorticoids: The Impact of the Use of Glucocorticoids on the Estimate by FRAX_« of the 10 Year Risk of Fracture: From Joint Official Positions Development Conference of the International Society for Clinical Densitometry and International Osteoporosis Foundation on FRAX_«. *Journal of Clinical Densitometry* 14:212-219.

[129] Teitelbaum, S.L., Seton, M.P., and Saag, K.G. 2011. Should bisphosphonates be used for long-term treatment of glucocorticoid-induced osteoporosis? *Arthritis & Rheumatism* 63:325-328.

[130] Saag, K.G., Shane, E., Boonen, S., Mar_Łn, F., Donley, D.W., Taylor, K.A., Dalsky, G.P., and Marcus, R. 2007. Teriparatide or Alendronate in Glucocorticoid-Induced Osteoporosis. *New England Journal of Medicine* 357:2028-2039.

[131] Sambrook, P.N. 2007. Anabolic Therapy in Glucocorticoid-Induced Osteoporosis. *New England Journal of Medicine* 357:2084-2086.

Chapter 3

CCKergic System, Hypothalamus-Pituitary-Adrenal (HPA) Axis, and Early-Life Stress (ELS)

Mingxi Tang, Anu Joseph, Qian Chen, Jianwei Jiao and Ya-Ping Tang

Additional information is available at the end of the chapter

1. Introduction

Early-life exposure to adverse experience or stress, simply termed early-life stress (ELS), is a worldwide problem that has a significantly negative impact in human health [1, 2]. In the United States, about 50% of adults had experienced some kind of stress before age 18 [3], and up to 15-25% of adults had traumatic ELS such as sexual abuse [4]. Most ELS is parents-originated, such as neglect, maltreatment, and abuse [5, 6]. In addition to the immediate, dreadful, and destructive effects on a child's life, ELS may produce a series of mental [7, 8], cardiovascular [9, 10], metabolic [11, 12], and many other types of disease [13, 14], at a later life stage. For example, adults who were sexually abused during childhood have a 5.7-fold increase in risk for drug abuse over those without ELS [7], and the prevalence of posttraumatic stress disorder (PTSD), a predominant form of anxiety disorders (ADs), is highly associated with ELS, with a 4-5 fold difference between adults with ELS and those without ELS [15]. Moreover, cognitive dysfunctions [16-18] such as learning and memory impairment [19-21] are also highly associated with ELS. Given that children, especially early adolescents, have a higher possibility to expose to a traumatic insult [22], adolescent trauma (AT) is an important risk factor for these post-ELS disorders.

Over the past decades, considerable insights have been gained into the molecular/neuronal mechanisms regarding how ELS impacts brain function and behavior [23-26]. Generally, it is now accepted that ELS can produce changes, most permanently, at multiple levels [25, 27]. Following ELS, for example, the overall volume of the hippocampus [28-30], corpus callosum [31-33], and cortex [34-36] all becomes smaller, compared to that of those brain regions in age-matched subjects. Besides these neuroanatomical changes, the neuronal activity and the synaptic function in the brain in ELS-victims are impaired [37-39], and most neurotransmitter systems are significantly affected too. By using positron emission tomography or fMRI, it has been found that a significantly increased release of dopamine in the ventral striatum is associated to ELS [40, 41]. The turnover rate of the serotonin (5-HT) metabolism or the 5-HT receptor density [42, 43] is altered following ELS. Similarly, the activity of the glutamatergic system [44, 45] and the cholinergic system [46, 47] are also altered in the brain of individuals following ELS. However, it should be emphasized that the changes in the hypothalamic-pituitary-adrenal (HPA) axis activity is of the most interest [48-52].

As the most important stress-related neuroendocrine system in the body, the HPA axis is anatomically and functionally composed of three major structures: the paraventricular nucleus of the hypothalamus (PVN), the anterior lobe of the pituitary gland, and the adrenal gland [53, 54]. The PVN contains magnocellular neurosecretory neurons that synthesize and release a corticotropin-releasing factor (CRF). CRF is a 41 amino acid peptide [55, 56], and can bind to three types of G-protein-coupled receptors: CRFR1, CRFR2, and CRFR3 [57-59]. In the mammalian brain, both CRF and CRFR1 are mainly distributed in the limbic system, while CRFR-2 is in the hypothalamus [60-62]. The essential role for the CRF system is to maintain the basal HPA axis activity as well as to trigger the HPA axis in response to stresses. After released from the PVN, the CRF binds to CRFR1 at the anterior pituitary and increase the release of adrenocorticotropic hormone (ACTH). The ACTH consequently stimulates the release of glucocorticoids from the adrenal gland [63]. Once released, glucocorticoids bind both high-affinity mineralocorticoid receptors and lower-affinity glucocorticoid receptors. The glucocorticoids, or cortisol in humans and corticosterone in rodents, play an essential role in energy metabolism, growth processes, immune function, and brain functions [63, 64].

In response to stress, CRF system plays an essential role in modifying peripheral physiological response to support "fight or flight" reactions, such as mobilizing energy stores, increasing blood sugar and heart rate, inhibiting digestive functions etc [65,66]. In addition, CRF itself may act on CRFR2 in the brain to directly regulate adaptive behavioral changes encountering stress [67-69]. Taken together, the CRF/HPA system plays a primary role in coordinating the endocrine, autonomic, immune, and behavioral response to stress. As stress, either real or imaged, is a necessary inducer for ADs, the CRF/HPA system must play a unique role in anxiety-related behaviors. Indeed, a huge body of evidence has documented this notion. For example, administration of CRF [70-72] or CRFR1 agonists [69,73,74] or overexpression of the CRF gene [75-77] produces Anxiety-like behaviors (ALBs) in the animals. On the other hand, CRFR1 antagonists exert significantly anxiolytic effects [78-80]. Knockout of CRF or CRFR1 in mice significantly reduces ALBs to stress and dramatically blunts stress-induced HPA axis activity [61,81,82]. Remarkably, previous chronic stress is able to enhance HPA axis activity in response to a novel acute stress, despite the negative feedback effects of increased glucocorticoids produced by the chronic stress [83-85]. For example, CCK-4-induced panic status in healthy volunteers significantly increases HPA axis activities [86]. Even the effects of early-life stress on HPA axis function are found to be associated with CCK sensitivity [130]. Most interestingly, interactions between the CCKergic system and the CRF/HPA system exist [88-90]. For example, the CCKergic system was found to be involved in this chronic stress-enhanced responsiveness, since chronic stress can specifically facilitate the release of CCK into the PVN, which directly projects to the pituitary, in response to acute stress [125]. All these findings have not only established the role of the CRF/HPA system in initiating behavioral responses to stresses, but also indicate that a significant interaction may exist between the CRF/HPA system and CCKergic system to regulate stress-related behaviors.

However, the vulnerability among different individuals to AT is different. This variability may at least partially attribute to a genetic variability [91]. A twin study of Vietnam veterans revealed that about 37.9% of vulnerability to PTSD was genetically related [92]. Further genetic evidence comes from clinical association studies, by which several candidate genes for ADs including PTSD have been associated, although a causative gene has not been yet established [91]. Among those candidate genes, cholecystokinin (CCK) receptor-2 (CCKR-2) has been linked to panic disorder, another major form of ADs [93,94].

As the most abundant neuropeptides, CCK distributes broadly in the brain and mainly in the limbic system [95,96]. CCK binds to CCK receptor-1 (CCKR-1) and CCKR-2, of which the CCKR-2 is predominantly found in the brain with the highest level in cortical area and the limbic system [97], a brain region that is critically involved in emotion response and behavior. Virtually, the CCKergic system has long been recognized as an anxiogenic factor for the animals [98], and this effect has been well validated in human populations as well [89,99,100]. Our recent study also showed that overexpression of CCKR2 in neurons of the forebrain of mice significantly enhanced ALBs [101]. At the same time, some candidate genes that are linked to ADs are also associated with HPA axis activity. For example, a common polymorphism at the serotonin transporter (5-HTT) gene, namely 5HTTLPR, is a strong candidate genetic variation for ADs and depression [102-103], and also is significantly implicated in HPA axis activity [104]. Similar to the CCKergic system, the HPA axis system has long been recognized as a stress hormone [105,106], and plays a critical role in the pathogenesis of ADs [107,108]. Indeed, following ELS, the activity of the HPA axis system is dysfunctional [109-111]. Moreover, given the overall role of both the HPA axis system [112-114] and the CCKergic system [115-117] in regulating neuronal, cardiovascular, and metabolic functions in the body, these two systems may play an integrative role in the pathogenesis of post-ELS disorders.

In this study, by using our previously engineered inducible forebrain-specific CCKR-2 transgenic (IF-CCKR-2 tg) mice [101], we demonstrated that the elevated CCKergic tone in the brain significantly facilitated the effect of AT on the impairment of the glucocorticoid negative feedback inhibition in response to a novel acute stressor during the adult stage in the mouse, providing direct evidence that reveals a molecular basis for this co-effect.

2. Materials and methods

2.1. Experimental animals

The procedures for the generation of IF-CCKR-2 tg (simply dtg) mice were described in our previous publication [101]. Briefly, we used the tTA/tetO-inducible gene expression system to produce these dtg mice. This system requires two independent transgenic mouse strains, tTA transgenic and tetO/CCKR-2 transgenic mice. Accordingly, two constructs were made. The first was for tTA transgenic mice, in which the expression of the tTA was under the control of an alpha-Ca^{2+} calmodulin kinase II (CaMKII) promoter. The tTA transgene cassette consists of

0.6 kb of exon-intron splicing signal (pNN265), 1.0 kb of tTA encoding sequence (pTet-Off, Clontech), and 0.5 kb of SV-40 poly-A signals (pTet-Off, CLONTECH). The other construct is for CCKR-2 transgenic mice, in which the expression of the CCKR-2 transgene was under the control of the tetO promoter. The CCKR-2 transgene cassette consisted of 1.3 kb of mouse CCKR-2 cDNA, an upstream 0.6 kb of splicing signal (pNN265), and a downstream 1.1 kb of b-globin poly-A signals. All these components were subcloned into the pTRE2 vector (CLONTECH). CCKR-2 cDNA was cloned by RT-PCR from the total RNA extracted from the brain of a male B6/CBA F1 mouse (The Jackson Laboratory) with the primers of 5'-CGG GAT CCA TGG ATC TGC TCA AGC TG-3' and 5'-GCT CTA GAT CAG CCA GGT CCC AGC GT-3'. A commercial RNA extraction kit (Invitrogen) and a reverse transcription kit (Stratagene) were used. The cloned cDNA was confirmed by sequencing. The plasmid constructs were then linearized with suitable enzymes and separately injected into the pronucleoli of B6/CBA F1 zygotes, as described [118]. Transgenic founders and the transgene copy numbers were determined by Southern blot analyses of the tail DNA. Founder mice with suitable gene copy numbers were backcrossed into B6/CBA F1 mice first to produce hemizygous single transgenic mice and then to produce double hemizygous transgenic mice. We have totally generated nine CaMKII-tTA transgenic founders and seven tetO-CCKR-2 transgenic founders. Southern blot analyses indicated that the gene copy numbers were from 2 to 70 for tTA transgenic founders and 2-150 for CCKR-2 transgenic founders (data not shown). To map the tTA expression pattern in the brain, we crossed a tetO-Lac-Z reporter mouse line (SJL-TgN-tetoplacZ, the Jackson Laboratory) into different independent CaMKII-tTA mouse lines to produce different tTA-LacZ double transgenic mouse lines. For Lac-Z staining, a commercial X-Gal staining kit (Invitrogen) and the recommended staining protocol were used with sagittal brain sections (30 μm), by which we identified a tTA transgenic line that was of the capacity to drive tetO/gene expression in almost all the neurons in the forebrain region (data not shown). Genotyping was determined by PCR analyses of both tTA (5'-AGG CTT GAG ATC TGG CCA TAC-3' and 5'-AGG AAA AGT GAG TAT GGT G-3') and the CCKR-2 (5'-ACG GTG GGA GGC CTA TAT AA-3' and 5'-GAG TGT GAA GGG CATG CAA-3') transgenes. Dtg mice used here were around 12-16 generations since they were generated, during which duration dtg mice were backcrossed into B6/CBA F1 mice in every 5-6 generations, in order to avoid an inbreed effect. Single transgenic (tTA or tetO-CCKR-2 only) and wild-type (wt) littermates of dtg mice were used as controls, and are collectively and simply called wt mice hereafter. Mice used here were kept in standard laboratory mouse cages under the standard condition (12 hours light/dark cycle, temperature at 22 ± 1 °C, humility at 75%) with food and water *ad libitum*. All experimental procedures for the use of animals were previously reviewed and approved by the institutional animal care and use committee at the Louisiana State University Heath Sciences Center at New Orleans, and all of the experiments were conducted in accordance with the Guide for the Care and Use of Laboratory Animals published by the US National Institutes of Health.

2.2. *In situ* hybridization

The hybridization was used to detect the expression level and pattern of the CCKR-2 transgene in the brain. Brains from both wt and dtg mice were collected by decapitation, and were frozen with powered dry ice immediately. Sagittal sections (20 µm) were made with a Cryostat (Leica, CM 1900, Richmond, IL). An oligo probe for tTA and a cRNA probe for the total CCKR-2 mRNAs were labeled with ^{35}S UTP (>1,000 Ci/mmol; NEN, Boston, MA) by a random labeling kit and *in vitro* transcription kit (Invitrogen, Carlsbad, CA), respectively. The hybridization was performed overnight at 55°C, and after washing, slides were exposed to Kodak BioMax film (NEN) for the same time.

2.3. Adolescent trauma (AT)

Both wt and dtg mice at the age of P25 were individually put into a small shock-box (4 X 4 X 10 inch in high) that was modified from the shock box from a fear-conditioning system (Coulbourn Instruments, Whitehall, PA), in order to ensure that the mice did not have much space for escaping during shocking. The current of the footshock was higher (1.0 mA) than it was commonly used in the fear-conditioning test (0.6-0.8 mA). The footshock was conducted for 5 times (trials), in total, during a period of 1 minute, and each trial lasted for 2 seconds, with an interval of 10 seconds between trials.

2.4. Acute stressor (AS)

Additional acute stressor (AS; 0.8 mA for 2 seconds for one trial) with a standard fear-conditioning paradigm as described previously [119], was used to trigger HPA axis reaction at the age of P60 (2 months).

2.5. ELISA

Commercially available kits for both the adrenocorticotropic hormone (ACTH) (MD Bioproducts, St. Paul, MN) and corticosteroid hormone (CORT) (R&D systems, Minneapolis, MN) were used to determine the serum level of these hormones. Experimental procedures followed the recommended steps. In order to have samples enough for triplicate measurements, blood was collected with a retroorbital eye bleeding method. In order to minimize non-specific effects, blood collection was conducted at 9:00 Am, and the procedure was completed within 30 seconds, by which time any possible charge that might be produced by the sampling procedure was not yet measurable.

2.6. Statistical analysis

Both female and male mice were almost equally distributed in each group. Data were analyzed with one-way ANOVA, followed by post-hoc tests. The p value less than 0.05 is considered significant.

3. Results

3.1. Expression of the CCKR-2 transgene in the brain of dtg mice

As shown in Fig 1, *in situ* hybridization revealed that the expression of the tTA was forebrain-specific in dtg mice (Fig. 1B), but was not detectable in wt mice (Fig. 1A). The expression pattern of the CCKR-2 transgene (data not shown) was the same as both the pattern of the tTA expression and the CCKR-2 transgene expression reported in our previous study [101].

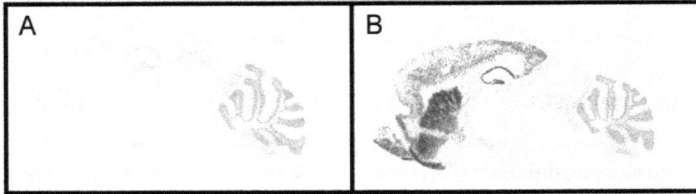

Figure 1. Expression pattern of the tTA mRNA detected by *in situ* hybridization with saggital brain sections in wt (A) and dtg (B) mice.

3.2. Dtg mice with AT exhibit an increased HPA axis activity in response to AS

Either wt (n = 60) or dtg mice (n = 60) were subjected to AT, and then were divided into 5 groups (n = 12) for a time-course study, in which both ACTH and CORT were examined before the AS for the basal level, and 1, 2, 4, and 8 hours following the AS. As shown in Fig. 2, although the difference in the basal level of ACTH (Fig. 2A) or CORT (Fig. 2C) between these mice was not significant, a tendency of a lower level ACTH (p = 0.0741) and CORT (p = 0.0648) was observed in dtg groups, compared to wt groups. Following the AS, an one-way ANOVA revealed a significant effect of the AT and CCKR-2 transgene on ACTH [F(1,8) = 6.781, p < 0.01] and CORT [F(1,8) = 9.201, p < 0.01]. Detailed post-hoc tests revealed that both ACTH (Fig. 2B) and CORT (Fig. 2D) in either wt or dtg mice reached the peak level at 1 hr after the AS, while a significant difference was observed at 1 and 2 hr in ACTH between wt and dtg groups (p > 0.05), and at 1 and 2 hr in CORT between wt and dtg groups (p > 0.05). In both wt and dtg mice, ACTH returned to the basal level at 4 hr (Fig. 2B), while CORT returned to the basal level at 4 hr (Fig. 2D). All these results indicate that the interaction between the AT and CCKR-2 transgene does not only increase the activity of the HPA axis following a novel stressor, but also impairs the CORT negative feedback in response this stressor.

3.3. Disassociation of the CCKR2 transgene expression and AT largely diminishes the effect of AT on HPA axis activity in response to AS

In this study, both wt and dtg mice were treated with doxycycline (doxy, 2 mg/100 ml in drinking water) for 5 days prior to AT, so that the transgene expression in dtg mice was inhibited during the episode of AT, and this inhibition lasted for about 3-5 days after the doxy treatment. At 2 months old, these mice were subjected to AS, and 1 hr later, which is the peak time of HPA axis response, as described in Fig. 2, the HPA axis activity was measured. Surprisingly, the levels of both ACTH and CORT were indistinguishable between wt and dtg mice, indicating that the coupling of AT and the transgene expression is critical for the AT to produce impaired glucocorticoid negative feedback inhibition in the animals.

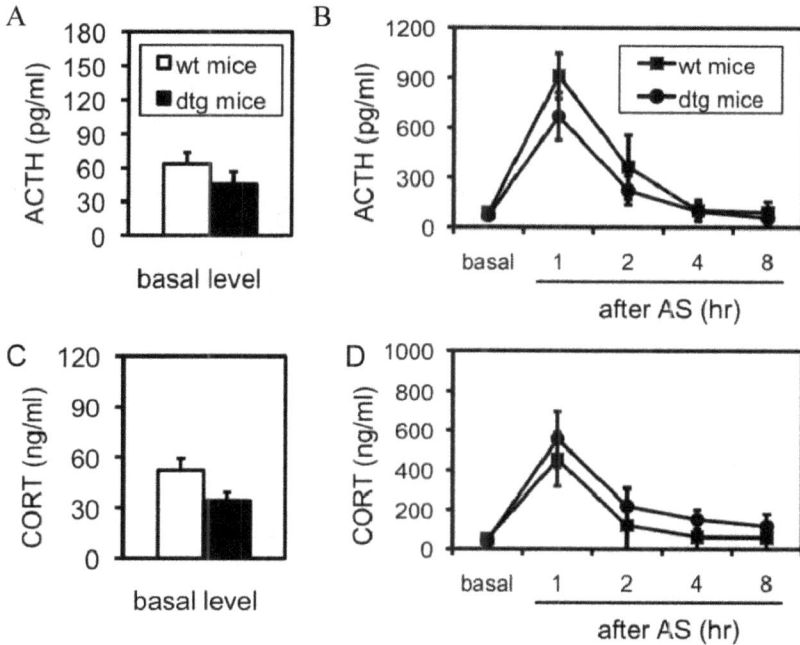

Figure 2. Increased HPA axis activity in dtg mice with AT/AS. A. Basal serum level of ACTH in naïve wt mice and naïve dtg mice. A tendency of a difference is shown, but it is not significant. Data are expressed as mean ± SEM. **B.** Time-course of ACTH response following the AS. **C.** Easal serum level of CORT in naïve wt mice and naïve dtg mice. A tendency of a difference is shown, but it is not significant. Data are expressed as mean ± SEM. **D.** Time-course of CORT response following the AS. The same groups of mice above were examined.

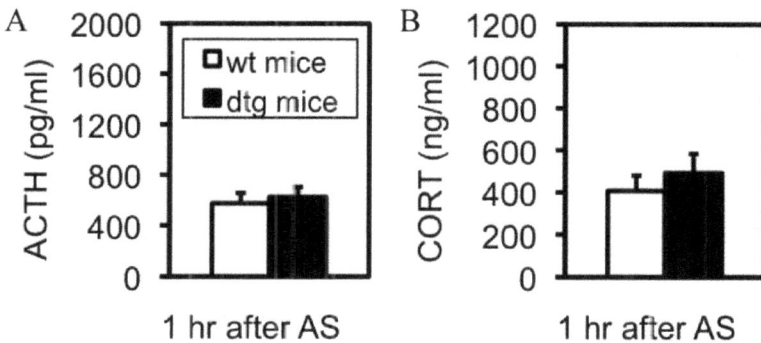

Figure 3. Level of ACTH (A) and CORT (B) in the mice after AT/AS. No significant difference was found between wt and dtg mice when the expression of the CCKR-2 transgene was suppressed during AT.

4. Discussion

We have for the first time demonstrated that a coupling of a higher CCKergic tone with an ELS event is a causative factor for the development of an impairment of glucocorticoid negative feedback inhibition in the animals in response to additional acute stressor at a later life stage.

This demonstration is achieved based on the technical merit in our transgenic mice, in which the transgene expression is inducible/reversible. The time resolution for this inducible/reversible feature is within 1 week, which is high enough for this time-coupling analysis. However, it is still not clear how this real-time coupling occurs, partially due to the fact that the functional significance of the CCKergic system is still not fully understood. As G protein-coupled receptors, CCKR are associated with Ca^{2+} release, PKC activation, PLA2 activity, and cAMP production [120]. In addition, there are robust interactions between the CCKergic system and other neurotransmitter systems including dopaminergic, serotonergic, and GABAergic systems at both the structural and functional levels [121,122], and therefore, the mechanism underlying this associative effect should be complicated, and need to be further studied.

An important finding in this study is the discovery of the change in the HPA axis activity, and these changes include (1) a slightly lower basal level of the HPA axis activity in dtg mice, compared to wt mice, (2) a synergistic effect of AT and the CCKR-2 transgene on the peak level of the HPA axis activity in response to the AS; (3) a prolonged decay time of the HPA axis activity following the AS in dtg mice with AT, and (4) a requirement of real-time coupling of the transgene expression and TA. It should be mentioned that it has been well established that a previous chronic stress in the animals down-regulates the HPA axis activity, but enhances their response to a novel acute stress, despite the negative feedback effects [83,123,124]. Because chronic stress can specifically facilitate the release of CCK into the PVN, which directly projects to the pituitary, in response to acute stress [88], the elevated CCKergic tone in our dtg mice may mimic the effect of a chronic stress by working as an "intrinsic stressor" for the animals. Therefore, this intrinsic stressor constitutes a basis for the higher vulnerability of dtg mice to AT. At the same time, the impaired AS-induced CORT negative feedback response may, in tern, significantly alter many other physiological functions, and eventually lead to a pathological condition.

As described above, following ELS, neuroanatomical changes were found in different brain regions. In addition, neuronal activity is altered too {125}. Consistent to the current study, the activity of the HPA axis system in the subject who experienced ELS was dysregulated [48-52]. Moreover, many other neurotransmitter systems were also affected by ELS [40, 126-128]. Therefore, the finding from the current study has provided additional evidence regarding how the CCKergic system and the HPA axis system are involved in the pathogenesis of post-ELS disorders.

The most important finding in this study is the demonstration of that if the transgene was temporally suppressed during the time of AT exposure, this impaired HPA axis inhibition in response to another acute stressor was largely diminished, indicating that the temporal association of the elevated CCKergic tone with AT is critically pathogenic. This finding has a potential translational significance. It is well know that the endogenous CCKergic activity, or the CCKR-2 level in the brain, plays a dominant role in the expression of anxiety. For example, the expression of anxiety was correlated with the increased CCKergic tone, which was evidenced by a higher CCK receptor-binding capacity in the brain of anxious animals, in comparison with non-anxious animals [129-131]. Different fear responses among different strains of the same animal species were attributed to different expression levels of CCKR-2 [132-134]. On the other hand, evidence also indicates that the CCKergic tone in the brain is dynamically regulated by stress. Following stress, for example, both CCK peptide immunoreactivity and CCK receptor density in the brain were significantly increased [135-139]. Social isolation, an anxiogenic stress, increased the CCK mRNA expression in the brain [140]. Especially, the effect of ELS on the HPA axis activity was associated with CCK activity [87]. Chronic stress could specifically facilitate the release of CCK into the PNV in response to acute stress [84,141]. Consistently, CCKR-2 agonists could only produce, or produce more pronounced, anxiogenic effect in stressed animals, but not in un-stressed animals [88, 142-144]. Patients with ADs were more sensitive to CCKR-2 agonists than normal controls [145-148]. Together with all these findings, it seems conclusive that the CCKergic system is dynamically involved in ELS-triggered mental disorders, and thus, an inhibition of the CCKergic tone timely associated with an ELS event might be useful to prevent the development of post-ELS disorder, especially ADs.

In summary, our study has revealed a Novel molecular underpinning for the development of post-ESL disorders, especially for mental disorders, and provide insightful information regarding how can we develop a preventive strategy for these post-ESL disorders in the humans.

Author details

Mingxi Tang
Department of Pathology, Luzhou Medical College, Sichuan, P. R. China

Anu Joseph , Qian Chen , Jianwei Jiao and Ya-Ping Tang [*]
Department of Cell Biology and Anatomy, Louisiana State University Health Sciences Center, New Orleans, LA, USA

Acknowledgement

This work was partially conducted in the University of Chicago. This study was partially supported by grants from National Institute of Mental Health (MH066243), Alzheimer's Association (NIRG-02-4368), National Science Foundation (0213112), and NARSAD, all to YPT.

---

[*] Corresponding Author

5. References

[1] Turecki G, Ernst C, Jollant F, Labonte B, & Mechawar N (2012) The neurodevelopmental origins of suicidal behavior. *Trends Neurosci* 35(1):14-23.

[2] McGowan PO & Szyf M (2110) The epigenetics of social adversity in early life: implications for mental health outcomes. *Neurobiol Dis* 39(1):66-72 .

[3] Green JG, *et al.* (2010) Childhood adversities and adult psychiatric disorders in the national comorbidity survey replication I: associations with first onset of DSM-IV disorders. *Arch Gen Psychiatry* 67(2):113-123 .

[4] Vogeltanz ND, *et al.* (1999) Prevalence and risk factors for childhood sexual abuse in women: national survey findings. *Child Abuse Negl* 23(6):579-592.

[5] Luecken LJ & Lemery KS (2004) Early caregiving and physiological stress responses. *Clin Psychol Rev* 24(2):171-191.

[6] Weich S, Patterson J, Shaw R, & Stewart-Brown S (2009) Family relationships in childhood and common psychiatric disorders in later life: systematic review of prospective studies. *Br J Psychiatry* 194(5):392-398.

[7] Kendler KS, *et al.* (2000) Childhood sexual abuse and adult psychiatric and substance use disorders in women: an epidemiological and cotwin control analysis. *Arch Gen Psychiatry* 57(10):953-959.

[8] Howell BR & Sanchez MM (2011) Understanding behavioral effects of early life stress using the reactive scope and allostatic load models. *Dev Psychopathol* 23(4):1001-1016 .

[9] Schooling CM, *et al.* (2011) Parental death during childhood and adult cardiovascular risk in a developing country: the Guangzhou Biobank Cohort Study. *PLoS One* 6(5):e19675.

[10] Nuyt AM & Alexander BT (2009) Developmental programming and hypertension. *Curr Opin Nephrol Hypertens* 18(2):144-152.

[11] Tarry-Adkins JL & Ozanne SE (2011) Mechanisms of early life programming: current knowledge and future directions. *Am J Clin Nutr* 94(6):1765S-1771S

[12] Portha B, Chavey A, & Movassat J (2011) Early-life origins of type 2 diabetes: fetal programming of the beta-cell mass. *Exp Diabetes Res* 2011:105076

[13] Rooks C, Veledar E, Goldberg J, Bremner JD, & Vaccarino V (2012) Early trauma and inflammation: role of familial factors in a study of twins. *Psychosom Med* 74(2):146-152.

[14] Entringer S, *et al.* (2011) Stress exposure in intrauterine life is associated with shorter telomere length in young adulthood. *Proc Natl Acad Sci U S A* 108(33):E513-518.

[15] Breslau N, Davis GC, & Schultz LR (2003) Posttraumatic stress disorder and the incidence of nicotine, alcohol, and other drug disorders in persons who have experienced trauma. *Arch Gen Psychiatry* 60(3):289-294.

[16] Pechtel P & Pizzagalli DA (2010) Effects of early life stress on cognitive and affective function: an integrated review of human literature. *Psychopharmacology (Berl)*.

[17] Majer M, Nater UM, Lin JM, Capuron L, & Reeves WC (2010) Association of childhood trauma with cognitive function in healthy adults: a pilot study. *BMC Neurol* 10:61.

[18] Hedges DW & Woon FL (2010) Early-life stress and cognitive outcome. (Translated from Eng) *Psychopharmacology (Berl)*

[19] Chu JA, Frey LM, Ganzel BL, & Matthews JA (1999) Memories of childhood abuse: dissociation, amnesia, and corroboration. *Am J Psychiatry* 156(5):749-755.

[20] Goodman GS, Quas JA, & Ogle CM (2010) Child maltreatment and memory. *Annu Rev Psychol* 61:325-351

[21] McCormick CM & Mathews IZ (2010) Adolescent development, hypothalamic-pituitary-adrenal function, and programming of adult learning and memory. (Translated from eng) *Prog Neuropsychopharmacol Biol Psychiatry* 34(5):756-765 (in eng).

[22] Costello EJ, Erkanli A, Fairbank JA, & Angold A (2002) The prevalence of potentially traumatic events in childhood and adolescence. (Translated from eng) *J Trauma Stress* 15(2):99-112 (in eng).

[23] Loman MM & Gunnar MR (2010) Early experience and the development of stress reactivity and regulation in children. (Translated from eng) *Neurosci Biobehav Rev* 34(6):867-876 (in eng).

[24] Fenoglio KA, Brunson KL, & Baram TZ (2006) Hippocampal neuroplasticity induced by early-life stress: functional and molecular aspects. (Translated from eng) *Front Neuroendocrinol* 27(2):180-192 (in eng).

[25] Gunnar M & Quevedo K (2007) The neurobiology of stress and development. (Translated from eng) *Annu Rev Psychol* 58:145-173 (in eng).

[26] Glaser R & Kiecolt-Glaser J (2005) How stress damages immune system and health. (Translated from eng) *Discov Med* 5(26):165-169 (in eng).

[27] Kiecolt-Glaser JK, *et al.* (2011) Childhood adversity heightens the impact of later-life caregiving stress on telomere length and inflammation. (Translated from eng) *Psychosom Med* 73(1):16-22 (in eng).

[28] Rao U, *et al.* (2010) Hippocampal changes associated with early-life adversity and vulnerability to depression. (Translated from eng) *Biol Psychiatry* 67(4):357-364 (in eng).

[29] Cohen RA, *et al.* (2006) Early life stress and morphometry of the adult anterior cingulate cortex and caudate nuclei. (Translated from eng) *Biol Psychiatry* 59(10):975-982 (in eng).

[30] Rao H, *et al.* (2010) Early parental care is important for hippocampal maturation: evidence from brain morphology in humans. (Translated from eng) *Neuroimage* 49(1):1144-1150 (in eng).

[31] Kitayama N, *et al.* (2007) Morphologic alterations in the corpus callosum in abuse-related posttraumatic stress disorder: a preliminary study. (Translated from eng) *J Nerv Ment Dis* 195(12):1027-1029 (in eng).

[32] Teicher MH, *et al.* (2004) Childhood neglect is associated with reduced corpus callosum area. (Translated from eng) *Biol Psychiatry* 56(2):80-85 (in eng).

[33] Jackowski A, *et al.* (2011) Early-life stress, corpus callosum development, hippocampal volumetrics, and anxious behavior in male nonhuman primates. (Translated from eng) *Psychiatry Res* 192(1):37-44 (in eng).

[34] van Harmelen AL, *et al.* (2010) Reduced medial prefrontal cortex volume in adults reporting childhood emotional maltreatment. (Translated from eng) *Biol Psychiatry* 68(9):832-838 (in eng).

[35] Tomoda A, *et al.* (2009) Reduced prefrontal cortical gray matter volume in young adults exposed to harsh corporal punishment. (Translated from eng) *Neuroimage* 47 Suppl 2:T66-71 (in eng).

[36] Hohmann CF, Beard NA, Kari-Kari P, Jarvis N, & Simmons Q (2012) Effects of brief stress exposure during early postnatal development in Balb/CByJ mice: II. Altered cortical morphology. (Translated from Eng) *Dev Psychobiol* (in Eng).

[37] Judo C, *et al.* (2010) Early stress exposure impairs synaptic potentiation in the rat medial prefrontal cortex underlying contextual fear extinction. (Translated from eng) *Neuroscience* 169(4):1705-1714 (in eng).

[38] Carrion VG, Haas BW, Garrett A, Song S, & Reiss AL (2010) Reduced hippocampal activity in youth with posttraumatic stress symptoms: an FMRI study. (Translated from eng) *J Pediatr Psychol* 35(5):559-569 (in eng).

[39] Korosi A, *et al.* (2010) Early-life experience reduces excitation to stress-responsive hypothalamic neurons and reprograms the expression of corticotropin-releasing hormone. (Translated from eng) *J Neurosci* 30(2):703-713 (in eng).

[40] Pruessner JC, Champagne F, Meaney MJ, & Dagher A (2004) Dopamine release in response to a psychological stress in humans and its relationship to early life maternal care: a positron emission tomography study using [11C]raclopride. (Translated from eng) *J Neurosci* 24(11):2825-2831 (in eng).

[41] Soliman A, *et al.* (2011) Limbic response to psychosocial stress in schizotypy: a functional magnetic resonance imaging study. (Translated from eng) *Schizophr Res* 131(1-3):184-191 (in eng).

[42] Huggins KN, *et al.* (2012) Effects of early life stress on drinking and serotonin system activity in rhesus macaques: 5-hydroxyindoleacetic acid in cerebrospinal fluid predicts brain tissue levels. (Translated from Eng) *Alcohol* (in Eng).

[43] Matsuzaki H, *et al.* (2011) Juvenile stress attenuates the dorsal hippocampal postsynaptic 5-HT1A receptor function in adult rats. (Translated from eng) *Psychopharmacology (Berl)* 214(1):329-337 (in eng).

[44] Martisova E, *et al.* (2012) Long lasting effects of early-life stress on glutamatergic/GABAergic circuitry in the rat hippocampus. (Translated from eng) *Neuropharmacology* 62(5-6):1944-1953 (in eng).

[45] Alexander GM, *et al.* (2012) Disruptions in serotonergic regulation of cortical glutamate release in primate insular cortex in response to chronic ethanol and nursery rearing. (Translated from eng) *Neuroscience* 207:167-181 (in eng).

[46] Aisa B, *et al.* (2009) Neonatal stress affects vulnerability of cholinergic neurons and cognition in the rat: involvement of the HPA axis. (Translated from eng) *Psychoneuroendocrinology* 34(10):1495-1505 (in eng).

[47] Lapiz MD, et al. (2003) Influence of postweaning social isolation in the rat on brain development, conditioned behavior, and neurotransmission. (Translated from eng) Neurosci Behav Physiol 33(1):13-29 (in eng).

[48] Carpenter LL, Shattuck TT, Tyrka AR, Geracioti TD, & Price LH (2010) Effect of childhood physical abuse on cortisol stress response. (Translated from Eng) Psychopharmacology (Berl) (in Eng).

[49] Gillespie CF, Phifer J, Bradley B, & Ressler KJ (2009) Risk and resilience: genetic and environmental influences on development of the stress response. (Translated from eng) Depress Anxiety 26(11):984-992 (in eng).

[50] Mirescu C, Peters JD, & Gould E (2004) Early life experience alters response of adult neurogenesis to stress. (Translated from eng) Nat Neurosci 7(8):841-846 (in eng).

[51] Cicchetti D, Rogosch FA, Gunnar MR, & Toth SL (2010) The differential impacts of early physical and sexual abuse and internalizing problems on daytime cortisol rhythm in school-aged children. (Translated from eng) Child Dev 81(1):252-269 (in eng).

[52] Gunnar MR, Frenn K, Wewerka SS, & Van Ryzin MJ (2009) Moderate versus severe early life stress: associations with stress reactivity and regulation in 10-12-year-old children. (Translated from eng) Psychoneuroendocrinology 34(1):62-75 (in eng).

[53] Smith SM & Vale WW (2006) The role of the hypothalamic-pituitary-adrenal axis in neuroendocrine responses to stress. (Translated from eng) Dialogues Clin Neurosci 8(4):383-395 (in eng).

[54] Koob GF (2010) The role of CRF and CRF-related peptides in the dark side of addiction. (Translated from eng) Brain Res 1314:3-14 (in eng).

[55] Vale W, Spiess J, Rivier C, & Rivier J (1981) Characterization of a 41-residue ovine hypothalamic peptide that stimulates secretion of corticotropin and beta-endorphin. (Translated from eng) Science 213(4514):1394-1397 (in eng).

[56] Liu J, et al. (2004) Corticotropin-releasing factor and Urocortin I modulate excitatory glutamatergic synaptic transmission. (Translated from eng) J Neurosci 24(16):4020-4029 (in eng).

[57] Dautzenberg FM & Hauger RL (2002) The CRF peptide family and their receptors: yet more partners discovered. (Translated from eng) Trends Pharmacol Sci 23(2):71-77 (in eng).

[58] Lewis K, et al. (2001) Identification of urocortin III, an additional member of the corticotropin-releasing factor (CRF) family with high affinity for the CRF2 receptor. (Translated from eng) Proc Natl Acad Sci U S A 98(13):7570-7575 (in eng).

[59] Perrin MH & Vale WW (1999) Corticotropin releasing factor receptors and their ligand family. (Translated from eng) Ann N Y Acad Sci 885:312-328 (in eng).

[60] Kostich WA, Grzanna R, Lu NZ, & Largent BL (2004) Immunohistochemical visualization of corticotropin-releasing factor type 1 (CRF1) receptors in monkey brain. (Translated from eng) J Comp Neurol 478(2):111-125 (in eng).

[61] Potter E, *et al.* (1994) Distribution of corticotropin-releasing factor receptor mRNA expression in the rat brain and pituitary. (Translated from eng) *Proc Natl Acad Sci U S A* 91(19):8777-8781 (in eng).

[62] Van Pett K, *et al.* (2000) Distribution of mRNAs encoding CRF receptors in brain and pituitary of rat and mouse. (Translated from eng) *J Comp Neurol* 428(2):191-212 (in eng).

[63] Dallman MF, Akana SF, Strack AM, Hanson ES, & Sebastian RJ (1995) The neural network that regulates energy balance is responsive to glucocorticoids and insulin and also regulates HPA axis responsivity at a site proximal to CRF neurons. (Translated from eng) *Ann N Y Acad Sci* 771:730-742 (in eng).

[64] Feek CM, Marante DJ, & Edwards CR (1983) The hypothalamic-pituitary-adrenal axis. (Translated from eng) *Clin Endocrinol Metab* 12(3):597-618 (in eng).

[65] Pecoraro N, Gomez F, & Dallman MF (2005) Glucocorticoids dose-dependently remodel energy stores and amplify incentive relativity effects. (Translated from eng) *Psychoneuroendocrinology* 30(9):815-825 (in eng).

[66] Dunn AJ & Berridge CW (1990) Physiological and behavioral responses to corticotropin-releasing factor administration: is CRF a mediator of anxiety or stress responses? (Translated from eng) *Brain Res Brain Res Rev* 15(2):71-100 (in eng).

[67] Kishimoto T, *et al.* (2000) Deletion of crhr2 reveals an anxiolytic role for corticotropin-releasing hormone receptor-2. (Translated from eng) *Nat Genet* 24(4):415-419 (in eng).

[68] Matys T, *et al.* (2004) Tissue plasminogen activator promotes the effects of corticotropin-releasing factor on the amygdala and anxiety-like behavior. (Translated from eng) *Proc Natl Acad Sci U S A* 101(46):16345-16350 (in eng).

[69] Rainnie DG, *et al.* (2004) Corticotrophin releasing factor-induced synaptic plasticity in the amygdala translates stress into emotional disorders. (Translated from eng) *J Neurosci* 24(14):3471-3479 (in eng).

[70] Butler PD, Weiss JM, Stout JC, & Nemeroff CB (1990) Corticotropin-releasing factor produces fear-enhancing and behavioral activating effects following infusion into the locus coeruleus. (Translated from eng) *J Neurosci* 10(1):176-183 (in eng).

[71] Sutton RE, Koob GF, Le Moal M, Rivier J, & Vale W (1982) Corticotropin releasing factor produces behavioural activation in rats. (Translated from eng) *Nature* 297(5864):331-333 (in eng).

[72] Salak-Johnson JL, Anderson DL, & McGlone JJ (2004) Differential dose effects of central CRF and effects of CRF astressin on pig behavior. (Translated from eng) *Physiol Behav* 83(1):143-150 (in eng).

[73] Valdez GR, Zorrilla EP, Rivier J, Vale WW, & Koob GF (2003) Locomotor suppressive and anxiolytic-like effects of urocortin 3, a highly selective type 2 corticotropin-releasing factor agonist. (Translated from eng) *Brain Res* 980(2):206-212 (in eng).

[74] Bale TL (2005) Sensitivity to stress: dysregulation of CRF pathways and disease development. (Translated from eng) *Horm Behav* 48(1):1-10 (in eng).

[75] Heinrichs SC, *et al.* (1997) Anti-sexual and anxiogenic behavioral consequences of corticotropin-releasing factor overexpression are centrally mediated. (Translated from eng) *Psychoneuroendocrinology* 22(4):215-224 (in eng).

[76] van Gaalen MM, Stenzel-Poore MP, Holsboer F, & Steckler T (2002) Effects of transgenic overproduction of CRH on anxiety-like behaviour. (Translated from eng) *Eur J Neurosci* 15(12):2007-2015 (in eng).

[77] Kasahara M, Groenink L, Breuer M, Olivier B, & Sarnyai Z (2007) Altered behavioural adaptation in mice with neural corticotrophin-releasing factor overexpression. (Translated from eng) *Genes Brain Behav* 6(7):598-607 (in eng).

[78] Rassnick S, Heinrichs SC, Britton KT, & Koob GF (1993) Microinjection of a corticotropin-releasing factor antagonist into the central nucleus of the amygdala reverses anxiogenic-like effects of ethanol withdrawal. (Translated from eng) *Brain Res* 605(1):25-32 (in eng).

[79] Takahashi LK (2001) Role of CRF(1) and CRF(2) receptors in fear and anxiety. (Translated from eng) *Neurosci Biobehav Rev* 25(7-8):627-636 (in eng).

[80] Kehne J & De Lombaert S (2002) Non-peptidic CRF1 receptor antagonists for the treatment of anxiety, depression and stress disorders. (Translated from eng) *Curr Drug Targets CNS Neurol Disord* 1(5):467-493 (in eng).

[81] Timpl P, *et al.* (1998) Impaired stress response and reduced anxiety in mice lacking a functional corticotropin-releasing hormone receptor 1. (Translated from eng) *Nat Genet* 19(2):162-166 (in eng).

[82] Nguyen NK, *et al.* (2006) Conditional CRF receptor 1 knockout mice show altered neuronal activation pattern to mild anxiogenic challenge. (Translated from eng) *Psychopharmacology (Berl)* 188(3):374-385 (in eng).

[83] Akana SF, *et al.* (1996) Clamped Corticosterone (B) Reveals the Effect of Endogenous B on Both Facilitated Responsivity to Acute Restraint and Metabolic Responses to Chronic Stress. (Translated from Eng) *Stress* 1(1):33-49 (in Eng).

[84] Bhatnagar S, *et al.* (2000) A cholecystokinin-mediated pathway to the paraventricular thalamus is recruited in chronically stressed rats and regulates hypothalamic-pituitary-adrenal function. (Translated from eng) *J Neurosci* 20(14):5564-5573 (in eng).

[85] Young EA, Akana S, & Dallman MF (1990) Decreased sensitivity to glucocorticoid fast feedback in chronically stressed rats. (Translated from eng) *Neuroendocrinology* 51(5):536-542 (in eng).

[86] Eser D, *et al.* (2005) Panic induction with cholecystokinin-tetrapeptide (CCK-4) Increases plasma concentrations of the neuroactive steroid 3alpha, 5alpha tetrahydrodeoxycorticosterone (3alpha, 5alpha-THDOC) in healthy volunteers. (Translated from eng) *Neuropsychopharmacology* 30(1):192-195 (in eng)

[87] Greisen MH, Bolwig TG, & Wortwein G (2005) Cholecystokinin tetrapeptide effects on HPA axis function and elevated plus maze behaviour in maternally separated and handled rats. (Translated from eng) *Behav Brain Res* 161(2):204-212 (in eng).

[88] Abelson JL, Khan S, Liberzon I, & Young EA (2007) HPA axis activity in patients with panic disorder: review and synthesis of four studies. (Translated from eng) *Depress Anxiety* 24(1):66-76 (in eng).

[89] Raedler TJ, *et al.* (2006) Megestrol attenuates the hormonal response to CCK-4-induced panic attacks. (Translated from eng) *Depress Anxiety* 23(3):139-144 (in eng).

[90] Abelson JL & Young EA (2003) Hypothalamic-pituitary adrenal response to cholecystokinin-B receptor agonism is resistant to cortisol feedback inhibition. (Translated from eng) *Psychoneuroendocrinology* 28(2):169-180 (in eng).

[91] Cornelis MC, Nugent NR, Amstadter AB, & Koenen KC (2010) Genetics of post-traumatic stress disorder: review and recommendations for genome-wide association studies. (Translated from eng) *Curr Psychiatry Rep* 12(4):313-326 (in eng).

[92] Chantarujikapong SI, *et al.* (2001) A twin study of generalized anxiety disorder symptoms, panic disorder symptoms and post-traumatic stress disorder in men. (Translated from eng) *Psychiatry Res* 103(2-3):133-145 (in eng).

[93] Kennedy JL, *et al.* (1999) Investigation of cholecystokinin system genes in panic disorder. (Translated from eng) *Mol Psychiatry* 4(3):284-285 (in eng).

[94] Maron E, *et al.* (2005) Association study of 90 candidate gene polymorphisms in panic disorder. (Translated from eng) *Psychiatr Genet* 15(1):17-24 (in eng).

[95] Dockray GJ (1976) Immunochemical evidence of cholecystokinin-like peptides in brain. (Translated from eng) *Nature* 264(5586):568-570 (in eng).

[96] Lotstra F & Vanderhaeghen JJ (1987) Distribution of immunoreactive cholecystokinin in the human hippocampus. (Translated from eng) *Peptides* 8(5):911-920 (in eng).

[97] Hill DR, Campbell NJ, Shaw TM, & Woodruff GN (1987) Autoradiographic localization and biochemical characterization of peripheral type CCK receptors in rat CNS using highly selective nonpeptide CCK antagonists. (Translated from eng) *J Neurosci* 7(9):2967-2976 (in eng).

[98] Della-Fera MA & Baile CA (1979) Cholecystokinin octapeptide: continuous picomole injections into the cerebral ventricles of sheep suppress feeding. (Translated from eng) *Science* 206(4417):471-473 (in eng).

[99] Katzman MA, Koszycki D, & Bradwejn J (2004) Effects of CCK-tetrapeptide in patients with social phobia and obsessive-compulsive disorder. (Translated from eng) *Depress Anxiety* 20(2):51-58 (in eng).

[100] Hebb AL, Poulin JF, Roach SP, Zacharko RM, & Drolet G (2005) Cholecystokinin and endogenous opioid peptides: interactive influence on pain, cognition, and emotion. (Translated from eng) *Prog Neuropsychopharmacol Biol Psychiatry* 29(8):1225-1238 (in eng).

[101] Chen Q, Nakajima A, Meacham C, & Tang YP (2006) Elevated cholecystokininergic tone constitutes an important molecular/neuronal mechanism for the expression of anxiety in the mouse. *Proc Natl Acad Sci U S A* 103(10):3881-3886.

[102] Gonda X, Rihmer Z, Juhasz G, Zsombok T, & Bagdy G (2007) High anxiety and migraine are associated with the s allele of the 5HTTLPR gene polymorphism. (Translated from eng) *Psychiatry Res* 149(1-3):261-266 (in eng).

[103] Neumeister A, et al. (2002) Association between serotonin transporter gene promoter polymorphism (5HTTLPR) and behavioral responses to tryptophan depletion in healthy women with and without family history of depression. (Translated from eng) Arch Gen Psychiatry 59(7):613-620 (in eng).

[104] Wust S, et al. (2009) Sex-specific association between the 5-HTT gene-linked polymorphic region and basal cortisol secretion. (Translated from eng) Psychoneuroendocrinology 34(7):972-982 (in eng).

[105] Udelsman R & Chrousos GP (1988) Hormonal responses to surgical stress. (Translated from eng) Adv Exp Med Biol 245:265-272 (in eng).

[106] Armario A, et al. (2012) What can We Know from Pituitary-Adrenal Hormones About the Nature and Consequences of Exposure to Emotional Stressors? (Translated from Eng) Cell Mol Neurobiol (in Eng).

[107] Tronche F, et al. (1999) Disruption of the glucocorticoid receptor gene in the nervous system results in reduced anxiety. (Translated from eng) Nat Genet 23(1):99-103 (in eng).

[108] van Santen A, et al. (2010) Psychological traits and the cortisol awakening response: results from the Netherlands Study of Depression and Anxiety. (Translated from eng) Psychoneuroendocrinology 36(2):240-248 (in eng).

[109] Essex MJ, et al. (2011) Influence of early life stress on later hypothalamic-pituitary-adrenal axis functioning and its covariation with mental health symptoms: a study of the allostatic process from childhood into adolescence. (Translated from eng) Dev Psychopathol 23(4):1039-1058 (in eng).

[110] Wilkinson PO & Goodyer IM (2011) Childhood adversity and allostatic overload of the hypothalamic-pituitary-adrenal axis: a vulnerability model for depressive disorders. (Translated from eng) Dev Psychcpathol 23(4):1017-1037 (in eng).

[111] Murgatroyd C & Spengler D (2011) Epigenetic programming of the HPA axis: early life decides. (Translated from eng) Stress 14(6):581-589 (in eng).

[112] Kudielka BM & Wust S (2011) Human models in acute and chronic stress: assessing determinants of individual hypothalamus-pituitary-adrenal axis activity and reactivity. (Translated from eng) Stress 13(1) 1-14 (in eng).

[113] Nieuwenhuizen AG & Rutters F (2008) The hypothalamic-pituitary-adrenal-axis in the regulation of energy balance. (Translated from eng) Physiol Behav 94(2):169-177 (in eng).

[114] Walker BR (2007) Glucocorticoids and cardiovascular disease. (Translated from eng) Eur J Endocrinol 157(5):545-559 (in eng).

[115] Benedetti F, Amanzio M, Vighetti S, & Asteggiano G (2006) The biochemical and neuroendocrine bases of the hyperalgesic nocebo effect. (Translated from eng) J Neurosci 26(46):12014-12022 (in eng).

[116] Lovick TA (2009) CCK as a modulator of cardiovascular function. (Translated from eng) J Chem Neuroanat 38(3):176-184 (in eng).

[117] Lee SY & Soltesz I (2011) Cholecystokinin: a multi-functional molecular switch of neuronal circuits. (Translated from eng) Dev Neurobiol 71(1):83-91 (in eng).

[118] Hogan B, Beddington R, Costantini F, & Lacy E (1994) Manipulating the mouse embryo, a laboratory manual. *(in eng)*.

[119] Im HI, *et al.* (2009) Post-training dephosphorylation of eEF-2 promotes protein synthesis for memory consolidation. (Translated from eng) *PLoS One* 4(10):e7424 (in eng).

[120] Wank SA (1995) Cholecystokinin receptors. (Translated from eng) *Am J Physiol* 269(5 Pt 1):G628-646 (in eng).

[121] Bradwejn J & de Montigny C (1984) Benzodiazepines antagonize cholecystokinin-induced activation of rat hippocampal neurones. (Translated from eng) *Nature* 312(5992):363-364 (in eng).

[122] Rasmussen K, Helton DR, Berger JE, & Scearce E (1993) The CCK-B antagonist LY288513 blocks effects of diazepam withdrawal on auditory startle. (Translated from eng) *Neuroreport* 5(2):154-156 (in eng).

[123] Hauger RL, Lorang M, Irwin M, & Aguilera G (1990) CRF receptor regulation and sensitization of ACTH responses to acute ether stress during chronic intermittent immobilization stress. (Translated from eng) *Brain Res* 532(1-2):34-40 (in eng).

[124] Ma S & Morilak DA (2005) Chronic intermittent cold stress sensitises the hypothalamic-pituitary-adrenal response to a novel acute stress by enhancing noradrenergic influence in the rat paraventricular nucleus. (Translated from eng) *J Neuroendocrinol* 17(11):761-769 (in eng).

[125] Mueller SC, *et al.* (2010) Early-life stress is associated with impairment in cognitive control in adolescence: an fMRI study. (Translated from eng) *Neuropsychologia* 48(10):3037-3044 (in eng).

[126] Ryan B, *et al.* (2009) Remodelling by early-life stress of NMDA receptor-dependent synaptic plasticity in a gene-environment rat model of depression. (Translated from eng) *Int J Neuropsychopharmacol* 12(4):553-559 (in eng).

[127] Coplan JD, *et al.* (2010) Early-life stress and neurometabolites of the hippocampus. (Translated from eng) *Brain Res* 1358:191-199 (in eng).

[128] Gatt JM, *et al.* (2010) Early Life Stress Combined with Serotonin 3A Receptor and Brain-Derived Neurotrophic Factor Valine 66 to Methionine Genotypes Impacts Emotional Brain and Arousal Correlates of Risk for Depression. (Translated from Eng) *Biol Psychiatry* (in Eng).

[129] Harro J, Kiivet RA, Lang A, & Vasar E (1990) Rats with anxious or non-anxious type of exploratory behaviour differ in their brain CCK-8 and benzodiazepine receptor characteristics. (Translated from eng) *Behav Brain Res* 39(1):63-71 (in eng).

[130] MacNeil G, Sela Y, McIntosh J, & Zacharko RM (1997) Anxiogenic behavior in the light-dark paradigm follwoing intraventricular administration of cholecystokinin-8S, restraint stress, or uncontrollable footshock in the CD-1 mouse. (Translated from eng) *Pharmacol Biochem Behav* 58(3):737-746 (in eng).

[131] Pavlasevic S, Bednar I, Qureshi GA, & Sodersten P (1993) Brain cholecystokinin tetrapeptide levels are increased in a rat model of anxiety. (Translated from eng) *Neuroreport* 5(3):225-228 (in eng).

[132] Farook JM, *et al.* (2004) The CCK2 agonist BC264 reverses freezing behavior habituation in PVG hooded rats on repeated exposures to a cat. (Translated from eng) *Neurosci Lett* 355(3):205-208 (in eng).

[133] Farook JM, *et al.* (2001) Strain differences in freezing behavior of PVG hooded and Sprague-Dawley rats: differential cortical expression of cholecystokinin2 receptors. (Translated from eng) *Neuroreport* 12(12):2717-2720 (in eng).

[134] Wang H, *et al.* (2003) Genetic variations in CCK2 receptor in PVG hooded and Sprague-Dawley rats and its mRNA expression on cat exposure. (Translated from eng) *Behav Neurosci* 117(2):385-390 (in eng).

[135] Harro J, Lofberg C, Rehfeld JF, & Oreland L (1996) Cholecystokinin peptides and receptors in the rat brain during stress. (Translated from eng) *Naunyn Schmiedebergs Arch Pharmacol* 354(1):59-66 (in eng).

[136] Harro J, Marcusson J, & Oreland L (1992) Alterations in brain cholecystokinin receptors in suicide victims. (Translated from eng) *Eur Neuropsychopharmacol* 2(1):57-63 (in eng).

[137] Nevo I, Becker C, Hamon M, & Benoliel JJ (1996) Stress- and yohimbine-induced release of cholecystokinin in the frontal cortex of the freely moving rat: prevention by diazepam but not ondansetron. (Translated from eng) *J Neurochem* 66(5):2041-2049 (in eng).

[138] Siegel RA, Duker EM, Pahnke U, & Wuttke W (1987) Stress-induced changes in cholecystokinin and substance P concentrations in discrete regions of the rat hypothalamus. (Translated from eng) *Neuroendocrinology* 46(1):75-81 (in eng).

[139] Zhang LX, *et al.* (1996) Changes in cholecystokinin mRNA expression after amygdala kindled seizures: an in situ hybridization study. (Translated from eng) *Brain Res Mol Brain Res* 35(1-2):278-284 (in eng).

[140] Del Bel EA & Guimaraes FS (1997) Social isolation increases cholecystokinin mRNA in the central nervous system of rats. (Translated from eng) *Neuroreport* 8(16):3597-3600 (in eng).

[141] Herman JP, Flak J, & Jankord R (2008) Chronic stress plasticity in the hypothalamic paraventricular nucleus. (Translated from eng) *Prog Brain Res* 170:353-364 (in eng).

[142] Widom CS (1999) Posttraumatic stress disorder in abused and neglected children grown up. (Translated from eng) *Am J Psychiatry* 156(8):1223-1229 (in eng).

[143] Cohen H, Kaplan Z, & Kotler M (1999) CCK-antagonists in a rat exposed to acute stress: implication for anxiety associated with post-traumatic stress disorder. (Translated from eng) *Depress Anxiety* 10(1):8-17 (in eng).

[144] Koks S, *et al.* (2000) Cholecystokinin-induced anxiety in rats: relevance of pre-experimental stress and seasonal variations. (Translated from eng) *J Psychiatry Neurosci* 25(1):33-42 (in eng).

[145] Bradwejn J, Koszycki D, & Shriqui C (1991) Enhanced sensitivity to cholecystokinin tetrapeptide in panic disorder. Clinical and behavioral findings. (Translated from eng) *Arch Gen Psychiatry* 48(7):603-610 (in eng).

[146] Brawman-Mintzer O, *et al.* (1997) Effects of the cholecystokinin agonist pentagastrin in patients with generalized anxiety disorder. (Translated from eng) *Am J Psychiatry* 154(5):700-702 (in eng).

[147] Kellner M, *et al.* (2000) Behavioral and endocrine response to cholecystokinin tetrapeptide in patients with posttraumatic stress disorder. (Translated from eng) *Biol Psychiatry* 47(2):107-111 (in eng).

[148] van Vliet IM, Westenberg HG, Slaap BR, den Boer JA, & Ho Pian KL (1997) Anxiogenic effects of pentagastrin in patients with social phobia and healthy controls. (Translated from eng) *Biol Psychiatry* 42(1):76-78 (in eng).

Chapter 4

Glucocorticoid-Induced Cardioprotection: A Novel Role for Autophagy?

Anna-Mart Engelbrecht and Benjamin Loos

Additional information is available at the end of the chapter

1. Introduction

Glucocorticoids (GC) are commonly used as anti-inflammatory and immunosuppressive therapy by approximately 1% of the total adult population. Glucocorticoid therapy has also been used in non-autoimmune and non-inflammatory conditions such as acute myocardial infarction, angina, endocarditis as well as in invasive cardiology, coronary interventions and cardiopulmonary- bypass surgery. Despite ample evidence for GC's role as a natural, physiologic regulator of the immune system, little is known about the molecular events induced by GCs during a stress response. Autophagy is a survival mechanism which is upregulated in response to stress in the cell. It has been described as the cell's major adaptive strategy in response to a multitude of extracellular stresses, such as nutrient deprivation, mitochondrial damage, endoplasmic reticulum stress or infection. Conserved in all eukaryotes, it is mediated by a unique organelle, the autophagosome, which, under inclusion of cytoplasmic cargo, fuses with lysosomes in order to yield recyclable nutrient metabolites. Basal autophagic activity plays a vital role in maintaining homeostasis during cellular stress. Its malfunction has been implicated with human pathologies such as heart disease, neurological storage disease and cancer.

It is known that GC-triggered autophagy plays a role in cell death during development. However, recent landmark studies also indicate that autophagy operates as a hub, integrating cellular stress, metabolism and glucocorticoid mediated anti-inflammatory action. Importantly, recent lines of evidence suggest that glucocorticoids impact on key signalling components, which control the activity of the autophagic machinery.

In this review we will focus on the connections between these key signaling components and autophagy, describing their central roles as modulators of GC-induced protection during a cellular stress response.

2. Glucocorticoid generation and metabolism

The understanding of the physiological regulation of glucocorticoid activity has considerably improved over the last few decades. The generation of glucocorticoids from cholesterol, which occurs in the zonae fasiculata and reticularis of the adrenal cortex, is tightly regulated by the hypothalamic-pituitary-adrenal (HPA) axis where glucocorticoids regulate its own generation through negative feedback inhibition. Glucocorticoids are produced de novo under this control and are released into the blood as required, with a definite circadian rhythm producing peak concentrations in the early morning [1]. When secreted into the blood, most (90-95%) of glucocorticoids are sequestered to corticosteroid-binding globulin and albumin with the unbound fraction available to interact with their receptors [2]. Metabolic inactivation of glucocorticoids occurs predominantly in the liver, but also in the kidney with inactive metabolites excreted in the urine.

3. Molecular actions of glucocorticoids: Genomic and non-genomic pathways

The classical mode of glucocorticoid-induced gene expression, i.e. the genomic effect involves ligand-dependent activation and release from chaperone proteins (heat shock protein-90 and others), translocation of the receptor-complex to the nucleus where binding of the glucocorticoid receptor to glucocorticoid response element (GRE) in the promoter of the target genes will lead to transcriptional activation of the genes within hours [3, 4]. Activation of glucocorticoid-responsive genes occurs via interaction between the DNA-bound GR and transcriptional co-activator molecules such as CREB-binding protein, which have intrinsic histone acetyltransferase activity and cause acetylation of core histones. This tags histones to recruit chromatin remodeling engines and subsequent association of RNA polymerase II resulting in gene activation [5]. Increasing evidence suggests that glucocorticoids can also cause rapid activation of signaling molecules prior to altering gene expression. These so called non-genomic effects occur within minutes of glucocorticoid exposure and are not affected by inhibiting RNA transcription [5, 6].

Metabolic effects of glucocorticoids represent most of the adverse effects of glucocorticoid therapy and are mainly ascribed to the transcriptional activity of the glucocorticoid receptor, whereas the therapeutically beneficial anti-inflammatory actions are thought to be predominantly caused by the mechanism of transrepression where the activated GR can selectively repress the transcription of specific inflammatory genes without binding to DNA itself but by a number of pleiotropic actions at the promoters of inflammatory genes. Inflammatory genes are regulated by the actions of proinflammatory transcription factors such as nuclear factor-κB (NF-κB), activator protein -1 (AP-1), and signal transducer and transcription proteins. Activated GR binds to these transcription factors, either directly or indirectly, and recruits co-repressor proteins that blunt the ability of these transcription factors to switch on inflammatory genes [7]. Furthermore, many pro-inflammatory genes are repressed by GC at post-transcriptional level via mRNA destabilization or inhibition of translation, however, this phenomenon cannot be accounted for by transrepression, therefore suggest the existence of an additional anti-inflammatory mechanism of GCs [8].

4. Ischemia/reperfusion-induced stress in the heart

Glucocorticoids play a key role in the response to stress in the heart where it can influence the regulation of blood pressure, inflammation, immune function and cellular energy metabolism [9-10]. These acute effects contribute to an adaptive response in the short term. Although the cardioprotective effects of glucocorticoids in the acute setting of ischemia/reperfusion have been experimentally demonstrated in animals [11-13] and humans [14], the molecular mechanisms still need to be fully elucidated.

Ischemia can be defined as an imbalance between the amount of oxygen, glucose and other substrates needed by the heart [15,16]. This leads to anaerobic metabolism and reduced contractile function. A biochemical imbalance occurs as the maintenance of the metabolism cannot be kept at a steady state due to inadequate coronary flow. A reduction in metabolite clearance also occurs during ischemia and intracellular pH levels drop as the acid by-products of glycolysis accumulate. The severity of ischemic injury depends on the duration of ischemia and subsequent reperfusion [15,16]. If, ischemia is maintained, reversible injury gradually transitions to irreversible injury and a myocardial infarct develops. Reperfusion with its reinforced oxygen and substrate availability is thus a prerequisite for myocardial salvage [16]. However, reperfusion after an ischemic period causes generation of free radicals and is associated with detrimental changes such as enzyme release, arrhythmias and intramyocardial haemorrhage which are known as reperfusion injuries [17]. Cardiomyocytes are highly dependent on a continuous supply of oxygen. During ischemia, cardiomyocyte capacity to generate sufficient ATP and creatine phosphate becomes depleted and multiple adaptive processes occur in response to these hypoxic environments created during ischemia. To reduce oxygen consumption, oxidative phosphorylation is limited and glycolysis is stimulated. This aids in ATP production, even under low oxygen supply [18]. Prolonged ischemia leads to cardiac failure which is characterized by the progressive death of myocytes [19]. Three major morphologies of cell death have been described, viz. apoptosis (type I), cell death associated with autophagy (type II) and necrosis (type III).

5. The basic mechanisms of Autophagy

Autophagy, from greek *self eating*, is a conserved degradation and recycling system for long-lived proteins and other sub-cellular constituents. This degradation system is inherent to all eukaryotes and is mediated by a unique organelle, the autophagosome, which, under inclusion of cytoplasmic cargo, fuses with lysosomes in order to yield recyclable nutrient metabolites. Although already described in 1966 by de Duve and Wattiaux [20], Autophagy has received significant renewed attention in the last years. This new interest is primarily based on the recently gained understanding of the molecular components of the autophagic machinery. Genetic analyses in yeast identified more than 30 autophagy-related genes (ATG), and their corresponding proteins (Atg) participating in the autophagic pathway [21].

Multiple mechanisms exist for the mode of delivery of cytoplasmic material to the lysosome, giving rise to different types of autophagy. While microphagy is characterized by cytoplasm engulfment directly at the lysosomal surface by invagination of its membrane, macroautophagy involves the synthesis of double-membrane vesicles, which sequester portions of the cytoplasm [22]. Chaperone mediated autophagy (CMA) on the other hand involves selective motif tagged protein translocation directly through the lysosomal membrane [23]. However, shared by all three mechanisms is the final step of lysosomal cargo degradation by hydrolases, allowing the recycling of degraded material. Here we will focus on macroautophagy (herein referred to as autophagy), as it is the primary mechanism for cytoplasm-to-lysosome delivery.

The autophagic process can be divided into distinct steps, which include the induction, cargo packaging, vesicle nucleation, vesicle expansion and protein retrieval, docking and fusion and finally vesicle degradation [21]. In brief, the first event is the formation of the isolation membrane of the autophagosome. The Atg1 kinase complex governs these early steps in autophagosome formation. Central to this regulation is the nutrient sensor kinase mTOR (TORC). When mTOR is suppressed due to nutrient starvation, Atg1 kinase activity is triggered and affinity for Atg13 increases [24], which leads to the recruiting of other Atg proteins to initiate autophagosome formation. Cellular sources for this autophagosome formation step have been shown to be Golgi, ER, mitochondria and the plasma membrane [25]. During this process, two strongly interdependent conjugation systems are coordinating the events leading to the formation, elongation and sealing of the isolation membrane [26]. In the first conjugation system, Atg proteins 5, 7, 10 and 12 undergo a multimerization step with Atg16, leading to the formation of an Atg16 homotetramer, which assembles with four Atg12-Atg5 conjugates [27]. In the second conjugation system, the protein Atg8 is Atg4 dependently conjugated with phosphatidylethanolamine (PE) [28]. Reactive oxygen species play a role in controlling this step, as Atg4 oxidization enables autophagosome formation to proceed [29]. Next, two kinase complexes, PI3 kinase and Atg1, participate in the late stages of autophagosome formation. Atg6 (the mammalian orthologue, beclin-1) belongs to the PI3 kinase (PI3-K) class III complex. When Atg1 interacts with Atg13, progression towards a complete autophagosome takes place [27]. Cytoplasmic cargo is now confined. Docking and fusion with a lysosome will allow acidification of the autophagosome lumen, leading to the complete and rapid degradation of cargo into constituent components that are released into cytoplasmic space via permeases (Figure 1).

6. Autophagy as a protective response during stress in the heart

The terminally differentiated nature of cardiomyocytes demands a strong molecular reliance upon a functional autophagic degradation system. In cardiomyocytes autophagy has been described already in the late 1970's where it was emphasized as an important repair mechanism of sublethal injury [30]. Sybers and coworkers demonstrated the occurrence of myocyte autophagy in a fetal mouse heart that was kept for 1 h in organ culture. In addition they observed that Autophagy was accelerated by oxygen and glucose deprivation, but the hearts function could be restored following resupply of glucose and oxygen. However, when the period of injury lasted for longer than four hours, necrotic cell death was induced [30]. To date, many models have produced clear evidence that upregulation of autophagy promotes cell survival under conditions of metabolic perturbations and energy deprivation [31-33]. In the ischaemic myocardium, autophagy is upregulated rapidly following 20 minutes of coronary artery occlusion, leading to an increased number in autophagosomes [34]. In isolated cardiomyocytes exposed to anoxia-reoxygenation it was shown that inhibition of autophagy leads to an increase in necrotic cell death, which was further increased by additional inhibition of apoptosis [35]. However, enhancing autophagic flux, as indicated by an increased rate of autophagosomal clearance, protects cardiac myocytes against ischaemic injury by reducing apoptosis [31]. Moreover, the homeostatic role of functional basal autophagic activity in the myocardium has been demonstrated by cardiac specific disruption of Atg5, manifesting in impaired contractility, hypertrophy, dilation and sarcomeric disarray [36-37].

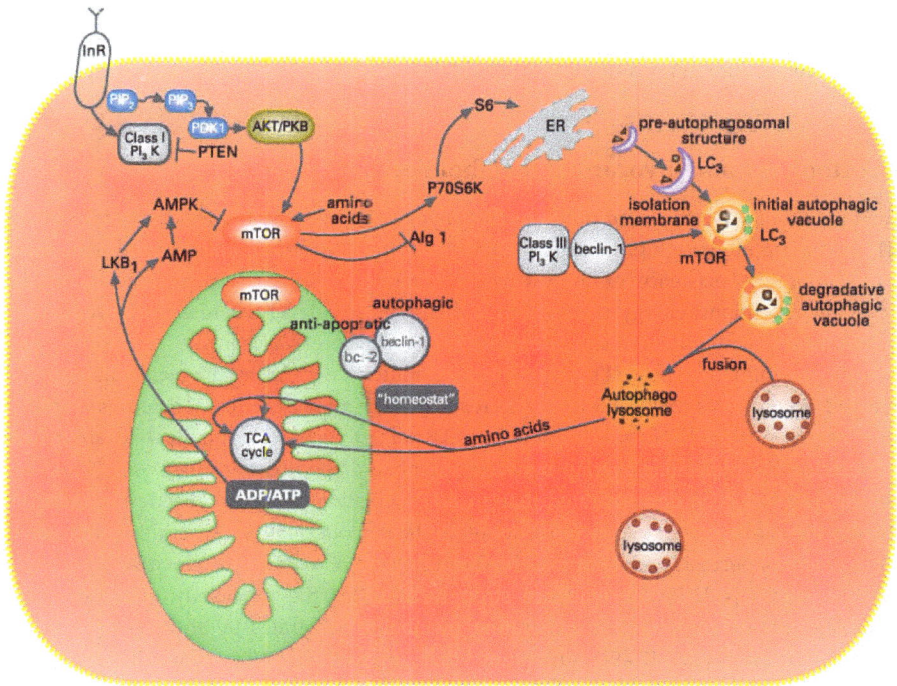

Figure 1. Schematic representation of the autophagic process, indicating the signalling network from induction to permease efflux with amino acid release, providing substrates for the TCA cycle.

7. Detrimental effects of Autophagy in the heart

Literature suggests that autophagy is uniquely controlled during ischemia and reperfusion. A large body of evidence indicates that upregulation of autophagy particularly during the reperfusion phase is detrimental and exacerbates myocyte death. Energy sensing mediated by the 5'-AMP-activated protein kinase (AMPK) appears to be central to this control mechanism. In glucose-deprived cardiac myocytes, autophagy resulting from ischemia has been shown to be accompanied by AMPK activation, and was inhibited by dominant negative AMPK, suggesting an AMPK dependent mechanism [34]. AMPK is rapidly activated during myocardial ischemia, and leads to an increase in glucose uptake and oxidation as well as fatty acid oxidation [38]. Autophagy is enhanced after reperfusion, which is accompanied by an inactivation of AMPK and an increase in beclin-1 [34]. As AMPK switches off ATP-dependent processes, [39] its inactivation at reperfusion may contribute to an unfavorable metabolic environment. Moreover, data indicate that energy sensing mediated by AMPK is also differentially controlled depending on the severity of the ischaemic insult [40]. These reports are strengthened by recent data derived from cultured myoblasts, where a differential induction of cell death was observed, which was dependent on the severity and duration of the ischaemic insult [33]. Only mild ischaemic injury induced autophagy and apoptosis, while severe injury led to primarily necrotic cell death.

8. Autophagy and myocardial metabolism

The total cellular ATP amount in the cardiac myocyte is consumed in less than one minute [41] indicating the very high metabolic demand of the myocardium, and at the same time highlighting the existence of an extremely efficient system of energy conversion. In ischaemic conditions, energy metabolism is disrupted to a level where energy production cannot meet the myocardial energy demand. However, there is a clear role for autophagy in ischemia to influence the cell's energy profile, indicative to maintain metabolic supply-demand homeostasis [33]. ATP levels decrease rapidly with ischemia and recover rapidly after reperfusion [42]. These dynamics of ATP depletion become highly relevant when considering the molecular overlap between autophagy, apoptosis and necrosis [32; 43-44, Figure 2]. It has been demonstrated that an ATP depletion of >50% is needed in order to change the mode of cell death from apoptotic to necrotic [45]. *Vice versa*, a progressive replacement of necrosis with apoptosis has been described, when intracellular ATP becomes available again [46]. Recent evidence strongly indicates the previously underestimated metabolic role of autophagy in generating metabolite substrates by shifting the cellular energetic balance [33; 47-49], suggesting that intracellular ATP availability may be controlled to a significant degree by the autophagic flux (Figure 2). These data strongly suggest that not only the magnitude of autophagic activity but also the cell's metabolic profile and microenvironment are crucial in controlling a favorable cellular response other than necrosis, and delaying apoptosis [32] (Figure 3).

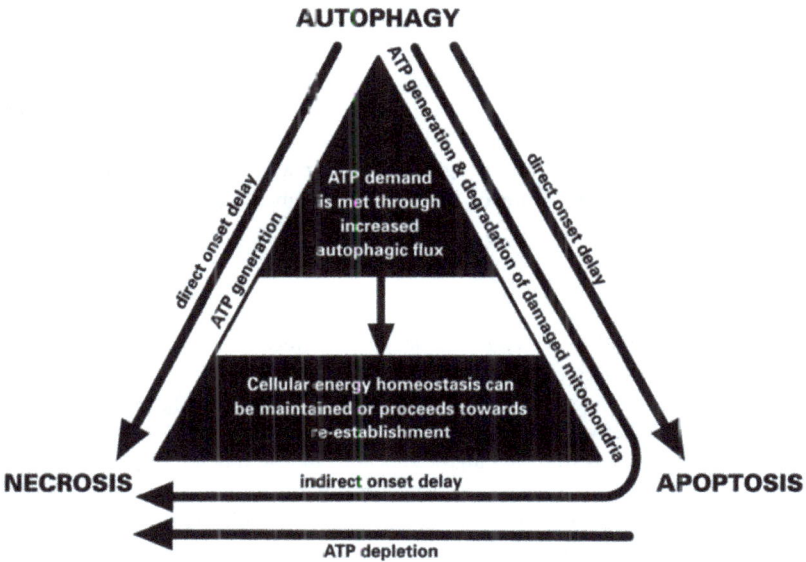

Figure 2. Recent evidence strongly indicates the previously underestimated metabolic role of autophagy in generating metabolite substrates and ATP by shifting the cellular energetic balance, with a direct and indirect effect on apoptosis and necrosis.

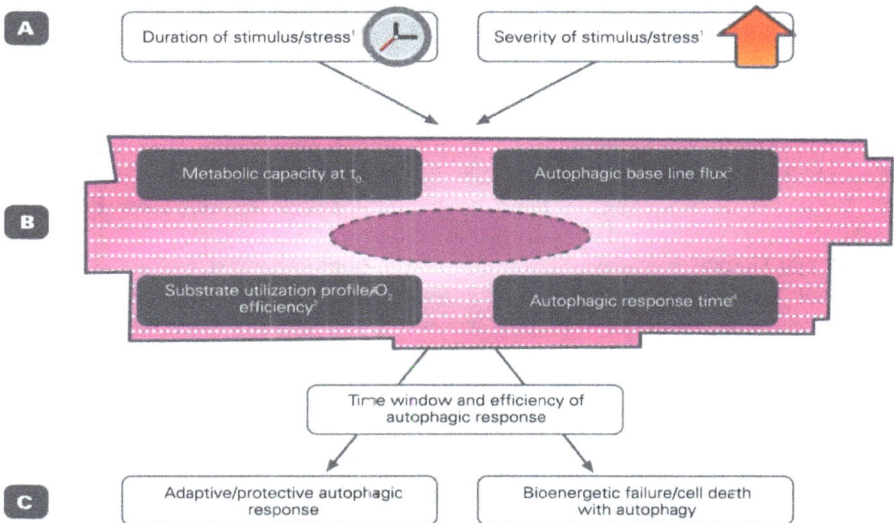

Figure 3. Whether autophagy may manifest in cytoprotection or type II programmed cell death is dependent on the severity and duration of the ischaemic insult, as well as autophagic flux- and metabolic parameters.

The above results also stress the significance of the severity and duration of the ischaemic event, to allow a sufficient induction of the autophagic machinery to take place. In fact, a direct relationship between autophagic flux and myocardial function has recently been proposed [50], indicating the strong need to measure autophagic activity accurately. Further characterization of the autophagic flux in clear context with myocardial injury will help to answer questions when autophagy functions as a primarily destructive pathway, manifesting in type II programmed cell death or when autophagy functions in a cytoprotective manner.

9. Autophagy and glucocorticoids-relationship and metabolic response

The multifaceted relationship between autophagy and glucocorticoids is already indicated in embryogenesis. Recent reports not only demonstrate an important metabolic role for autophagy during embryogenesis and postnatal development [51,52], but also indicate a likely molecular link between autophagic programmed cell death and steroids during development [53]. Embryos from the atg5$^{-/-}$ knockout mouse model die perinatally due to energy depletion, leading to a reduced plasma- and tissue amino acid concentration [54]. Moreover, increased apoptosis is displayed in various embryonic tissues derived from such embryos, supporting a role for autophagy in the removal of apoptotic bodies or in delaying the onset of apoptotic cell death [54]. Targeted disruption of beclin 1 in mice also leads to early death in embryogenesis [55]. Many examples of autophagy as a mode of programmed cell death during embryogenesis exist, suggesting that an important role for autophagic cell death in development. It has been shown that autophagic cell death requires the genes ATG7 as well as beclin 1 and can be induced by caspase-8 inhibition [56]. In addition, embryonic fibroblasts from Bax/Bak double knockout mice undergo autophagic cell death, which can be suppressed by inhibitors of autophagy and which is dependent on ATG5. These data suggest a role for Bcl-2 family proteins controlling also non-apoptotic cell death in addition to regulating apoptosis [57]. Especially in lower eukaryotes, the rise in steroid titers can elicit a transcription regulatory hierarchy that results in synchronous autophagic cell death [53]. Such steroid triggered programmed autophagic cell death has been observed in larval salivary gland cells [53] as well as motorneurons [58]. These findings suggest that steroids can play a governing role in very specific scenarios, controlling autophagic activity and the duration of increased flux, which in turn can control the synchronous induction of cell death. It is however not known, whether a robust increase in cortisol release in humans following psychological stress, trauma, sepsis or starvation can elicit similar effects on autophagic activity during embryogenesis. Such studies deserve a great deal of attention.

Although limited data are available, similarities exist between the role of the autophagic pathway as a response mechanism to metabolic perturbations and glucocorticoids in the regulation of metabolic responses. Chronic excessive activation of glucocorticoid receptors leads to major cellular metabolic rearrangements such as insulin resistance, glucose intolerance and dyslipidaemia. Obesity and metabolic syndrome, which are characterized by a nutrient overload, have been associated with a hyperactivation of tissue mTOR, indicating a blunted autophagic response [59]. The systemic glucocorticoid excess is associated with an increase in cardiovascular risk factors [60]. One of the major causes of impact on these risk factors is thought to be the glucocorticoid mediated intravascular volume overload [60]. As the access of glucocorticoids to their receptors is controlled by the isozymes of 11-β-hydroxysteroid dehydrogenase in a tissue specific manner, makes manipulation of this pathway an attractive therapeutic target. By selective isozyme inhibitors, the glucocorticoid activity can be modulated locally, keeping systemic glucocorticoid concentrations within homeostatic range.

Also in the acute setting a relationship exists between glucocorticoid availability and autophagy induction. In the treatment of acute lymphoblastic leukemia, glucocorticoids are used as crucial therapeutic agent, due to their effect on inducing G1 phase cell cycle arrest and apoptosis. Recently it was shown that dexamethasone treatment induces cell death and involves the induction of autophagy before the onset of apoptosis [61]. Moreover, another level of interaction has been demonstrated as the role of autophagy in innate immunity has recently become clear. Both the ATG16L1 risk allele as well as ATG5 are selectively important for the function of the Paneth cell, a specialized epithelial cell in the small intestine [62]. Through genome-wide association screenings it was shown that the autophagic pathway plays a fundamental role in the predisposition to the inflammatory bowel condition Chron's disease [63]. Taken together, these data indicate the dynamic relationship between glucocorticoid-induced metabolic perturbations, autophagy induction, inflammation and cell death susceptibility. Further investigations are likely to provide new insights into this complex relationship to treat cardiovascular disease more effectively by exploiting the modulation of the autophagic machinery in context with controlling local glucocorticoid activity.

10. The role of the mitogen-activated protein kinases (MAPKs) during ischemia/reperfusion-induced stress in the heart

Great efforts have been made to disentangle the intricate relationship between signalling pathways and the stress response of the heart during ischemia/reperfusion-induced injury. Analysis is complicated due to the fact that several pathways can be activated simultaneously with differential effects. It has become however evident that the MAPKs are major mediators of I/R-induced injury. Recent data pin point the MAPK's as one of the crossroads between autophagy and glucocorticoid signalling events.

Three major classes of MAPKs (Figure 4), which include the extracellular signal regulated protein kinase (ERK)/p42/44, c-Jun NH2-terminal protein kinase (JNK)/stress activated protein kinase (SAPK) and p38 MAPK families have been identified [64,65]. The ERK pathway has been depicted as a pro-survival pathway and is activated by a variety of mitogens and phorbol esters [66,67]. The JNK and p38 MAPK pathways are regarded as pro-apoptotic pathways and are mainly activated by environmental stress and inflammatory cytokines [67,68].

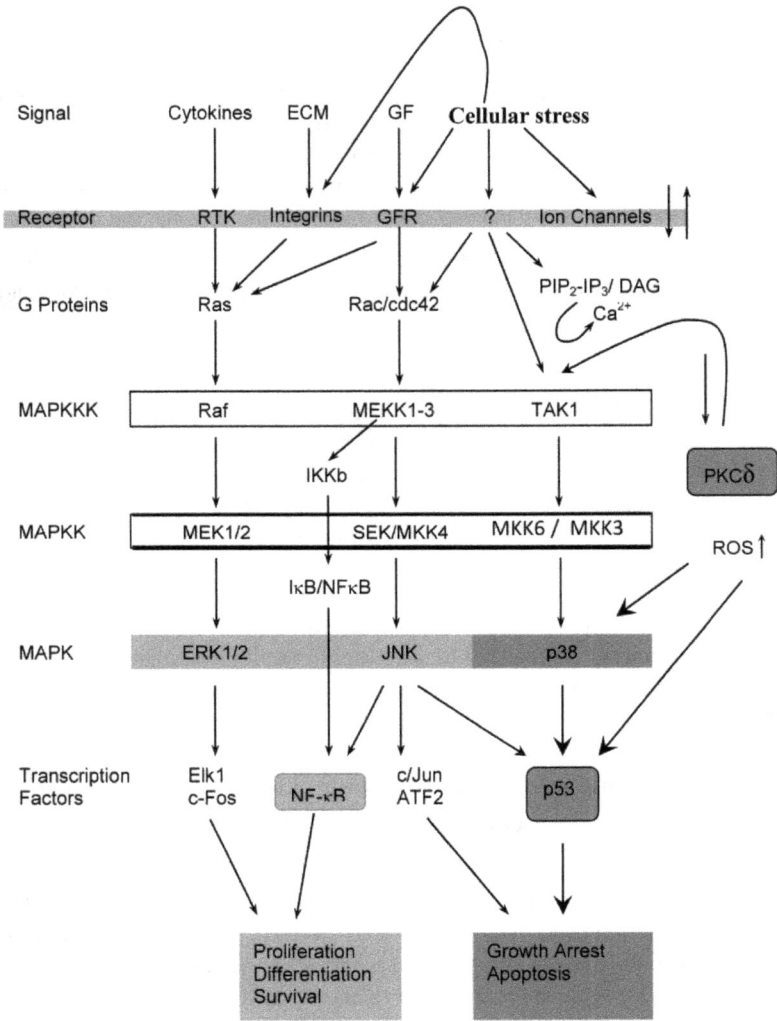

Figure 4. MAPK activation in stress-induced signalling in the heart. A variety of stress signals can activate the MAPKs directly or indirectly. MAPKs comprise a family of tyrosine/threonine kinases. Receptor activation initiates a cascade of phosphorylation events involving sequential activation of G proteins, MAPK kinase kinase (MAPKKK), MAPK kinase (MAPKK) and finally MAPK. Activated MAPK, in turn, is responsible for the phosphorylation and activation of various other regulatory proteins and transcription factors, which induce the expression of genes involved in the regulation of cell proliferation and apoptosis. ERK kinases mediate cell survival and proliferation, whereas JNK and p38 induce growth arrest and apoptosis (modified from Wernig and Xu, 2002).

Studies using chemical inhibitors have led to the conclusion that activation of the p38-MAPK promotes cardiac myocyte death during extended periods of ischaemia [69-71]. In a cultured neonatal rat cardiac myocyte model, inhibition of p38-MAPK protects against ischaemic injury by decreasing LDH release [69,70]. In addition, Barancik and co-workers (2000) reported that a specific inhibitor of p38-MAPK, SB203580, protected pig myocardium against ischaemic injury in an *in vivo* model by reducing infarct size [71]. Several studies indicated that p38-MAPK plays a pivotal role in promoting myocardial apoptosis [69,72-73]. Ma and co-workers (1999) demonstrated that in isolated perfused rabbit hearts, ischemia alone caused a moderate but transient increase in p38-MAPK activity [72]. Ten minutes' reperfusion further activated p38-MAPK, which remained elevated throughout reperfusion (20 minutes). Administration of SB203580 before ischemia and during reperfusion completely inhibited p38 MAPK activation and exerted significant cardioprotective effects, characterized by decreased myocardial apoptosis and improved post-ischaemic function, as well as attenuated myocardial necrotic injury. In contrast, administering SB203580 10 minutes after reperfusion (a time point when maximal MAPK activation had already been achieved), failed to convey significant cardioprotection. Mackay and Mochly-Rosen (1999) indicated that in neonatal rat cardiac myocytes, two distinct phases of p38 activation were observed during ischemia: the first phase began within 10 minutes and lasted less than 1 hour, and the second began after 2 hours and lasted throughout the ischaemic period [69]. They demonstrated that SB203580 also protected cardiac myocytes against ischemia by reducing activation of caspase-3, a key event in apoptosis. However, the protective effect was seen even when the inhibitor was present during only the second, sustained phase of p38 MAPK activation. Subsequent studies by Yue and co-workers (2000), exposing rat neonatal cardiomyocytes to ischemia showed a rapid and transient activation of p38-MAPK and JNK [73]. On reoxygenation, further activation of SAPKs was noted. With pretreatment of the cells with SB203580 apoptotic cells were reduced, suggesting p38 MAPK activation mediates apoptosis in rat cardiac myocytes subjected to ischemia/reoxygenation. In addition, Yue and co-workers (2000) also showed that SB203580 improved cardiac contractile function in rat isolated ischaemic hearts. Inhibition of p38 MAPK activation, therefore, correlated with cardioprotection against ischemia/reperfusion injury in cardiac myocytes as well as in isolated hearts [73].

Zechner and co-workers (1998) also reported that overexpression of MKK6 (Figure 4), an upstream activator of p38 MAPK, resulted in protection of cardiac myocytes from apoptosis induced either by anisomycin or MEKK1, an upstream activator of the JNK pathway [74]. In addition, expression of MKK6 elicited a hyperthrophic response, which was enhanced by co-infection of p38β [75]. Therefore, a distinct isoform of p38 MAPK, p38β, may participate in mediating cell survival. In contrast, over expression of MKK3 in mouse cardiomyocytes led to apoptosis, which was increased by co-infection of p38α [75]. Therefore differential activation of p38-MAPK isoforms may exert opposing effects: p38α is implicated in cell death, while p38β may mediate myocardial survival.

To determine whether p38 MAPK activation was isoform selective, rat neonatal cardiomyocytes were infected with adenovirus encoding wild-type p38α or p38β [70]. They showed that transfected p38α and p38β were differentially activated during sustained ischemia, with p38α remaining activated but p38β deactivated. Furthermore, cells expressing a dominant negative p38α, which prevented ischemia-induced p38 MAPK activation, were resistant to sustained ischaemic injury. Therefore, activation of p38α MAPK isoform is detrimental during ischemia.

11. MAPK inactivation by phosphatases

Dephosphorylation of either the threonine or tyrosine residue within the MAPK activation loop TxY motif alone can result in their enzymatic inactivation. In intact cells, dephosphorylation and inactivation of MAPK occur, within minutes to several hours depending on the cell type and activating stimulus. In endothelial cells, exposure to serum leads to ERK activation that is sustained at high levels for over 2 h. In contrast, different patterns can be observed in the a PC12 cell line where EGF-stimulated ERK activation is transient, with inactivation initiated within 5 min and nearly complete within 15-30 min, whereas this MAPK displays prolonged activation for several hours on stimulation with NGF [76]. It is believed that different patterns of ERK activation elicited by EGF and NGF underlie their differential effects to drive either cellular proliferation of differentiation, respectively [77]. Using PC12 cells as a model system to identify key phosphatases suppressing ERK activation, biochemical studies revealed that early rapid inactivation of these MAPKs reflects, in part, threonine dephosphorylation by the serine/threonine protein phosphatase PP2A [76].

In addition to threonine dephosphorylation, these studies also indicated that tyrosine-specific protein phosphatases (PTPs) also contribute to ERK inactivation [76]. Currently, 50 or more PTPs have been characterized [78-80], and although the PC12 cell PTPs were not identified molecularly [76], recent studies in other cell types have identified a possible role for three related PTP gene family members [81-84]. Notwithstanding the importance of these early reports on PP2A and tyrosine-specific PTPs inactivating ERKs, little is known about their general importance in terminating MAPK signaling, of the molecular mechanisms that may control phosphatase catalytic activity, or of their specificity for inactivating different MAPK isoforms.

In contrast to these protein phosphatase classes, there has been significant and rapid progress in our understanding of the role played by a subclass of PTP that possess activity for dephosphorylating both phosphotyrosine and phosphothreonine residues, known as the dual specificity phosphatases (DSPs).

The first mammalian DSP was identified as the mouse immediate early gene 3CH134 or its human orthologue CL100, which is induced rapidly after exposure to growth factors, heat shock, or oxidative stress [85-87]. Recombinant CL100/3CH134 was shown to dephosphorylate threonine and tyrosine residues of ERK, which was paralleled by its inactivation. These studies showed that CL100/3CH134 was specific for dephosphorylation of ERK when compared to a number of other unrelated phosphoproteins [76]. A correlation between 3CH134 levels and ERK inactivation was also found in mammalian cells, leading to its renaming as MAPK phosphatase-1 (MKP-1) [88]. Despite this important early work, the relevance of MKP-1 in ERK inactivation remains to be elucidated. Firstly, ERK activity is apparently normal after deletion of the MKP-1 gene in mice [89]. Secondly, it has also become evident that MKP-1 is at least as effective in inactivating JNK and p38 when compared to the ERKs [90-91]. Thirdly, newly identified members of the DSP gene family appear highly selective for ERK and may represent the true physiological regulators of this MAPK isoform. Since the initial cloning of MKP-1, eight additional mammalian DSP gene family members have been identified and characterized, which include MKP-2, MKP-3, MKP-4, MKP-5, MKP-X, PAC1, M3/6 and B59. These DSPs all appear to be effective in mediating inactivation of MAPKs.

The following model for MAPK inactivation by DSP is suggested (Figure 5). Stimulation by growth factors, cytokines, cellular stresses or some active oncogenes leads to rapid transcription of one or a subset of DSP genes. Increased DSP transcription may reflect activation of specific MAPK, although alternative pathways are not excluded. After translation of the DSP mRNA into protein, the catalytically inactive DSP translocates to a specific subcellular compartment within either the nucleus or the cytosol. Upon encountering its target MAPK, the DSP binds tightly through its amino terminus, which in turn triggers activation of the phosphatase catalytic domain. If the bound MAPK is already activated, then this will result in its rapid inactivation. Conversely, if the MAPK is not

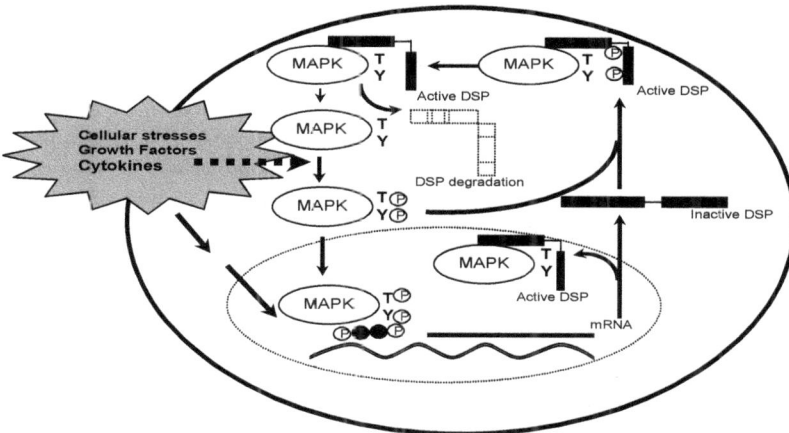

Figure 5. Cell exposure to growth factors, cytokines and cell stresses leads to induction of a subset of DSP genes. Increased expression is likely to reflect activation of transcription factors (black circles) via both MAPK-dependent and independent pathways. Newly synthesized DSPs translocate to specific subcellular compartments as dictated by anchorage and/or localization motifs not yet identified. Specific binding to target MAPKs through regions within the DSP amino terminus then triggers activation of the phosphatase catalytic domain. Bound MAPKs are in turn inactivated by dephosphorylation on threonine and tyrosine residues localized within the "activation loop" motif of TxY. Inactive MAPKs then dissociate, leaving the DSP free to bind and inactivate another MAPK molecule. In the absence of continued DSP gene transcription and protein synthesis, rapid degradation may limit their duration of activity in cells (Camps et al., 1999).

active, then its tight interaction with an active DSP is expected to block any possibility of kinase activation by a subsequent stimulus. MAPKs that fail to bind the DSP within its amino terminus remain active or susceptible to activation after extracellular stimulation. Depending on their cellular localization, these regulatory effects allow for selected inhibition of MAPK activities in specific subcellular compartments. Some DSPs have been shown to possess short half-lives [76], suggesting that in the absence of continued gene transcription and protein synthesis, their rapid turnover limits their duration of action in cells. Overall, tight control of DSP gene induction, combined with their differential binding and catalytic activation by a specific repertoire of MAPKs, provides a sophisticated mechanism for rapid targeted inactivation of selected MAPK activities.

12. MAP kinase phosphatase-1 (MKP-1): A mediator of the beneficial effects of glucocorticoids during ischemia/reperfusion-induced stress in the heart

It is noteworthy that many genes that are positively regulated at post-transcriptional level by p38-MAPK, are negatively regulated at the same level by glucocorticoids. Lasa and co-workers investigated the effects of GCs on the p38-MAPK pathway and have shown that dexamethasone destabilized cyclooxygenase-2 (COX-2) mRNA by inhibiting the function, but not the expression of p38-MAPK [92]. The inhibition of p38-MAPK was then shown to be mediated by MKP-1. We and others have also demonstrated that dexamethasone induces the expression of MKP-1 which potently inactivated p38-MAPK [93-94].

Wu and Bennet (2005) demonstrated that MKP-1 promotes cell survival in fibroblasts through the attenuation of stress responsive MAPK-mediated apoptosis [95]. Upregulation of MKP-1 has also been shown to be associated with cardioprotection by long-chain polyunsaturated fatty acids [93]. It has also been reported that transgenic mice overexpressing MKP-1 were protected, whereas knock-out mice show greater injury after ischemia/reperfusion [96]. The exact mechanism of the beneficial effects of glucocorticoids on the heart during ischemia/reperfusion-induced stress still remain to be established. In view of the significant contribution of apoptosis, necrosis and autophagy during ischemia/reperfusion-induced stress, it is expected that GC-induced cardioprotection to be associated with reduced apoptosis and necrosis. Indeed, Fan and co-workers have demonstrated that dexamethasone, administered intraperitoneally or added directly to the perfusate, significantly improved post-ischemic functional recovery and reduced infarct size compared to untreated controls [94]. These were associated with associated with upregulation of MKP-1 protein expression [94]. Furthermore, it was also shown by us that upregulation of MKP-1 during simulated ischemia/reperfusion is associated with an attenuation of apoptosis in neonatal cardiomyocytes [93].

13. Conclusions

It has been suggested that upregulation of MKP-1 during ischemia/reperfusion-induced stress attenuates myocardial injury [93,94]. MKP-1, found predominantly in the nucleus, is a dual specific phosphatase which dephosphorylates phosphotyrosine and phosphothreonine-containing protein kinases such as the MAPKs. MAPKs are known to be involved in intracellular signalling pathways that regulate gene expression in response to a variety of extracellular signals. MAPKs are activated during ischemia/reperfusion-induced stress in the heart. It was also demonstrated that glucocorticoids act via MKP-1 induction and subsequent p38-MAPK inhibition to induce cardioprotection during ischemia/reperfusion-induced stress [94].

MAPKs have been found to be involved in autophagic, apoptotic and necrotic cell death during stress responses of the heart [97-102]. Autophagy is foremost a survival mechanism which is activated in cells subjected to nutrient or growth factor deprivation. However, when the cellular stress continues, cell death may occur via autophagy, or becomes associated with features of apoptotic or necrotic cell death [103]. Apoptosis is essential for removal of specifically targeted cells, through the process of apoptotic body formation and phagocytosis [104]. Necrosis is a pathological cellular response requiring no ATP. Necrotic cells are morphologically characterized by disrupted membranes, cytoplasm and mitochondrial swelling, disintegration of organelles and complete cell lysis [105]. Cell death following ischemia/reperfusion-induced stress is thought to manifest in morphological features indicative for all three, apoptotic, necrotic and autophagic cell death [106].

MKP-1 has been shown to be involved in the regulation of apoptosis [107] and it was also very recently demonstrated that MKP-1 may lead to autophagy induction in cancer cells [108]. We have recently demonstrated that inhibition of MKP-1 and subsequent increased p38-MAPK phosphorylation during ischemia/reperfusion-induced stress is associated with attenuated autophagy and increased apoptosis and necrosis in the heart (unpublished data). We thus propose the following mechanism of GC-induced protection in the heart: During ischemia/reperfusion-induced stress in the heart, p38 MAPK is activated, GCs sustain/upregulate autophagy via an increase in MKP-1 and subsequent dephosphorylation of p38 MAPK which ultimately protects the heart from apoptosis and necrosis, driven by the effects of autophagy on the metabolic balance sheet of the heart.

Author details

Anna-Mart Engelbrecht* and Benjamin Loos
Dept of Physiological Sciences, Stellenbosch University, Stellenbosch, South Africa

14. References

[1] Dallman MF, Strack AM, Akana SF, Bradbury MJ, Hanson ES, Scribner KA (1993) Feast and famine: critical role of glucocorticoids with insulin in daily energy flow. Fron Neuroendocrinol 14: 303-347.

---

* Corresponding Author

[2]   Hammond GL, Smith CL, Paterson NAM, Sibbald WJ (1990) A role for corticosteroid-globulin in delivery of cortisol to activated neutrophils. J Clin Endocrinol Metab 71: 34-39.

[3]   Buttgereit F, Scheffod A (2002) Rapid glucocorticoid effects on immune cells. Steroids 6: 529-534.

[4]   Stellato C (2004) Port-transcriptional and nongenomic effects of glucocorticoids. Proc Am Thorac Soc 1: 255-263.

[5]   Limbourg FP, Liao JK (2003) Nontranscriptional actions of the glucocorticoid receptor. J Mol Med 81: 168-174.

[6]   Wehling M (1997) Specific, nongenomic actions of steroid hormones. Annu Rev Physiol 59: 365-393.

[7]   Ito K, Chung KF, Adcock IM (2006) Update on glucocorticoid action and resistance. J Allergy Clin Immunol 117: 522-543.

[8]   Clark AR, Dean JL, Saklatvala J (2003) Post-transcriptional regulation of gene expression by mitogen-activated protein kinase p38. FEBS Letters 546: 37-44.

[9]   Sapolsky RM, Romero LM, Munck AU (2000) How do glucocorticoids influence stress responses? Integrating permissive, suppressive, stimulatory, and preparative actions. Endocr Rev 21: 55-89.

[10] Libby P, Maroko PR, Bloor CM, Sobel BE, Braunwald E (1973) Reduction of experimental myocardial infarct size by corticosteroid administration. J Clin Invest 52: 599-607.

[11] Valen G, et al (2000) Glucocorticoid pre-treatment protects cardiac function and induces cardiac heat shock protein 72. Am J Physiol Heart Circ Physiol 279: H836-H843.

[12] Varga E, et al (2004) Inhibition of ischemia/reperfusion-induced damage by dexamethasone in isolated working rat hearts: the role of cytochrome c release. Life Sci 75: 2411-2423.

[13] Skyschally A, et al (2004) Glucocorticoid treatment prevents progressive myocardial dysfunction resulting from experimental coronary microembolization. Circulation 109: 2337-2342.

[14] Giugliano GR, Giugliano RP, Gibson CM, Kuntz RE (2003) Meta-analysis of corticosteroid treatment in acute myocardial infarction. Am J Cardiol 91: 1055-1059.

[15] Dennis SC, Gevers W & Opie LH (1991) Protons in ischemia: where do they come from: where do they go to? J Mol Cell Cardiol 23: 1077-1086.

[16] Zong WX & Thompson SB (2006) Necrotic death as a cell fate. Genes Dev 20: 1-15.

[17] Murry CE, Jennings RB & Reimer KA (1986) Preconditioning with ischemia: a delay of lethal cell injury in ischemic myocardium. Circulation 74: 1124-1136.

[18] Nishida K, Kyoi S, Yamaguchi O, Sadoshima J & Otsu K (2009) The role of autophagy in the heart. Cell Death Differ 16: 31-38.

[19] Olivetti G, Abbi R, Quaini F, Kajstura J, Cheng W, Nitahara JA, Quaini E, Di Loreto C, Beltrami CA, Krajewski S, Reed JC & Anversa P (1997) Apoptosis in the failing human heart. N Engl J Med 336: 1131-1141.

[20] De Duve C & Wattiaux R (1966) Functions of Lysosomes. Ann Rev Physiol 28: 435-92.

[21] Mizushima N, Levine B, Cuervo AM, Klionsky DJ (2008) Autophagy fights disease through cellular self-digestion. Nature 451(7182):1069-75.

[22] Baba M, Takeshige G, Baba N and Ohsumi Y (1994) Ultrastructural analysis of the autophagic process in yeast: Detection of autophagosomes and their characterization. J Cell Biol 6:903-13.

[23] Dice FJ (2007) Chaperone-Mediated Autophagy. Autophagy 4:295-9.

[24] He C, Klionskly DJ (2009) Regulation mechanisms and signaling pathways in autophagy. Annu Rev Genet 43 67-93.

[25] Cuervo AM (2010) The plasma membrane brings autophagosomes to life. Nat.Cell Biol12: 735-737.

[26] Cuervo AM (2004) Autophagy: Many paths to the same end. Mol Cell Biochem 263:55-72.

[27] Yorimitsu T and Klionsky DJ (2005) Autophagy: molecular machinery for self-eating. Cell Death Differ 12:1542-1552.

[28] Fass E, Amar N and Elazar Z (2007). Identification of essential residues for the c-terminal cleavage of mammalian LC3. Autophagy 3:1:48-50.

[29] Scherz-Shouval R, Shvets E, Elazar Z (2007) Oxidation as a post-translational modification that regulates autophagy. Autophagy 4:371-3.

[30] Sybers HD, Ingwall J, DeLuca M (1978) Autophagy in cardiac myocytes. Recent Adv Stud Cardiac Struct Metab 12:453-463.

[31] Hamacher-Brady A, Brady NR, Gottlieb RA (2006) Enhancing macroautophagy protects against ischemia/reperfusion injury in cardiac myocytes. J Biol Chem 281: 29776-29787.

[32] Loos B, Engelbrecht AM (2009). Cell death: a dynamic response concept. Autophagy 5(5):1–14.

[33] Loos, B; Genade, S.; Ellis, B.; Lochner, A.; Engelbrecht, A. M (2011). At the core of survival: Autophagy delays the onset of both apoptotic and necrotic cell death in a model of ischemic cell injury. Exp Cell Res 317: 1437-1453.

[34] Matsui Y, Takagi H, Qu X, Abdellativ M, Sakoda H, Asano T (2007) Distinct roles of autophagy in the heart during ischemia and reperfusion: roles of AMP-activated protein kinase and beclin 1 in mediating autophagy. Circ Res100: 914-922.

[35] Dosenko VE, Nagibin VS, Tumanovska LV and Moibenko AA (2006) Protective effect of autophagy in anoxia-reoxygenation of isolated cardiomyocytes? Autophagy 2(4): 305-306.

[36] Yue Z, Jin S, Yang C, Levine AG. Heintz N (2003). Beclin 1, an autophagy gene essential for early embryonic development, is a haploinsufficient tumor suppressor. Proc Natl Acad Sci USA; 100: 15077-15082.

[37] Nakai A, Yamaguchi O, Takeda T, Higuchi Y, Hikoso S, Taniike M (2007) The role of autophagy in cardiomyocytes in the basal state and in response to hemodynamic stress. Nat Med 13: 619-624.

[38] Gustafsson ÅB, Gottlieb RA (2009). Autophagy in ischemic heart disease. Circ Res 104:150-158.

[39] Lam A, Lopaschuk GD (2007) Anti-anginal effects of partial fatty acid oxidation inhibitors. Curr Opin Pharmacol 7:179-185.

[40] Altarejos JY, Taniguchi M, Clanacham AS, Lopaschuk GD (2005). Myocardial ischemia differentially regulates LKB1 and an alternate 5'-AMP-activated protein kinase kinase. J Biol Chem 280:183-190.

[41] Jafri MS, Dudycha SJ, O'Rourke B (2001). Cellular energy metabolism: models of cellular respiration. Annu Rev Biomed Eng 3:57–81.

[42] Takagi H, Matsui Y, Sadoshima J (2007). The role of autophagy in mediating cell survival and death during ischemia and reperfusion in the heart. Antioxid Redox Signal 9:1373-1381.

[43] Grover GJ, Atwal KS, Sleph PG, Wang FL, Monshizadegan H, Monticello T (2004) Excessive ATP hydrolysis in ischemic myocardium by mitochondrial F1F0 ATPase: effect of selective pharmacological inhibition of mitochondrial ATPase hydrolase activity. Am J Physiol Heart Circ Physiol 287: 1747-1755.

[44] Kunapuli S, Rosanio S, Schwarz ER (2006) "How do cardiomyocytes die?" Apoptosis and autophagic cell death in cardiac myocytes. J Card Fail 12:381-391.

[45] Leist M, Single B, Castoldi AF, Kuhnle S, Nicotera P (1997) Intracellular adenosine triphosphase (ATP) concentration: A switch in the decision between apoptosis and necrosis. J Exp Med 185: 1481-6.

[46] Tatsumi T, Shiraishi J, Keira N, Akashi K, Mano A, Yamanaka S (2003) Intracellular ATP is required for mitochondrial apoptotic pathways in isolated hypoxic rat cardiac myocytes. Cardiovasc Res 59: 428-40.

[47] Singh R and Cuervo AM (2011). Autophagy in the cellular energetic balance. Cell Metabolism 13: 495-504

[48] Mizushima N and Klionsky DJ (2007) Protein turnover via autophagy: implications for metabolism. Annu Rev Nutr 27:19-40.

[49] Singh R , Kaushik S, Wang Y, Xiang Y, Novak I, Komatsu M, Tanaka K, Cuervo AM and Czaja MJ (2009) Autophagy regulates lipid metabolism. Nature 458: 1131-1135.

[50] Nemchenko A, Chiong M, Turer A, Lavandero S, Hill JA (2011). Autophagy as therapeutic target in cardiovascular disease. JMCC 51: 584-593.

[51] Juhász G, Csikós G, Sinka R, Erdélyi M, Sass M (2003) The Drosophila homolog of Aut1 is essential for autophagy and development. FEBS Lett 543: 154-8.

[52] Levine B and Klionsky DJ (2004). Development by self-digestion: molecular mechanisms and biological functions of autophagy. Developmental Cell 6: 463-477.

[53] Martin DN, Balgley B, Dutta S, Chen J, Rudnick P, Cranford J, Kantartzis S, DeVoe DL, Lee C, Baehrecke EH (2007) Proteomic analysis of steroid-triggered autophagic programmed cell death during Drosophila development. Cell Death Differ 14: 916-23.

[54] Kuma A, Hatano M, Matsui M, Yamamoto A, Nakaya H, Yoshimori T, Ohsumi Y, Tokuhisa T, Mizushima N (2004) The role of autophagy during the early neonatal starvation period. Nature 432: 1032-6.

[55] Yue Z, Jin S, Yang C, Levine AG, Heintz N (2003). Beclin 1, an autophagy gene essential for early embryonic development, is a haploinsufficient tumor suppressor. Proc Natl Acad Sci USA 100: 15077-15082.

[56] Yu L, Alva A, Su H, Dutt P, Freundt E, Welsh S (2004) Regulation of an ATG7-beclin 1 program of autophagic cell death by caspase-8. Science 304: 1500-1502.

[57] Shimizu S, Kanaseki T, Mizushima N, Mizuta T, Arakawa-Kobayashi S, Thompson CB and Tsujimoto Y (2004) Role of Bcl-2 family proteins in a non-apoptotic programmed cell death dependent on autophagy genes. Nature Cell Biology 6: 1221 – 1228.

[58] Kinch G, Hoffman KL, Rodrigues EM, Zee MC, Weeks JC (2003) Steroid-triggered programmed cell death of a motorneuron is autophagic and involves structural changes in mitochondria. J Comp Neurol 17: 384-403.

[59] Khamzina L, Veilleux A, Bergeron S, Marette A (2005). Increased activation of the mammalian target of rapamycin pathway in liver and skeletal muscle of obese rats: possible involvement in obesity-linked insulin resistance. Endocrinology 146:1473-1481.

[60] Hadoke PWF, Iqbal J, Walker BR (2009). Therapeutic manipulation of glucocorticoid metabolism in cardiovascular disease. Brit J Pharmacol 156: 689-712.

[61] Laane E, Tamm KP, Buentke E, Ito K, Khariza P, Oscarsson J, Corcoran M, Bkörklund AC, Hultenby K, Lundin J, Heyman M, Söderhäll S, Mazur J, Porwit A, Pandolfi PP, Zhivotovsky B, Panaretakis T and Grandér D (2009). Cell death induced by dexamethasone in lymphoid leukemia is mediated through initiation of autophagy. Cell Death Differ 16: 1018-1029.

[62] Cadwell K, Liu JY, Brown SL, Miyoshi H, Loh J, Lennerz JK, Kishi C, Kc W, Carrero JA, Hunt S, Stone CD, Brunt EM, Xavier RJ, Sleckman BP, Li E, Mizushima N, Stappenbeck TS, Virgin HW (2008) A key role for autophagy and the autophagy gene Atg16 in mouse and human intestinal Paneth cells. Nature 13(456): 259-63.

[63] Deretic V (2009) Links between autophagy, innate immunity, inflammation and Chron's disease. Dig Dis 27:246-251.

[64] Begum N, Ragolia L, Rienzie J, McCarthy M & Duddy N (1989) Regulation of mitogen-activated protein kinase phosphatase-1 induction by insulin in vascular smooth muscle cells. Evaluation of the role of the nitric oxide signalling pathway and potential defects in hypertension. J Biol Chem 273: 25164-25170.

[65] Cowan KJ & Storey (2003) Mitogen-activated protein kinases: new signalling pathways functioning in cellular responses to environmental stress. J Exp Biol 206: 1107-1115.

[66] Marczin N, El-Habashi N, Hoare GS, Bundy RE & Yacoub M (2003) Antioxidants in myocardial ischemia-reperfusion injury: therapeutic potential and basic mechanisms. Arch Biochem Biophys 420: 222-236.

[67] Junttila MR, Li SP, Wetermarck J (2008) Phosphatase-mediated crosstalk between MAPK signalling pathways in the regulation of cell survival. Faseb J 22: 954-965.

[68] Weston CR & Davis RJ (2007) The JNK signal transduction pathway. Curr Opin Cell Biol 19: 142-149.

[69] Mackay K, Mochly-Rosen D (2001) Arachidonic acid protects neonatal rat cardiac myocytes form ischaemic injury through ε protein kinase C. Cardiovasc Res 50: 65-74.

[70] Saurin AT, Martin JC, Heads RJ, Foley C, Mockridge JW, Wright MJ, Wang Y, Marber S (2000) The role of differential activation of p38 mitogen activated protein kinases in preconditioned ventricular myocytes. Faseb J 14: 2237-2246.

[71] Barancik M, Htun P, Strohm C, Killian S, Schaper W (2000) Inhibition of the cardiac p38-MAPK pathway by SB20350 delays ischemic cell death. J Cardiovasc Pharmacol 35: 474-483.

[72] Ma XL, Kumar S, Gao F, Louden CS, Lopez BL, Christopher TA, Wang C, Lee JC, Feuerstein GZ, Yue TL (1999) Inhibition of p38 mitogen-activated protein kinase decreases cardiomyocyte apoptosis and improves cardiac function after myocardial ischemia and reperfusion. Circulation 99: 1685-1691.

[73] Yue TL, Wang C, Gu J-L, Ma XL, Kumar S, Lee JC, Feuerstein GZ, Thomas H, Maleeff B, Ohlstein EH (2000) Inhibition of extracellular signal-regulated kinase enhances ischemia/reoxygenation-induced apoptosis in cultured cardiac myocytes and exaggerates reperfusion injury in isolated perfused hearts. Circ Res 86: 692-699.

[74] Zechner D, Craig R, Hanford HS, McDonough PM, Sabbadini RA, Glembotski CC (1998) MKK6 activates myocardial cell NF-kappaB and inhibits apoptosis in a p38 mitogen-activated protein kinase-dependent manner. J Biol Chem 273: 8232-8239.

[75] Wang X, Martindale JL, Liu Y, Holbrook NJ (1998) The cellular response to oxidative stress: influences of mitogen-activated protein kinase signalling pathways on cell survival. Biochem J 333: 291-300.

[76] Alessi DR, Gomez N, Moorhead G, Lewis T, Keyse SM, Cohen P (1995) Inactivation of p42 MAPK kinase by protein phosphatase 2A and a protein tyrosine phosphatase, but not CL 100, in various cell lines. Curr Biol 5: 283-295.

[77] Marshall CJ (1995) Specificity of receptor tyrosine kinase signalling: transient versus sustained extracellular signal-regulated kinase activation. Cell 80: 179-185.

[78] Neel BG, Tonks NK (1997) Protein tyrosine phosphatases in signal transduction. Curr Opin Cell Biol 9: 193-204.

[79] Hooft van Huijsduijnen R (1998) Protein tyrosine phosphatases: counting trees in the forest. Gene 225: 1-8.

[80] Denu JM, Dixon JE (1998) Protein tyrosine phosphatases: mechanisms of catalysis and regulation. Curr Opin Chem Biol 2: 663-641.

[81] Wurgler-Murphy SM, Maeda T, Witten EA, Saito H (1997) Regulation of the Saccharomyces cerevisiae HOG1 mitogen activated protein kinase by PTP2 and PTP3 protein tyrosine phosphatases. Mol Cell Biol 15: 1289-1297.

[82] Shiozaki K, Russel P (1995) Cell-cycle control linked to extracellular environment by MAP kinase pathway in fission yeast. Nature 378: 739-743.

[83] Millar JB, Buck V, Wilkinson MG (1995) Pyp1 and Pyp2 PTPases dephosphorylated an osmosensing MAP kinase controlling cell size at division in fission yeast. Genes Dev 9: 2117-2130.

[84] Zhan X-L, Deschenes RJ, Guan KL (1997) Differential regulation of FUS3 MAP kinase by tyrosine-specific phosphatases PTP2/PTP3 and dual-specificity phosphatase MSG5 in Saccharomyces cervisiae. Genes Dev 11: 1690-1702.

[85] Keyse SM & Emslie EA (1992) Oxidatives stress and heat shock induce a human gene encoding a protein-tyrosine phosphatase. Nature 359: 644-646.

[86] Charles CH, Sun H, Lau LF, Tonks NK (1993) MKP-1, an immediate early gene product is a dual specificity phosphatase that dephosphorylates MAP kinases in vivo. Cell 75(3): 487-493.

[87] Noguchi T, Metz R, Chen L, Mattei MG, Carasco D, Bravo R (1993) Structure, mapping and expression of erp, a growth factor-inducible gene encoding a nontransmembrane

protein tyrosine phosphatase, and effect of ERP on cell growth. Mol Cell Biol 13: 5195-5205.

[88] Sun H, Charles CH, Lau LF, Tonks NK (1993) MKP-1 (3Ch134), an immediate early gene product, is a dual specificity phosphatase that dephosphorylates MAP kinase in vivo. Cell 75: 487-493.

[89] Dorfman K, Carrasco D, Gruda M, Ryan C, Lira SA, Bravo R (1996) Disruption of the erp/mkp-1 gene does not affect mouse development: normal MAP kinase activity in ERP/MKP-1-deficient fibroblasts. Oncogene 13: 925-931.

[90] Chu Y, Solski PA, Khosravi-Far R, Der CJ, Kelly K (1996) the mitogen-activated protein kinase phosphatases PAC1, MKP-1 and MKP-2 have unique substrate specificities and reduced activity in vivo towards ERK2 sevenmaker mutation. J Biol Chem 271: 6497-6501.

[91] Franklin CC, Kraft AS (1997) Conditional expression of the mitogen-activated protein kinase (MAPK) phosphatase MKP-1 preferentially inhibits p38 MAPK and stress-activated protein kinase in U937 cells. J Biol Chem 272: 16917-16923.

[92] Lasa M, Abraham SM, Boucheron C, Saklatvala J, Clark AR (2002) Dexamethasone causes sustained expression of mitogen-activated protein kinase (MAPK) phosphatase 1 and phosphatase-mediated inhibition of MAPK p38. Mol Cel Biol 22: 7802-7811.

[93] Engelbrecht A-M, Engelbrecht P, Genade S, Niesler C, Page C, Smuts M, Lochner A (2005) Long-chain polyunsaturated fatty acids protect the heart against ischemia/reperfusion-induced injury via a MAPK dependent pathway. J Mol Cell Cardiol 39: 940-954.

[94] Fan WJ, Genade S, Genis A, Huisamen B, Lochner A (2009) Dexamethasone-induced cardioprotection: a role for the phosphatase MKP-1? Life Sci 84: 838-846.

[95] Wu JJ & Bennett AM (2005) Essential role for mitogen-activated protein (MAP) kinase phosphatase-1 in stress-responsive MAPK and cell survival signalling. J Biol Chem 280: 16461-16466.

[96] Kaiser RA, Bueno OF, Lips DJ, Doevendans PA, Jones F, Kimball TF, Molkentin JD (2004) Targeted inhibition of p38 mitogen-activated protein kinase antagonizes cardiac injury and cell death following ischemia-reperfusion in vivo. J Biol Chem 279: 15524-1530.

[97] Lee TH, Huang Q, Oikemus S, Shank J, Ventura JJ, Cusson N, Vaillancourt RR, Su B, Davis RJ, Kelliher MA (2003) The death domain kinase RIP1 is essential for tumor necrosis factor alpha signalling to p38 mitogen-activated protein kinase. Mol Cell Biol 23: 8377-8385.

[98] Khan TA, Bianchi C, Ruel M, Voisine P, Sellke FW (2004) Mitogen-activate protein kinase pathways and cardiac surgery. J Thorac Cardiovasc Surg 127: 806-811.

[99] Lee TH, Cusson N, Kelliher MA (2004) The kinase activity of Rip1 is not required for tumor necrosis factor alpha-induced IkappaB kinase or p38 MAP kinase activation or for ubiquitination of Rip1 by Traf2. J Biol Chem 279: 33185-33191.

[100] Codongo P & Meijer AJ (2005) Autophagy and signalling: Their role in cell survival and cell death. Cell Death Differ 12(2): 1509-1518.

[101] Park KJ, Lee SH, Lee CH, Jang JY, Chung J, Kwon MH, Kim YS (2009) Upregulation of beclin-1 expression and phosphorylation of Bcl-2 and p53 are involved in the JNK-mediated autophagic cell death. Biochem Biophys Res Commun 382: 762-729.

[102] Yang LY, Wu KH, Chiu WT, Wang SH & Shih CM (2009) The cadmium-induced death of mesangial cells results in nephrotoxicity. Autophagy 5: 571-572.

[103] Maiuri MC, Zalckvar E, Kimchi A, Kroemer G (2007) Self-eating and self-killing: crosstalk between autophagy and apoptosis. Nat Rev Mol Cell Biol 8: 741-752.

[104] Peter C, Waibel M, Radu CG, Yang LV, Witte ON, Schulze-Osthoff K, Wesselborg S, Lauber K (2008) Migration to apoptotic "find-me" signals is mediated via the phagocyte receptor G2A. J Biol Chem 283: 5296-5305.

[105] Zong WX & Thompson CB (2006) Necrotic death as a cell fate. Genes Dev 20: 1-15.

[106] Murphy E & Steenbergen C (2008) Mechanisms underlying acute protection from cardiac ischemia-reperfusion injury. Physiol Rev 88: 581-609.

[107] Morisco C, Marrone C, Trimarco V, Crispo S, Monti MG, Sadoshima J, Trimarco B (2007) Insulin resistance affects the cytoprotective effect of insulin in cardiomyocytes through an impairment of MAPK phosphatase-1 expression. Cardiovasc Res 76: 453-464.

[108] Lu HH, Kao SY, Liu TY, Liu ST, Huang WP, Chang KW, Lin SC (2010) Areca nut extract induced oxidative stress and upregulated hypoxia inducing factor leading to autophagy in oral cancer cells. Autophagy 6: 725-737.

Chapter 5

Glucocorticoids and the Intestinal Environment

Hümeyra Ünsal and Muharrem Balkaya

Additional information is available at the end of the chapter

1. Introduction

For thousands, perhaps millions of years, human have marveled to understand how the body is formed and function, how it maintains its wholeness and healthy state, and how disordered states occur. In frame of holistic philosophy of ancient eastern cultures, a person had been accepted as physical, emotional, mental, and spiritual ones. In this concept, the balance of the body, mind and spirit were accepted as the healthy state of an individual [1,2]. The ancient Greeks defended the concept of the four humors doctrine; blood, black bile, yellow bile, and phlegm. *Ad modum* this doctrine these four humors in a healthy person were believed to be balanced, and the reason why a person fell ill was due to the fact that these fluids were disturbed [3,4]. With the separation of medicine from superstition, magic and religion by famous Greek physician Hippocrates in around 5th century B.C., more realistic and relevant approaches could be developed to better understanding the life, structures of living creatures and their healthy and diseased conditions. These and the time-dependent innovative developments in technology and science throughout the following centuries led to more concrete observations, mainly on animals. Gathered evidences and additive knowledge base from these observations mankind led mankind to make realistic definitions on the subjects "the structure, integrity and functions" of the animal and human body. In 19th century Louis Pasteur, a French chemist and microbiologist, stated the germ theory of diseases. He believed that micro-organisms (bacteria) infect animals and humans, thus they cause diseases [5]. At the same times, a French Physiologist Claude Bernard tried to understand how living creatures maintain their integrity, and how it is regulated, and defeated. He discriminated the internal environment from the external environment and was in opinion that living creatures maintain their internal milieu relatively constant under continuously changing environmental conditions. Claude Bernard [6] attributed also an important role to nervous system in the maintenance of internal environment in physiological ranges in human and animal organisms and remarked the substantial differences between animals and plants in this respect. Since that time, the interest of the researchers in different fields worldwide is mainly focused on possible regulation mechanisms of various living species. Thus, it can be said that the philosophical roots of the concept "stress" and "stress physiology" is going back to the early observations that living creatures are exposed continuously to the effects of various environmental challenges against which they have to defend their integrity, and following statement from Claude Bernard that living creatures strive to maintain their internal environments relatively constant *via* various homeokinetic mechanisms even if their environmental conditions are changing, thereby keep their normal physiological functioning and prerequisite for a free, independent live or shortly *'la fixité du miliéu interieur est la condition d'une vie libre et indépendante'* as defined by him *"Il y a pour l'animal deux milieux: un milieu extérieur dans lequel est placé l'organisme, et un milieu intérieur dans lequel vivent les éléments des tissus"*. However, Hans Selye, one of the Pioneers and founders of stress from 1930's, was the first who introduced the term "stress" as the real or perceived physical or psychological events which are threaten the homeokinesis in medical terminology. *Ad modum* Selye the stress is somewhat like living, not so easy to define, although there is no doubt about its presence [7]. The environmental challenges affecting a living creature, thus causing stress, can vary from physical, to chemical and bio-psycho-social factors, while all the reactants, their contra- and/or co-players within the living systems are of chemical nature at the last instance; intracellular or intra-bodily signaling elements as either hormones including glucocorticoids and catecholamines or neurotransmitters, cytokines and chemokines, etc., or a group or all of them functioning simultaneously within the body for the same purposes.

Stress and the glucocorticoids are associated or interweaving concepts with each other. Indeed, to physiologists the term "stress" has come to mean any event that elicits increased cortisol secretion [8]. However, as it is well known, glucocorticoids are not only mediators of the stress responses; they take a part in peripheral components of stress responses. The stress response is mediated by the stress system which is composed of two components; central nervous system and the peripheral part. The central, greatly interconnected effectors of this system include the hypothalamic hormones arginine vasopressin, corticotropin-releasing hormone/factor (CRH/CRF) and pro-opiomelanocortin-derived peptides, and the locus ceruleus and autonomic norepinephrine centers in the brainstem. The peripheral components of the stress system include (*a*) the peripheral limbs of the hypothalamic-pituitary-adrenal (HPA) axis; (*b*) the efferent sympathetic-adrenomedullary system, and (*c*) components of the parasympathetic system [9-11]. There are also bidirectional positive feedback regulation between the CRF secreted paraventricular nucleus of hypothalamus and central noradrenergic system [9,11,12].

Stressors activate different physiological processes. The first classical response is the secretion of adrenalin and noradrenalin hormones from the adrenal medulla *via* activation of sympathetic nervous system. This response is called "fight or flight syndrome", because adrenaline and noradrenalin increase the respiratory rate, the heartbeat, the concentration of glucose in circulating blood and the blood flow to the skeletal muscles. This fast response is primarily related to survival. Stressors also activate the HPA axis. The activation of this axis begins with the stimulation of parvocelular neurons of hypothalamus and secretion of CRH. CRH stimulates the secretion of adrenocorticotrophic hormone (ACTH) from the adenohypophsis and the ACTH acts on cortex of adrenal glands and stimulates the release of glucocorticoid hormones. GC hormones (corticosterone in rodents and cortisol in humans), which are the ultimate product of HPA axis activation, act on multiple bodily systems to maintain homeokinesis. They stimulate protein catabolism, gluconeogenesis and release of glycerol and fatty acids into the blood, maintain the vasoconstructive effect of norepinephrine, inhibit glucose uptake and oxidation by many body cells except the brain (insulin antagonism) and also inhibit inflammation and specific immune response [8-11].

The secretion of ACTH, and therefore of cortisol or corticosterone, is stimulated by several hormones and molecules in addition to hypothalamic CRH. Depending on the stressor, substances such as vasopressin, epinephrine, angiotensin II, various cytokines (tumor necrosis factor (TNF)-α, interleukin (IL)-1, and IL-6), and lipid mediators of inflammation affect the hypothalamic, pituitary, and/or adrenal components of the HPA axis and potentiate its activity. Glucocorticoids play an important role in the regulation of basal activity of the HPA axis, as well as in the termination of the stress response by acting at extra-hypothalamic centers, the hypothalamus, and the pituitary gland. The negative feedback of glucocorticoids on the secretion of CRH and ACTH serves to limit the duration of the total tissue exposure of the organism to glucocorticoids, thus minimizing the catabolic, lipogenic, anti-reproductive, and immunosuppressive effects of these hormones [8,10,11].

The activation of the HPA is a longer-term adjustment by the humans or animals to the changes in their micro- or surrounding environments. Selye [7] called it as the 'general adaptation syndrome' (GAS). The process of adaptation, also known as "allostasis" (literally "maintaining stability, through change"), supports the homeokinesis [13]. In acute stress, the activation of both sympathetic system and HPA axis are essential for survival of individual and they help to re-establish or maintain homeokinesis through adaptation. However, in chronic periods, prolonged or repeated activation of stress systems can result in cumulative biological changes (known as allostatic load) and can alter adaptive mechanism. If the ability of the organisms to maintain their integrity is poor or not strong enough to compensate the effects of environmental challenges, they can also harm the living creatures *via* various mechanisms. Excessive or inappropriate, inadequate adaptive responses to stress may play a causal role in development of certain diseases [10,11,14,15]. Indeed, depending on the stressors and their severity as well as the capability of living creatures to respond them, the reactions of living creatures to the stressors can be systematic, also reflecting itself throughout the whole body, or mainly local or regional, reflecting self at the organel/celluler/organ or system levels [11,14]. Similarly, the application of glucocorticoids for a long time can also cause events with serious consequences [16].

The gastrointestinal tract and the immune system are particularly responsive to different stressors. This system has many cellular targets for the stress mediators such as catecholamines, glucocorticoids and CRF [17-19]. The association between stress and various gastrointestinal diseases, including functional bowel disorders, inflammatory bowel disease (IBD), peptic ulcer disease and gastroeosophageal reflux disease, is being actively investigated [15,17]. However, there is a parodox that the chronic stress plays a role in inflammatory bowel disease while the glucocorticoid therapy is widely used to cure the same disease.

Gastrointestinal system (GIS) is the biggest surface area (~ 200 m^2) of the body that is binding the organism to the external environment. This system is continuously exposed to various antigens from consumed foods and resident bacteria and also from potentially harmful pathogens, such as viruses, bacteria, fungi or parasites. Besides digestion and absorption processes, it forms a barrier between the internal and external environments [20]. Intestinal barrier is composed of various components such as tight junction conformation between the intestinal epithelial cells, mucosal immune system, mucin secretion, and intestinal microbiota. The barrier function is quite critical process because of the barrier should confirm the hyporesponsiveness or tolerance towards commensal bacteria while maintaining the ability to fight pathogenic microorganisms. The breakdown of this critical balance usually results in inflammation-associated damages. Gastrointestinal system is rather complex system, which has own nervous and endocrine system. The enteric nervous system is connected bidirectionally to the brain by parasympathetic and sympathetic pathways forming the brain–gut axis. The description of stress-induced alterations in this axis is thought to be important for the solving problems of many stress-related gastrointestinal disorders [17,20]. A number of paracine acting endocrine cells have important functions for the regulation of digestion processes. These hormones exist in both central nervous system and gastrointestinal plexus neurons where they function as neurotransmitters or neuromodulators [8]. Recent findings suggest that glucocorticoid hormones may also be synthesized from extra-adrenal tissues such as brain, skin, vascular endothelium and intestine. These tissues express steroidogenic enzymes and were claimed to be potential extra-adrenal sources of glucocorticoids [21]. It is emphasized that intestinal glucocorticoid synthesis might be of potential importance in regulation of mucosal immune responses and information of inflammatory bowel disease [22].

Gastrointestinal system hosts also a large number of microorganisms. They all together are called as gastrointestinal microbiota, and form the great part of the system. The microbiota–host interactions play an active role in many physiologic and pathophysiologic processes of the host [19,23,24]. While gastrointestinal microbiota could affect the stress response [25] and intestinal structure and functions of the host [23,24], stress hormones of the host organism such as the catecholamines can also alter directly growth, motility, biofilm formation and/or virulence of pathogens and commensal bacteria [19,26,27] or they may affect their microbiota indirectly by changing the intestinal environment [20].

The effects of stress on important physiological functions of the gut include; motility, secretion and absorption, visceral sensitivity, mucosal integrity, permeability, immune system, blood flow, microbiota and microbiota-host interactions [17,20]. Some stress-related alterations in gut physiology also can be induced by exogenous glucocorticoids [28-30]. However; recent findings using central and peripheral CRF administration showed that CRF and their receptor subtypes (CRF1 and CRF2) are playing important roles in many stress-related alterations of the gut. The stress-related alterations including intestinal permeability, mast cell activity [20], goblet cell and mucin formation [31], and motility alterations [32] can be mimicked by the CRF agonists and inhibited by CRF receptor antagonists. Therefore; CRF have been suggested as a target to treat stress-induced functional gastrointestinal disorders.

In this chapter, the effects of stress and stress-related hormones, especially glucocorticoids on the components of intestinal environment suc as intestinal epithelium, mucin formation, mucosal immune system, intestinal microbiota and microbiota-host interactions, and also the role of corticosteroids and stress in bacterial colonization and intestinal diseases were reviewed.

2. Stress models for gastrointestinal studies

A great number of animal models of stress (acute/chronic, early life/adult, physical/ psychological or both physical and psychological) have been described for studying the effects of stress on gastrointestinal functions. For this purpose, rather naturally (Wistar-Kyoto rats) or genetically modified stress susceptible animals were also used. As denoted by Soderholm and Perdue [20], stress models that psychological effects are more powerful than the physical effects are preferred for mimicking the effects of the life and environmental stress on several pathologies. However, the kind and duration of stressors and other factors including genetic or perinatal environment, etc. might be a key factor in the evaluation of the stress effects on specific gastrointestinal functions such as stress-induced visceral hyperalgesia. Depending on the characteristics of the stressors and the time-course of their effects, alterations caused by stress can be immediate, delayed, transient or sustained or never be seen [33,34]. For example, the small intestinal transit was significantly inhibited by restraint stress, but not by footshock stress although plasma corticosterone levels were significantly elevated to the same extent by restraint stress and foot-shock stress [33].

Williams et al [35] reported that acute mild restraint (wrap restraint) elevated plasma levels of adrenocorticotropic hormone and beta-endorphin, and caused analgesia. Gastric ulcer did not form, gastric emptying was not affected, however, small intestinal transit was inhibited, and large intestinal transit was stimulated by wrap restraint stress, and there was an associated increase in fecal excretion. Because of neither adrenalectomy nor hypophysectomy have prevented the response of the intestine to stress, they suggested that adrenal or pituitary-derived factors are not responsible for mediating the effects of stress on the gut.

Restraint stress is most widely used as an acute stress model. Restraining can be supplied with restraint devices or by wrap restraint for times varying from 30 min to 4 hours. This model could be modified with a cold environment (cold restraint stress) or water immersion (water immersion restraint stress) for creating both physical and psychological stress [20]. Cold enhanced the changes in rat intestine caused by restraining. However, plasma corticosterone levels increased in both restraint and cold restraint stressed rats in same extent compared with fasted unstressed rats. Fasting corticosterone levels also increased compared with the fed rats [36].

The acute (one time) and chronic (1 hour/day for 10 consecutive days) models of water avoidance stress are also preferred potent psychological models in determination of stress-induced gastrointestinal functions. These models result in elevations of ACTH and corticosterone within 30 min [37], and induce enlargement of the adrenal glands [38]. Recently, Vicario et al [39,40] reported that crowding stress (8 rats/cage) or sham-crowding (2 rats/cage) for up to 15 consecutive days triggers reversible inflammation, mast cell-mediated barrier dysfunctions, persistent epithelial dysfunction, and colonic hyperalgesia. Crowding-stressed rats showed higher plasma corticosterone levels than sham-stressed animals from day 1 and up to day 15. After 15 days of crowding stress, corticosterone levels decreased %38 (slightly adaptation), but HPA reactivity to incoming stressors was preserved. Crowding stress, differently from the stress models induced in laboratory, is actualized in natural environment of animals and may reflect life stress well for humans. Thus, this model has been also suggested as a suitable animal model to unravel the complex pathophysiology underlying to common human intestinal stress-related disorders, such as IBS.

Early life stress models such as maternal deprivation of pups from the dams have also been widely used [31,41,43,44], because stressful events in the early period of life (in the form of abuse, neglect or loss of the primary caregiver) have been shown to modify adult immune and gastrointestinal tract functions [12].

3. Intestine and its microenvironment

The gastrointestinal system is a tubular organ and the part 'intestine' extends downwards from the pyloric sphincter. With its many loops and coils, small and large intestines fill much of the abdominal cavity. Microscopically, both the small and large intestine are composed of four distinct layers; the mucosa covering the internal site of the tube, the submucosa, the muscularis externa and the serosa. The mucosa consists of layer of epithelia, loose connective tissue layer (lamina propia) containing blood vessels, lymphatics, and some lymphoid tissue, and muscularis mucosa. They both have different types of cells as building blocks; however, some of them are especially important in relation to luminal challenges *via* different agents including undigested or partly digested dietary proteins, gut microbiota and its metabolites. Located among the enterocytes are goblet cells secreting mucin which *per se* build a barrier; scattered enteroendocrine cells with paracrine and endocrine actions; Paneth cells characterized by their granules containing lysozyme, tumor necrosis factor-α and defensins have antibacterial roles; M cells with their well-known roles in antigen sampling and transportation; and the intestinal subepithelial myofibroblasts located in proximity to the mucosal epithelium and produce growth factors including hepatocyte growth factor promoting the proliferation of the intestinal epithelial stem cells, thus responsible for regeneration and maintaining of the integrity of the intestinal mucosa; and dendritic cells (DCs) highly specialized for antigen presentation which can capture non-self proteins and recognize microbial products [45-55].

Intestinal epithelial cells continuously contact with two different environments; first, luminal environment, which include intestinal secretions, food antigens, commensal bacteria, and also noxious or pathogenic materials, and second, the interstitial fluid surrounding the cells at the basolateral side. The single layer intestinal epithelium along the small and large intestine has a number of physiologic functions; it forms a barrier between the external (luminal) and internal environments besides its digestive and absorptive functions, and this epithelial barrier limits the space for bacterial growth. The ability of the epithelium to control uptake of molecules into the body is denoted as the intestinal barrier function [20,56,57]. The characteristics of intestinal epithelium for participation to the barrier function include; tight junction adherence between the epithelial cells, fluid and mucin secretions, secretions of numerous antimicrobial peptides, transepithelial transport of secretory IgA and the antigen presenting cell activity. However, intestinal epithelium is not only component of the intestinal barrier. Mucosal immune system, microbiota and microbiota-host interactions exist in major components of intestinal barrier [23,24]. All these components of intestinal barrier are controlled by the mediators of neuro-endocrine-immune network, and stress and stress mediators have significant impact on these components and regulatory network [20,24].

4. The effects of stress and glucocorticoids on intestinal barrier function

Intestinal mucosal epithelium is very sensitive against different types of stress because of the half-time of mucosal epithelia which may be as short as one and half day in certain parts. In other words, compared to many other tissues in the human and animal body, it is not well differentiated and very fragile [8,57]. The effects of acute or chronic stress on intestinal barrier function or intestinal permeability does not appear very different from each other in animal models of stress. However, the duration and repetition of stressors may influence severity, and the alterations may be temporary or permanent [34,58]. Generally, intestinal ion secretion [40,59], macromolecular permeability [60,61], inflammation [40,59], visceral hypersensivity and colonic motility increased [40], while gastric motility decreased in various animal models of stress [62-64]. These stress responses have been also described in IBD patients and involve dysregulation of HPA axis [12,15,17]. They are mediated by stress-related neuropeptides such as CRF, neural mechanisms and mast cells [18,20,65]. Various stress factors including heat, nutritional alterations, overcrowding, physical restraints and transporting also destroy the microbial balance and their microenvironment in the gut [66,67]. When the stressful events cause a decrease in beneficial bacteria, they generally increase the pathogenic species within the gut microenvironment [67-69]. In following sections, the effects of stress mediators on each component of barrier were discussed in details.

5. The physical barrier of epithelium

Cell-cell and cell–basement membrane interactions of intestinal epithelial cells control the transcellular and paracellular transports of luminal macromolecules and prevent bacteria from translocating into the subepithelial layer. Tight junctions (TJ) are primary physical components of intestinal barrier, located at the most apical part of lateral membranes of epithelial cells and restrict paracellular passage. The breakdown of tight junctions during bacterial infections results in gut barrier failure, often termed "leaky gut" [20,23]. Proteins that constitute the TJ complex include transmembrane proteins such as occludin, claudin, junction adhesion molecules and intracytoplasmic proteins zonula occludens 1 and 2 (ZO1-ZO2) and members of the membrane-associated guanylate kinase (MAGUK) protein family [70]. Tight junctions are highly dynamic structures, and their permeability is regulated by several physiological and pathophysiological conditions. Signals from intestinal microbiota may promote integrity of the epithelial barrier and have been shown to regulate tight junctions and protect intestinal epithelial cells (IECs) from injury by controlling the rate of IEC proliferation and inducing cytoprotective proteins [23]. Inflammatory cytokines can disrupt tight junctions and impair gut barrier integrity. Treating epithelial monolayers with TNF-α or IL-1b increased the permeability of tight junctions by stimulating transcription and activation of myosin light chain kinase (MLCK) [71-73]. The acute partial wrap restraint stress increased colonic permeability and rectal hypersensitivity *via* epithelial cell cytoskeleton contraction through myosin light chain kinase activation [74]. Acute immobilization stress also induced an increase in TJ permeability in the rat terminal ileum. These changes were mainly due to irregularly distribution of TJ transmembrane protein occludin and of the plaque protein ZO-1 which were seen after 2 hours from the stress induction and returned to a normal pattern within 24 hours [70]. Mazzon and Cuzzocrea [75] also suggested that TNF-α has active roles in the increase of tight junction permeability during acute restraint stress. They demonstrated *in vivo* in a TNF-α R1 knock-out mouse (TNF-α R1KO) model of restraint stress that the inhibition of TNF-α attenuates the development of TJ alteration in the ileum. Restraint stress caused the increase of heat shock protein-70 expression and associated decrease in the expression of type 1 (ZO-1) protein in the colonic epithelium of mice. These stress-induced changes can be inhibited by the glucocorticoid receptor antagonist mifepristone [76]. However, Boivin et al. [77] reported that glucocorticoids enhanced epithelial barrier function by suppressing transcription of myosin light chain kinase. Bacterial pathogens target tight junctions and breach epithelial integrity to promote colonization, obtain nutrients and access the underlying tissues [23]. So, alterations in gastrointestinal microbiota induced by several stressors or exogenous glucocorticoids might be an important threat for the barrier disruption.

6. Fluid and ion secretion

Due to their diluting and flushing effects, fluid and ion secretion of epithelial cells is another protective mechanism contributing to the barrier function [20]. In humans, the jejunal net water and sodium chloride absorption decreased during both psychological (induced by dichotomous listening) [78] and physical stress (induced by cold pain) [79], and also ion absorption is changed toward secretion in psychological form [78]. Both acute and chronic stress inductions increased short circuit current (an *in vitro* technique used for measuring the secretory response of intestines) in several parts of rodent intestines [36,41,59,80]. In addition, the peripheral non-selective CRF antagonists astressin or α-helical CRF9-41 abolished stress- induced alterations [41,80,81]. Intraperitoneal injection of a newly developed selective CRF(1) peptide agonist cortagine also induced an increase in defecation and watery diarrhea in mice and rats [82]. The effects of mineralocorticoids and glucocorticoids on intestinal water and ion movements are well known. Methylprednisolone for 3 days increased Na^+K^+adenosinetriphosphatase activity and Na^+ absorption [83]; it also increased guanylate cyclase activity and Cl^- secretion in the jejunum and ileum 6 h after administration [84,85]. However, there is no direct information about the increase of water and ion secretion related with increased glucocorticoid secretions in different stressful conditions.

7. Intestinal permeability and mast cell functions

An increase in intestinal permeability was reported in animals [61,86] and humans [87] submitted to acute or chronic stress, and in IBD and IBS patients [88,89]. Increase of intestinal permeability or macromolecular permeability also involves mucosal inflammation, mucosal damage, and mast cell hyperactivity. The barrier properties of the intestinal epithelium are usually studied by assessing the permeability to various probe/marker molecules (such as horseradishperoxidase, ^{51}Cr-EDTA, mannitol) in vivo or in vitro with intestinal segments mounted in Ussing-type chambers [20]. Bagchi et al [90] investigated the effects of acute (90 minute by water immersion) and chronic (15 min/day for 15 consecutive days by water immersion) stress on the production of reactive oxygen species (ROS) and oxidative tissue damage in gastric and intestinal mucosa. Both acute and chronic stress increased ROS production, lipid peroxidation and DNA fragmentation in both gastric and intestinal mucosa, but acute stress produced greater injury when compared to chronic stress. Colonic myeloperoxidase, mucosal mast cell activity and colonic permeability increased (as assessed with macroscopic damage and bacterial translocation to mesenteric lymph nodes, liver and spleen) at 12 weeks-period in maternally deprived rat pups induced by separation from their mothers on 2-14 days period for 3 hours a day [91]. Besides, the responses of maternally deprived rats to the TNBS-induced colitis were more prominent compared with the control rats. Both acute and chronic cold stress could cause oxidative stress of duodenum and a change in iNOS, which was related to the intestinal damage process in broiler chicks [92]. There are also evidences about the bacterial production of iNOS [93]. Boudry et al [58] suggested that both apoptosis in the crypts and an immature epithelium covering the villus surface can be responsible for a barrier defect in rats submitted to WAS (1 h/day) for 5 or 10 days. Morphologic [39,94] and enzymatic alterations [40] in mitochondria of the intestinal epithelium can also participate to promotion of intestinal dysfunctions in stress-induced animals.

Mast cell activity of gastrointestinal mucosa has altered in both acute and chronic stress models. They contain inflammatory and immunmodulating mediators such as prostaglandins, histamine and serotonin that directly alter epithelial transport properties [80] and nerve and muscle functions [95]. So it has a pivotal role in visceral hypersensivity [34], intestinal inflammation, intestinal mucin secretion [96] and epithelial barrier disruption [20,61]. Castagliuolo et al. [96] found that mast cells are essential for the colonic mucin and prostaglandin secretions in immobilization stressed mice, because of these secretions were absent in mast-cell deficient animals. Even, reconstitution of bone marrow with mast cells reversed that response to normal stress values [96]. Mast cell-deficient rats (Ws/Ws) and their normal mast cell-containing littermates (1/1) were submitted to water avoidance (1 h/day) or sham stress for 5 consecutive days. Stress increased baseline jejunal epithelial ion secretion, ionic permeability, macromolecular permeability [61,94], and the number and proportion of mucosal mast cells [94] in 1/1 rats but not in Ws/Ws rats, compared with non-stressed controls. Morphological, inflammatory and permeability changes were not seen in ileum and colon of mast cell-deficient rats in a chronic stress model [42]. Kim et al [97] reported that acute stress increased mast cell number and mucosal proteinase-activated receptor-2 (PAR2) expression (G-protein coupled receptor which can be activated by mast cell tryptase and modulate gastrointestinal functions) in the rat colon. Because of CRF-antagonist astressin inhibited these alterations, they suggested that CRF can be mediator of these events. Dexamethasone treatment improves PAR-2 agonist-induced visceral hypersensitivity, but does not prevent PAR-2 agonist-induced increase in colonic permeability in rats. This effect is coupled with a reduction of colonic mast cell numbers and RMCP-II contents [98]. Chronic stressful stimulus also caused greatest numbers of degranulated mast cells [99] and mast cell hyperplasia in the intestine of rats [100]. In our unpublished study, we found that while acute cold swimming stress (swimming in 18 ^{0}C water, for 15 min) increased the mucosal mast cell numbers in ileum, dexamethasone decreased their numbers significantly. It has been reported that mast cell numbers and their protease II activity were decreased in different dexamethasone treatments [98,101,102]. Wrap restraining stress in rats for 2 hours increased histamine content in colonic mast cells without degranulation, and this was found to be mediated by interleukin I and CRF [103]. Santos et al [80] reported that CRH, when injected intraperitoneally, mimicked the effects of acute restraint stress on colon epithelium such as increased colonic ion secretion, macromolecular permeability *via* cholinergic and adrenergic nerves and mast cells. Because CRH-induced alterations in colon epithelium inhibited by CRH-antagonist, adrenergic, nicotinic and muscarinic receptor antagonists and mast cell stabilizing agent doxantrazole, but not by aminoglutethimide (mineralcorticoid and glucocorticoid synthesis blocker, they suggested that steroids have no role in CRH-induced colonic pathology. They also denoted that stimulatory effects of CRH on mast cells can be mediated by direct or indirect neural pathways. Also in humans, CRH mediates transcellular uptake of HRP in colonic mucosal biopsy samples *via* CRH receptor subtypes R1 and R2 on subepithelial mast cells [104].

8. Mucin – Physicochemical barrier

Mucin secretion is also a major component of intestinal barrier which protects the mucosa by forming a coating layer over the epithelium against bacterial penetration. In addition to providing a biophysical barrier, mucus forms a matrix that allows the retention of high concentrations of specific and nonspecific antimicrobial molecules, such as secretory IgA and defensins in close proximity to the epithelial surface [23,105,106]. The secreted mucus forms two layers, a thinner inner layer that is accepted to be sterile and difficult to dislodge and an outer layer that is not sterile and is more easily removed. Mainly MUC2 type mucin is synthesized from goblet cells in small and large intestines. Epithelial cells and Paneth cells secrete antimicrobial peptides that help preventing of bacteria to penetrate the inner mucus layer. Both the physicochemical structure and thickness of mucin coating show differences through the gastrointestinal canal. It was suggested that mucus thickness is increased and the increase was correlated with luminal bacterial concentrations of related parts of gastrointestinal canal. The inner layer is ~15–30 μm and the outer layer is 100–400 μm in small intestine and it is thickest in ileum because there are approximately 10^5–10^7 bacteria per gram of faeces in the lumen. Otherwise, the inner layer of ~100 μm and a thick outer layer of ~700 μm in large intestine where 10^{10}–10^{12} bacteria per gram of luminal content resides [106]. Mucin is not only a barrier against the bacteria but also nutritional source for bacteria. In addition, bacteria capable of colonizing mucus can avoid rapid expulsion *via* peristalsis of the intestine and take an advantage for transmitting their signaling pathway to the host [107]. Microbiota can stimulate mucin secretion *via* bacterial products and increase MUC2 expression *via* activation of TLRs and NOD-like receptors or other signaling pathways at transcriptional level. Mucin secretion is also influenced by hormones, inflammatory mediators, several signaling peptides, growth factors and infectious bacteria [106,107]. Castagliuolo et al. [108] reported that acute stress caused a depletion of goblet cells and an increase of mucin secretion related with decrease of mucin containing goblet cell numbers *via* an increase of CRF secretion [20]. They proposed that although rapid mucin release during acute stress would increase the barrier properties and provide a degree of protection against invasion of a leaky epithelium, goblet cell depletion would be deleterious in a longer time period because of the reduced capacity to respond to ongoing or new threats. A 10-day chronic stress model was resulted in barrier dysfunction in the ileum and colon (increased macromolecular permeability and depletion of mucus) and ultrastructural changes in epithelial cells (enlarged mitochondria and presence of autophagosomes) associated with bacterial adhesion and their penetration into enterocytes [42]. Studies revealed that CRF signaling can activate mucin secretion because goblet cells have CRF1 receptors and stress and peripheral injection of CRF induces mucus depletion in rat distal colon [18]. On the other hand, maternal separation stress increased mucus secretion and thus caused an elevation in the number of mucosal goblet cells in rats [109]. In our unpublished study, both acute cold swimming stress and dexamethasone injection increased the goblet cell counts in the ileum within six hours, but the effects of dexamethasone were more prominent than the swimming stress. Further, while the effect of the dexamethasone on goblet cells maintained in 24 hours period that of swimming stress was disappeared [Ünsal et al., unpublished data]. Finnie et al. [110] reported that exogenous prednisolone and hydrocortisone also increased the mucin secretion significantly in left slightly and in right uninvolved colonic biopsies of patients with ulcerative colitis. They suggested that therapeutic effects of corticosteroids in ulcerative colitis may be related partly with their stimulatory effects on mucin synthesis.

As partly mentioned above, most stress-induced gastrointestinal (GI) dysfunctions can be induced by peripheral CRF agonists and prevented by CRF receptor antagonists [18]. In a review article Larauche et al [18] reported about "CRF signaling" and emphasized that peripheral injection of CRF or urocortin stimulates colonic transit, motility, Fos expression in myenteric neurons, and defecation through activation of CRF1 receptors, whereas it decreases ileal contractility *via* CRF2 receptors. Additionally, intraperitoneal administration of CRF induces colonic mast cells degranulation *via* both CRF1 and CRF2 receptors and increases ion secretion and mucosal permeability to macromolecules, which can in turn promote intestinal inflammation and alters visceral sensitivity. Furthermore, CRF peptides can reproduce secretomotor and mucosal alterations *in vitro*. Although there are a lot of events that CRF is primary mediator in stress-induced alterations of GIS in animals and humans [17,18,32,80-82,111], similar reports for the glucocorticoids are limited [28-30]. Meddings and Swain [28] reported that stress-induced increases in gastrointestinal epithelial permeability seemed to be mediated by adrenal corticosteroids and disappeared after adrenalectomy or pharmacologic blockade of glucocorticoid receptors. Besides, dexamethasone treatment of control animals increased gastrointestinal permeability and mimicked the effects of stress. Spitz et al. [29,30] evaluated the effects of dexamethasone on intestinal barrier functions in various conditions such as starvation and after bacterial contamination. They found that starvation significantly impairs secretory IgA, promotes bacterial adherence to the mucosa and increases intestinal permeability to f-MLP in rats given 0.8 mg/kg dexamethasone intraperitoneally. These effects are significantly attenuated by the feeding of rat chow [30]. In other study, they also found out that dexamethasone administration increased intestinal permeability and bacterial adherence to the mucosa [29]. However, antibiotic decontamination of the intestine completely abrogated the intestinal permeability defects observed in this model. Basing these findings they concluded that bacterial-mucosal cell interactions may be responsible for alterations in intestinal permeability after dexamethasone administration.

9. Intestinal immune system

Intestinal homeokinesis depends on complex interactions between the microbiota, the intestinal epithelium and the host immune system. Innate and acquired immune cells of the intestine have critical roles in barrier function because of they should tolerate the antigens belonging to the food and commensal microbiota as well as they should protect the body against pathogen microorganisms [20,57]. Systemic nonresponsiveness to antigens that are introduced orally is a phenomenon known as "oral tolerance". Oral tolerance is typically characterized by the suppression of the systemic T helper 1 (Th1) response to antigens and elevated levels of IL-I0, TGF-β and antigen-specific sIgA at the mucosal surface. The T helper 2 (Th2) response also promotes the induction of tolerance in the gut. Production of IL-4 and IL- 5 during Th2 response acts synergistically to enhance IgA production. These cytokines also act further to inhibit the Th1 response [57]. The cells of the innate immunity discriminate potentially pathogenic microbes from harmless antigens through pattern recognition receptors (PRR). Toll-like receptors (TLRs) are a family of pathogen-recognition receptors of the innate immune system. TLRs are present on a variety of cell types such as intestinal epithelium, monocytes, and dendritic cells. They recognize conserved molecular motifs on microorganisms called pathogen associated molecular patterns (PAMPS). TLRs are activated by various components of microorganisms, e.g. TLR4 binds lipopolysaccharide (LPS) in gram-negative bacteria. Besides, TLR5 binds to flagellin, TLR2/6 binds to fungal zymosan and TLR7 binds single stranded RNA (ssRNA) from viruses. Activation of the TLRs by either pathogenic ligands or host factors results in downstream activation or inhibition of pathways involved in inflammation. Toll-like receptor activation by commensal bacteria plays an essential role in maintaining colonic homeostasis and controlling tolerance in the gut [57,112,113,114]. However, inappropriate activation of their signaling pathways may lead to deleterious inflammation and tissue injury. TLRs have been implicated in the pathogenesis of many GI disorders [57,114]. Although intestinal immune system is thought to have a critical role in stress-induced alterations of GIS functions, the studies about this situation are limited as this also the case for other functions of GIS such as motility, secretion and permeability [18,115,116]. McKernan et al. [116] investigated for the first time the regulation of TLR expression in the colonic mucosa in two distinct chronic stress models; Wistar-Kyoto (WKY) rats and maternally separated rats where Sprague Dawley rats were used as controls. Significant increases are seen in the mRNA levels of TLR3, 4 and 5 in both the distal and proximal colonic mucosa of MS rats compared with controls. No significant differences were noted for TLR 2, 7, 9 and 10 while TLR 6 could not be detected in any samples in both rat strains. The WKY strain showed increased levels of mRNA expression of TLR3, 4, 5, 7, 8, 9 and 10 both in the distal and proximal colonic mucosa compared to the control animals of Sprague-Dawley strain. No significant differences in expression were found for TLR2 in all samples of both strains. These authors suggested that the up-regulation of TLR 4 and 5 may indicate increases in cytokine production in response to the increases in sensitivity to gut bacteria. In addition, they suggested that the observed differences in TLR expression activity between MS and WKY rats might be related with their different neuroendocrine responses or microbiota. In spleens isolated from mice subjected to chronic 12-hour daily physical restraint for two days, TLR-4 expression significantly increased, T helper 1 (Th1) cytokine IFN-γ and IL-2 levels were found to be decreased, but Th2 cytokine and IL-4 increased. They suggested that stress modulates the immune system through a TLR4-dependent mechanism, because TLR4-deficient mice are resistant to stress-induced lymphocyte reduction and the restraint stress significantly inhibits changes of Th1 and Th2 cytokines in TLR4-deficient mice compared with the wild type mice [117]. Repeated social defeat stress (SDR) has been shown to increase the expression of TLR2 and TLR4 [118] and can activate dendritic cells for enhanced cytokine secretion in response to TLR specific stimuli. Besides, glucocorticoid resistance was determined in CD11+ dendritic cells isolated from spleens of SDR mice, whereas under baseline conditions DCs are highly sensitive to glucocorticoids [119]. Glucocorticoids and catecholamines appear to be able to regulate the expression of certain TLRs [116]. Toll-like receptor agonist-induced cytokine (IL1b, IL6, IL8 and TNF-α) release was markedly enhanced in stimulated whole blood samples from IBS patients compared with healthy controls. Plasma levels of cortisol, IL-6 and IL-8 were also significantly increased in IBS patients [120].

Chronic stress (induced by water avoidance stress for 1 hour/day for 10 consecutive days) induced the infiltration of neutrophils and mononuclear cells, and increased myeloperoxidase (MPO) activity in ileum and colon mucosa, but these changes were not shown in mast cell deficient rats [42]. Similary, jejunal inflammatory cells such as neutrophils, eosinophils and mononuclear cells and expression of IL-4 (TH2 type cytokine) increased, while interferon–γ (IFN- γ) (TH1 type cytokine) decreased in same chronic stress model of rats. Treatment of stressed rats with an antagonist to CRH eliminated the manifestations of intestinal hypersensitivity [121].

Velin et al [122] evaluated the M cell-containing follicle associated epithelium (specialized in antigen uptake) in acute and chronic stress conditions. Acute stress increased horseradish peroxidase (HRP) flux in villus as well as in follicle-associated epithelium (FAE), and chronic stress increased E. coli passage in follicle-associated epithelium whereas there was no significant increase in villus epithelium. In patients with Crohn's disease (CD), transmucosal uptake of non-pathogenic E. coli across the FAE increased in ileum, despite unchanged macromolecular permeability, but these changes were not observed in patients with ulcerative colitis [123]. Recently, Keita [124] showed that application of CRF agonist increased HRP and E. coli passage, stress-induced increases in uptake across FAE of HRP, and E. coli were reduced by CRF antagonist, mast cell stabilizer and atropine. Chronic restraint stress increases eosinophils expressing CRF in the jejunum, which participate to the recruitment of mast cells and epithelial barrier dysfunction [125]. The influence of CRF signaling on intestinal mast cell activity is detailed above. However, the information about their effects on other immune components of intestine (such as intestinal epithelial cells, TLR expression or intraepithelial lymphocytes) is limited. Larauche et al [82] reported that treatment of mice with CRF-1 agonist cortagine exhibits a dose-related interferon-γ (IFNγ) response indicating T cell and/or natural killer (NK) cell activation, which is followed by tight junction deregulation and dose dependent apoptotic loss of different cell populations in ileum.

IECs participate in initiating adaptive immune responses in the gut by transporting luminal antigens to underlying immune cells for presentation by professional antigen presenting cells or can present antigen themselves [57]. intraepithelial lymphocyte (IEL) and paneth cells (specialized IEC located at the base of intestinal crypts in small intestine) do also synthesis the antimicrobial peptides such as lysozymes, alpha defensins, cathelicidins, lipocalins, and C-type lectins such as RegIIIγ [126]. Production of RegIIIg [127] and alpha-defensins [128] as well as that of secretory IgA [129] are induced by commensal bacteria. Nutritional and infection stress affected the secretory activity of Paneth cells in human [130]. In women, acute cold stress induced the release of α-defensin in the jejunum [131]. Evidences suggested that dysfunction of Paneth cells and impaired defensin secretion may contribute to IBD susceptibility [57,105].

Corticosteroids and catecholamines are well recognized and accepted powerful regulators and players of the body in its response to environmental challenges including biological factors of stress. Stress or corticosteroid applications are known to have also profound effects on intestinal wall structure and functioning. Intestinal submucosa is the place where lymphocytes, eosinophils and mast cells reside in men and animals under normal conditions. Jarillo-Luna et al. [115] investigated the effects of chronic restraint stress in mice submitted to different procedures (adrenalectomy, chemical sympathectomy, and treatment with a glucocorticoid antagonist (RU486), dexamethasone, and epinephrine) on intraepithelial lymphocyte (IEL) numbers. They found that chronic restraint-stress reduced the IEL population in the small intestine and adrenal catecholamines and glucocorticoids are essential in preserving IEL population because adrenalectomy, treatment with RU-486 and chemical sympathectomy decreased the number of γδ, CD4+ and CD8+ T cells in non-stressed groups. They also found that adrenalectomy did not buffered the stress-induced reduction in CD8 lympocytes, but glucocorticoid receptor antagonist RU-486 buffered stress-induced decrease in γδ and CD8+, but not in CD4+ T cells. Besides, low and high doses of dexamethasone (5 and 50 mg/kg BW) significantly reduced the number of γδ and CD8+ T cells, and epinefrin (0.1-0.5 mg/kg) reduced the number of γδ, CD4+ and CD8+ T cells in intact mice. Also many other studies reported that both stress-related endogen rises of glucocorticoids [115,132-134] and exogenous glucocorticoid administrations [135,136] induce decreases in intraepithelial lymphocytes and/or those in ileal Peyer patches. Pretreatment with glucocorticoid receptor antagonist mifepristone significantly reduced apoptosis in both T- and B-cell populations in intraepithelial lymphocytes after the burn injury [133]. Experimental studies also suggested that single or repeated parenteral applications of cortisone cause a decrease in eosinophil concentration in all parts of examined gastrointestinal wall from stomach up to colon [137,138]. Immunosuppressive effects of glucocorticoids are explained mainly by an increase of apoptosis and a decrease of cytokine production. Corticosterone impaired the maturation of DCs and cytokine production and reduced the ability of DCs to prime naive CD8+ T cells *in vivo*; there was no reduction in surface TLR4 expression in CORT-treated DCs [139]. However, McEwen et al. [140] proposed that although glucocorticoids are mainly known with and used widely for their immunsuppressive aspects, adrenal steroids play also different roles as important modulators of the immune system. Pharmacological as well as physiological changes in glucocorticoids result in a decrease in lymphocyte, monocyte and eosinophil numbers and an increase in neutrophil numbers in the blood of men and rodents. These changes are not related with the glucocorticoid-induced leukocyte deaths. The nonspecific stress and glucocorticoid administration cause redistribution of leukocytes from peripheral blood into various tissues and organs, such as bone marrow, spleen and lymph nodes [140-142].

10. Intestinal microbiota

One of the important groups of the environmental biological stressors belongs to the microbiota, and it is associated with every multicellular organism on earth. It is estimated that in humans and many animals reside at least 10^{14} microorganisms, making approximately 1.5 kg biomass, in various parts of the body, most abundant of them residing the distal part of the gut in humans and animals with exception of ruminants [143-146]. These parts of the body lined by the skin or mucous membranes and all are in direct contact with the environment. Although the microorganisms are preferable grouped as pathogenic, while they harm the multicellular organisms, and saprophytic, while they seemingly do not harm their hosts instead they build symbiotic relationships, but possibly this depends only on the balance or imbalance among numerous groups of microorganisms constituting the microbiota in a definite part of the body and between the microbiota and its host, in general.

The first days, weeks, months or years, the time spent in mothers' womb or in egg-shall of the metazoan life is the only time which they are free of microbes. The delivery into the outside exposes them to an enormous range of microbes from diverse environments. This is the first encounters with life forms with different morphology and functions. The studies have shown that within a short time following delivery, the microrganisms are present on the skin and mucosal surfaces of the body. With time, a dense, complex gastrointestinal microbiota develops [147,148]. Due to the unique properties of microorganisms including their small size, metabolic versatility and genetic plasticity, microorganisms can tolerate and easily adapt to unfavorable and immense variety of continuously changing environmental conditions [149]. However, although a wide variety of microorganisms were exposed to representative individuals from start up throughout the life periods, only a limited numbers of species are able to colonize permanently in available body surfaces of man and animals. The microorganisms display a tissue tropism; e.g., they colonize predominantly only certain body sites. Consequently, each side is inhabited by only certain species of microorganisms. The microorganisms found at a particular body site constitute what is known as the indigenous or normal microbiota of this site, wherein the term 'indigenous' include all of viruses, protozoa, archae, and fungi [150,151]. The GIT is inhabited with 10^{13}–10^{14} microorganisms, approximately 500 to over 1000 different species and more than 7000 strains. Their counts exceed ten times the numbers of somatic cells of their hosts [144,151-154].

The very complex and diverse gastro-intestinal microbiota differs from species to species, in dependence of nutritional habits with some geographic motives. Besides, it varies from one segment to another and varies over time in the same individual, because the environment of the GIT varies considerable along its length and with the lifetime of an individual [144]. Thus, the composition and intensity of the microbiota of a newborn is quite different from those of an adult which are in turn quite different from that of an elderly individual [155,156]. Colonization begins at birth with facultative bacteria and the colonization of anaerobic bacteria which are composed of more than %90 of GIS microbiota develops later. In humans, the microbiota has a stable adult-like signature by 1 year of age [113,154]. Similarly, the composition and intensity of the microbiota varies along the gastrointestinal tract where they are attached to the mucosa or are present in the contents. In stomach and duodenum of humans, microorganism numbers is 10^3CFU/ml and include more lactobacilli, streptococci and yeasts species. In jejunum (10^4CFU/ml) and ileum (10^{7-8} CFU/ml) *Lactobacillus, Bacteroides, Enterobacteriaceae,* Streptococci, *Bifidobacterium and Fusobacteria species* are more existent. The highest numbers of bacteria (10^{11-12} CFU/ml) displaying enormous diversity are found in colon, predominant species being *Bacteroides, Fusobacterium, Eubacterium,Peptococcus, Peptostreptococcus, Veillonella, Bifidobacterium, Escherichia, Clostridium, Lactobacillus* and others [147,154]. Although only 40-45% part of GI microbiota could be growth with classical microbial culture tecniques, recently developed moleculer techniques allow the definition of non-culturable members of microbiota. The vast majority of microorganisms belong to the phyla of *Firmicutes, Bacteroidetes, Actinobacteria,* and *Proteobacteria* while *Fusobacteria, Verrucomicrobia and TM7* are represent in relatively lower numbers [144,145,157,158]. There are also some fungi and *Archaea* present in the gastrointestinal tract [144,159,160], but they comprise less than 1% of total inhabitants. The majority of the intestinal bacteria are composed of gram-negative anaerobes [143].

With the acquisition and establishment in the intestinal lumina with various microbial populations bidirectional interactions between microbiota and host organism starts [161,162]. There are symbiotic relationships between the host and its GI microbiota in steady-state conditions. The gastrointestinal tract serves a natural habitat for a dynamic microbial community of different origins while the microbiota is very essential for both gastrointestinal integrity [163] and general health of host organisms [113]. Comparison between the conventional and germ-free animals has allowed obtaining information about the effects of microbiota on morphologic, functional and metabolic characteristics of host organisms [23,113,154,160]. Germ free animals have enlarged cecum [164], they have thinner gut wall, smaller total surface area and more cubic epithelium than the columnar, increased enterochromaffin cell area and smaller Peyer's patches, and intestinal epithelium has slower turnover rate compared with the conventional animals [160,165]. The materiality of the gut microbiota also for many gut functions such as motility, immune and barrier functions are reviewed by several authors [23,113].

Complex association between the host and its microbiota collectively extends the processing indigestible parts of food to the benefits of the host organisms *via* metabolic capacities which are not coded in host genomes like mammalian and avian species [166-168]. They digest the unusable parts of the diets; metabolites reach to the intestinal lumina within various secretions and desquamated cells of their hosts for growth and proliferation. At the same time, they also supply the host organisms with a considerable amount of nutrients, which makes this ecosystem an invaluable, essential metabolic organ, which contributes significantly to the homeokinesis of the host organisms [23,113,152,169]. They produce substances including vitamins, volatile or short-chain fatty acids (SCFAs) and polyamines which are absorbed throughout the intestinal wall and used directly by intestinal epithelial cells or other cells of the body [170,171]. SCFA profoundly influence gut barrier functions, host immunity, epithelial proliferation and bacterial pathogenesis [172]. Zheng et al. [171] showed extensive gut microbiota modulation of host systemic metabolism involving short-chain fatty acids, tryptophan and tyrosine metabolism, and possibly a compensatory mechanism of indole-melatonin production. All these metabolites have also many regulatory functions in host organisms. Tryptophan and tyrosine are precursors of neurotransmitters acting directly at the central nervous system level [113]. Thus, the gut microbiota enhances the host's metabolic capacity for processing nutrients and modulates the activities of multiple pathways in a variety of organ systems, including the brain.

Microbiota acts as a luminal barrier against incoming pathogens; this phenomenon has been described as colonization resistance [23,154]. Beneficial and pathogen microorganism compete with each other for the attachment sites and for nutrients, so microbiota and their products can prevent pathogen colonization directly. On the other hand, microbiota acts on barrier functions also indirectly by stimulating mucosal immune system [172]. The abundant antigenic stimulus supplied by microbiota and their products are essential for the stimulation of immune system cells locally and systemically [173-175]. In germ-free animals, besides the poor developed Peyer's patches, altered compositions of CD4+ T cells and IgA-producing B cells in the lamina propria [165], TH 17 cells, which is a subset of the T cells and contribute to resistance against colonization by pathogens were virtually absent in germ free animals [176,177]. Chow and Mazmanian [177] denoted that although Th17 cells are essential for immunity, they have also been implicated in the pathogenesis of many autoimmune diseases, including IBD, arthritis, psoriasis, and experimental autoimmune encephalomyelitis (EAE).

The gut microbiota has recently been identified as the main source of highest biological variability confined in an individual [178]. Because the metazoan life-forms and the inhabitation of their gastrointestinal tract with microorganisms evolved together, there are close links between any host or its epi-genome and its very complex diverse gastrointestinal microbiota with their multitude genomes. It is estimated that this microbial community has 70–140 times more total genes than the human host. These functional inter-relationships between host and microbiota or two different genomes determine the health or disease state of the metazoan hosts and the balance among different microorganism populations [113,172,179]. It is well accepted that the intestinal microbiota involves in metabolome of the host, thus promotes actively fat accumulation and weight gain and sustains indirectly a low-grade systemic inflammation especially when imbalanced, and consequently, enhances the risk for complex, multifactorial diseases such as insulin resistance, diabetes, obesity and cardiovascular diseases. The search of global obesity epidemic led to the growing evidences about the possible roles of intestinal microbiota in these respects [180,181,182]. Claus et al. [170] has noted that the colonization of the gut microbiota was associated with a rapid increase in body weights of animals up to 4% within 5 days of colonization. Findings of various studies also revealed that gut microbiota profile of obese and diabetic individuals differ by phylum level both in its quantity and quality from that of lean and nonobese individuals [182,183]. Recent evidences exhibit that the composition of the gut microbiome may influence body weight of the host by various mechanisms including enhancing the ability of intestines to extract energy from food [184], regulating fat storage in tissues [185] and affecting satiety by modulating the levels of local hormones that regulate satiety and by direct effects in central nervous system [186].

There is a growing appreciation of the critical roles played by the commensal microbiota, both in general well-being of the hosts and in the specific functioning of the brain–gut axis [113]. Bidirectional communications of brain–gut–enteric microbiota axis simply actualized by through signals from the brain can influence the motor, sensory, and secretory modalities of the gastrointestinal tract and conversely, visceral messages from the gastrointestinal tract can influence brain functions [187]. Sudo and colleagues [25] showed that gut microbiota effect the stress responses of host organisms. They compared the response of the HPA axis to stress in GF, specific pathogen free (SPF) and gnotobiotic mice that were mono-associated with a single bacterium. Restraint stress caused an exaggerated ACTH and corticosterone elevation in GF rather than SPF mice. This hyper-response of the HPA axis was reversed by mono-association with *Bifidobacterium infantis*. They also showed in following experiments that the levels of brain-derived nerve factor (BDNF), norepinephrine and 5- 5-hydroxytryptamine (5-HT) in the cortex and hippocampus were significantly lower in GF mice than in SPF mice [188]. Improvements of stress-related symptoms by probiotic administration also support the possible regulatory effects of microbiota on HPA axis and brain functions [44,189]. Gareau et al [44] reported that probiotic treatments improved colonic dysfunction and corrected the higher corticosterone levels in stressed rats induced by maternal seperation. L. rhamnosus (JB-1) reduced stress-induced corticosterone and anxiety- and depression-related behavior in mice. In different region of brain, this therapy also altered GABA receptor expression implicated in the pathogenesis of anxiety and depression, which are highly comorbid with functional bowel disorders. Due to the neurochemical and behavioral effects were not found in vagotomized mice, they suggested that vagus could be a major modulatory constitutive communication pathway between the bacteria exposed to the gut and the brain [189]. The roles of probiotics and gut microbiota in modulation of visceral and even somatic pain perception and their possible roles in alterations of mood and behavior were reviewed by Forsythe et al. [190] and Grenham et al. [113].

As mentioned above, intestinal dysbiosis can adversely influence gut physiology both by direct effects to the surrounding gut wall and by leading to inappropriate brain–gut axis signaling and associated consequences for CNS functions and disease states. Stress at the level of the CNS can also impact on gut functions and lead to perturbations of the microbiota [113].

11. Stress and intestinal microbiota

Intestinal microbiota have once been seen as potential treat for the host organisms, but recently accepted as an integral part of metazoan life and even as an organ with a huge variety of building blocks which mainly cooperate with each other and with the host for maintaining the health and survival [113,144]. However, various stress factors such as heat, cold, nutritional alterations, overcrowding, physical restraints and transporting or fouled or contaminated foods can destroy the microbial balance in the gastrointestinal system [66,67,191-195] and alter their relationships with each other and with their hosts. Stressful stimuli can affect gastrointestinal microbiota directly, for example *via* limited availability of food ingredients or direct actions of stress mediators such as adrenaline or noradrenaline on microbiota [27,196], and indirectly *via* altering the intestinal environment of bacteria such as intestinal secretion, motility, permeability and immune functions as reviewed above.

The effects of several stressors and stress mediators on intestinal microbiota were given in Table 1. Bailey et al [197] induced social disruption stress (SDR) in mice to determine whether the microbiome contributes to stressor-induced immune enhancements. They analyzed bacterial populations in the cecum with using bacterial tag-encoded FLX amplicon pyrosequencing (bTEFAP) and found that microbiota significantly changed immediately after stressor exposure as summarized in Table 1, and stress also increased circulating levels of IL-6 and MCP-1, which were significantly correlated with stressor-induced changes to three bacterial genera (i.e., *Coprococcus, Pseudobutyrivibrio,* and *Dorea spp*). However in antibiotic treated mice, exposure to SDR failed to increase IL-6 and MCP-1. Bailey et al [191] reported that restraint stress also significantly change the composition of the intestinal microbiota in mice and disruption of the microbiota increased susceptibility to murine enteric pathogen *Citrobacter rodentium* which can be associated with reduced competitive exclusion of commensal bacteria and increased tumor necrosis factor alpha (TNF-α) gene expression in colonic tissue. Reduction in bifidobacteria and lactobacilli numbers in fecal samples of infant monkeys whose mother had been exposed to stress in either early or late pregnancy period showed that maternal pregnancy conditions affect infant health and can enhance susceptibility to infection [68]. Similarly, early life stress induced by maternal separation altered fecal microbiota with concomitant increases in corticosterone and also visceral hypersensitivity and systemic immune response to *in vitro* lipopolysaccharide challenges in rats [198]. Knowles et al [199] reported that non-extreme 'every day' stress events such as exam stress can affect the integrity of the indigenous gastrointestinal microflora of humans but these changes are not supported by cortisol responses. Maternal separation of rhesus macaques also caused to decrease of lactobacilli at 3th days post-separation but significant differences in the cortisol responses did not predict the magnitude of the reduction of lactobacilli numbers. These authors suggested that more than one neuro-hormone can modulate microbiota changes.

Because of their immune-suppressive or stress-mediating effects, some studies have been focused on the effects of glucocorticoids on intestinal microbiota. These studies showed that exogenous glucocorticoid applications to the host organisms are also able to cause changes in gastrointestinal microbiota. We [200,Ünsal et al., unpublished study] and others [29,30,201] demonstrated that exogenous glucocorticoid administrations can also affect gut microbiota by enhancing total aerobe and gram negative enteric bacteria and their translocation to extraintestinal tissues [201]. We compared the effects of different doses of dexamethasone on ileal microbiota and found, in contrast to well-known stress effects, that 5mg/kg dexamethasone injection also increased the numbers of total anaerobe and lactobacilli in ileal content of rats [200]. However, their number did not change in lower doses of dexamethasone. Also in our unpublished study acute cold swimming stress decreased the numbers of lactobacilli, while dexamethasone in dose of 5 mg/kg increased total aerobe, gram-negative enteric bacteria and lactobacilli. Thus, the evidences available suggest that several stressors reduce the number of lactobacilli, while on the contrary, they increases growth, epithelial adherence and mucosal uptake of Gram-negative pathogens. Lactobacilli may possible be defined as stress indicator bacteria of the gut microbiota which is sensible to the effects of various stressors, in general. Although it is known that exogenous glucocorticoids increase the counts of gram negative enteric bacteria [29,30,201], no other information about their effects on the lactobacilli in the gut could be found.

The roles of stress and stress-related hormones in the pathogenesis of infectious diseases are beyond any argument. Microbial endocrinology is a new research area which appeared from the demand how stress influence the bacterial infections, how neuro-endocrine-immune secretions of host organisms influence their harboring microbiota and how infectious microbes can actively use the neurohormonal products of the stress to their own advantages [202,203]. Recently, several *in vitro* studies have focused on direct effects of stress hormones on bacterial growth and their virulence in an effort to explore and understand the interactions of so-called stress hormones and infections. These studies gathered the evidence that catecholamines stimulate the growth of a wide variety of gram-negative bacterial species, including those of medical importance [27,196,204-209]. Furthermore, catecholamines were also found to be able to induce *E.coli* to produce a heat-stable autoinducer of growth [19,27,204,210] as well as for adhesion required K99 pilus and shigella-like toxins I and II, which may have important roles in its pathogenic activity [210].

The effects of norepinephrine and its receptor antagonists on mucosal bacterial adherence were also determined in sheets obtained from different parts of the gut, mounted in Ussing chamber. Norepinephrine increased the adherence of enterohemorrhagic *Escherichia coli* O157:H7 (EHEC) to colonic epithelium through interactions with α-2 adrenergic receptors [211-213] and it increased the internalization of enterohemorrhagic E. coli O157:H7 (EHEC) and S. enterica serovar Choleraesuis in jejunal mucosa containing Peyer's patch follicles [214,215]. Parallel studies related to the direct actions of other stress mediators such as cortisol or CRF on bacterial growth could not be found. However, Kakuno et al. [216] suggested that hydrocortisone enhance intracellular colonizations of E. coli and Schreiber and Brown [217] reported that ACTH increased EHEC adherence to the porcine colonic mucosa.

Many factors participate in the pathology of inflammatory bowel disease (IBD) such as genetic and immune status of host organism, the gut microbiota, and environmental triggers [218]. Some scientific events support that the enteric microbiota is involved in abnormal inflammatory responses observed in diverse animal models for inflammatory bowel disease [219,220]. These events reviewed by the authors [219,220] are arranged as the reduction or absence of intestinal inflammation in animal models of colitis in antibiotic-treated or germ-free animals; colitis formation with some bacterial inoculations to germ free rats or not to formation with other bacterial species; and beneficial effects of probiotics and prebiotics in IBD patients or animal models of IBD. However, although microbiota has been thought to play an active role in etiopathogenesis of inflammatory bowel disease, it is not clear whether they are cause or outcome. In other words, whether alterations in intestinal microenvironment of microbiota such as mucin secretion, immune modifications and epithelial dysfunctions cause to changes in commensal microbiota or microbial alterations cause to inflammatory responses of intestinal mucosa in stressful conditions is not clear yet [221].

Although the reports in microbiome composition of IBD-patients or models show differences, changes in microbiota composition are characterized more likely by decreases in lactobacilli and bifidobacteria, and increases or unchange in aerobe and facultative anaerobic bacteria [222]. Molecular analysis of the microbiota of IBD patients have shown that temporal stability and diversity of the gut microbiota composition in IBD patients decreased compared to non-IBD controls [223], and commensal bacteria, particularly members of the phyla *Firmicutes* and *Bacteroidetes* decreased and *Proteobacteria* and *Actinobacteria* increased [224]. These changes look alike to those that seen following effects of stress on intestinal microbiota.

Stress and/or Stress Mediators	Microbiota	Method	References
Social disruption stress (SDR) in mice (total of 6, two-hour cycles of SDR)	Decrease in *Bacteroides* spp., tended to decrease in *Lactobacillus* spp., tended to increase in *Clostridium* spp. and changes in *Coprococcus, Pseudobutyrivibrio,* and *Dorea spp. in cecal content*	(bTEFAP)	197
Restraint stress for 7 days in mice (between 18.00- 08.00 h)	Overgrowth of facultatively anaerobic microbiota, reduction in family *Porphyromonadaceae,and* genus *Tanneralla,*reducing microbial richness and diversity in the ceca	both culture technique and bTEFAP	191
Prenatal stress induced by acoustical startle paradigm for 6 weeks in early or late pregnancy in Rhesus Monkey	prenatal stress reduced the overall numbers of bifidobacteria and lactobacilli in fecal cultures of infants	culture technique	68
Maternal separation in rhesus macaques *(Macaca mulatta)*	Decrease of lactobacilli in fecal samples at 3th days postseparation, not correlated with cortisol responses	culture technique	26
Academic stress in undergraduate students	Reduction in fecal lactic acid bacteria, unsignificantly cortisol enhancement	culture technique	199
Food, water and bedding deprivation in mice	Decrease in lactobacilli in stomach, increase of coliforms in jejunum, ileum and cecum, reduction in fusiform-shaped bacteria associated with mucosal epithelium of cecum and colon	culture technique	192
Dexemethasone (0.8 mg/kg) Dexamethosone (0.8 mg/kg)+ starvation for 48 h in Fischer rat	impairs secretory IgA, promotes bacterial adherence to the mucosa, increase of intestinal permeability		29,30,225

Stress and/or Stress Mediators	Microbiota	Method	References
Dexamethasone 5 mg/kg in rats	Increase of total aerobe bacteria and lactobacilli in ileum	culture technique	200, Ünsal et al., unpublished study
Methylprednisolone (3 mg/kg) in rats subjected to temporary liver inflow occlusion	Increase of intestinal *Klebsiella spp* and *Proteus spp* and of translocation to multiple organs.	culture technique	201
Pregnant rats were treated with either cortisone acetate or normal saline on days 18-21 of gestation	Total bacteria and gram-negatives found in association with the mucosa were significantly lower in pups prenatally treated with steroids.	culture technique	226
Norepinephrine action on porcine or murine cecum/ colon/jejunum explants	Increases cecal-colonic adherence of E. coli O157:H7; changes Salmonella and E. coli uptake into Peyer's patches		211-215
ACTH action on explants of porcine distal colonic mucosa	Increases adherence of E. coli O157:H7 to colonic mucosa		217

Table 1. The effects of some different type stressors and/or stress mediators on intestinal microbiota

12. Nutritional stress

Nutrition and nutrients of metazoans play very important multifunctional key roles both for metazoan host and for its gastrointestinal microbiota. They are essential not only in colonization, growth and survival of the microbiota in intestinal system but also in maintaining the balance among different species and their localization within its lumina [67,192,227,228]. Nutrition plays an important role as stressor for host organisms and their gastrointestinal tract *via* three mechanisms. Firstly, foods supply nutrients for intestinal microbiota and also serve as carriers of various microorganisms into gastrointestinal tract which may under circumstances lead to imbalances among different species; secondly, nutritional deficiencies or imbalances are perceived from the organisms as stressors setting them to the state of well-known alarm reaction of stress; and thirdly, certain food ingredients in their undigested forms as foreign substances accepted as non-self from organisms and stimulate a stress situation. In cases of carrying the microorganisms into gastrointestinal tract or acting as antigens, the foreign treats come into direct contact with the wall of gastrointestinal tract. A great part of microorganisms stay in gastrointestinal canal for a short time period, while others colonize its lumina permanently and their genera can be life-long present there, mostly in a symbiotic relationship with the host organisms.

Dietary ingredients, which are not digestible for the host organisms or which are digestible but escape from the intestinal digestion can be utilized as substrate for growth from microbiota colonized in the following sections of the gut [229,230]. All microorganisms residing in gastrointestinal tract needs the nutrients that necessary for their growth and proliferation are continuously supplied *via* foods of their hosts and from host organisms in secretions of digestive organs including saliva, gastric juice, pancreatic, hepatic (bile) and intestinal wall secretions and desquamated epithelial structures. The composition and amount of the food, even the compositions of these secrets may undergo substantial changes. This is why the hosts' balanced nutrition and physiological state exerts a strong controlling effect on its microbiota [160,181,192,231-237]. Thus, any nutritional deficiency or imbalance of their hosts serve the most important challenge for the growth, survival and balance of different microbial species within the intestinal lumina.

Malnutritions in different nature or nutritional imbalances had always been and are still very widespread health problems of men and animals worldwide and frequently seen in infants and elderly, and those subjects having malignancies, getting chemotherapy and/or radiotherapy or infected with human immunodeficiency virus. Very common forms of malnutrition are protein, calorie and protein calorie deficiencies which almost always are complicated with deficiencies of other nutrients, especially that of minerals and vitamins [238]. As mentioned above, deficiencies of calories, proteins, minerals or vitamins in hosts' food can influence the indigenous microbiota both directly *via* the restricted availability of the metabolites and their indigestible parts for hosts and indirectly by inducing a stress response within the host organism and affecting the compositions of gastrointestinal morphology and secretions as well as by impairing the general and local immune responses and neuro-endocrine-immune network leading to an imbalance between the host organism and its microbiota, in general. These changed milieus offer possibilities to certain new species of the microbiota for adaptation in gastrointestinal tract or cause their dispersion from their localization areas to others. In protein calorie malnutrition, colonic type microbiota known to spread to and proliferate in the upper small intestine which may cause a variety of metabolic disturbances including steatorrhea, vitamin deficiencies, nutrient malabsorbtions, and consequently water leakage into lumina and diarrhea [160,239-241]. Generally, pathogenic microorganisms including Enterobacteriaceae, Pseudomonas, Klebsiella and Candida were increased [240,241]. In such clinical cases of complicated protein and/or calorie malnutrition, pathogenic microorganisms often cause endotoxemia and infection in addition to intestinal disruptions including diarrhea and metabolic diseases [242,243]. Thus, they all affect the composition of the intestinal digesta and its passage time, which in turn may influence the composition of the indigenous intestinal microbiota and their relationships with the intestinal wall [244-246].

Generally, experimental studies use deficiencies or excesses of a definite dietary component or several components, and animals are held under more hygienic, defined conditions throughout the rearing and experimental periods than their counterparts, whereas clinical cases develop spontaneously in man and animals. Thus, they give the possibility to detect the possible effects of a certain dietary component on the behavior of the gastrointestinal microbiota. However, such experimental evidences from studies using deficiencies or imbalances of definite nutrients in this respect are very sparse. So, an almost protein-free diet disrupted the cecal microbiota, and made mice more susceptible to bacterial translocation than those mice nourished adequately [227,236,247]. The counts of cecal total aerobic bacteria and Gram-negative enteric bacilli were found to be increased time-dependently when CD-1 mice were fed an almost N-free diet for 21 days [236]. The results of another study on adult female Crl:CD-1[CR]BR mice also showed that both the feeding an almost protein-free and 20% fat containing diet for 14 days and starvation for 3 days resulted in an increase in counts of Gram-negative enteric bacilli and a decrease in counts of lactobacilli and strict anaerobes [227]. In certain studies the effects of dietary manipulations combined and/or compared with those of endotoxemia were investigated. So, Deitch et al. [227] studied the effects of starvation and malnutrition alone or in combination with endotoxemia and found that the spread of bacteria from the gut could not be controlled nor translocated bacteria be cleared in protein malnourished mice as effectively as in the controls. However, no association between protein malnutrition and bacterial translocation could be found by Katayama et al. [247]. Instead, these authors determined that the total numbers of Gram-negative enteric bacilli adherent to the mucosa of ileum and cecum were less in protein malnourished rats than in their adequately nourished controls. Further, there was also a significant negative correlation between the duration of protein malnutrition and bacterial adherence to the intestinal mucosa. Only, *E. coli* binding to insoluble ileal mucus was increased in the rats receiving endotoxin. Tannock and Savage [192] reported that the deprivation of food and water and bedding for 48 hours increased the counts of coliform bacteria while they decreased the counts of cecal lactobacilli of CD-1 and C57BL mice strainsIn a preliminary study, we found that feeding an almost protein-free diet to male Wistar rats for 35 days affected especially the total aerobe microorganisms and lactobacilli while total anaerobe and *Enterobacteriaceae* remained relatively unaffected. Compared to controls with balanced nutrition, both dietary qualitative and quantitative protein malnutrition decreased mean lactobacilli counts. Also, the quality and quantity of the dietary protein made a difference in their effects on intestinal microbiota; compared to gelatin-fed animals, lower aerobe and higher lactobacilli counts could be observed in cecal samples of rats given an almost protein-free diet. Furthermore, it could also be shown that the actual immune status (e.g. suppression of neutrophils) of the host can modify the effects of the qualitative and quantitative protein malnutrition on the intestinal microbiota [193].

Human cultural characteristics may also have implications on the compositions of the gastrointestinal microbiota. Living on a high carbohydrate diet caused also the presence of fewer bacteriodes and more enterococci in feces of the people than those living on a Western diet with more fat and animal proteins [231].

After all, the mechanisms *via* which different type of diets or dietary manipulations affect the host and its guest organ 'gut microbiota' are still not exactly cleared. The effects of dietary qualitative and/or quantitative protein malnutrition on regulatory systems in men and animals are well characterized and are the topic of numerous texts. Earlier studies with definite protein malnutrition were summarized by Aschkenasy [248] and suggest that protein malnutrition of different types or amino acid imbalances generally result in increases of adrenalin and glucocorticoid concentrations in man and animals. Torún and Viteri [249] also noted that in protein and/or protein-calorie malnutrition, the concentrations of adrenalin and glucocorticoids are either increased or showed no important change while many other hormones with exceptions of aldosterone and growth hormone decreased significantly. However, such studies have very important drawbacks as they look only one aspect of the regulators such as their concentrations in blood. Generally, the concomitant expression status of the enzymes which interconvert active and inactive forms of a given hormone and their receptors in target tissues or cells are ignored or not evaluated concurrently. A study conducted by Marroqui et al. [250] on mice demonstrated that during a protein malnutrition plasma glucagon concentration increased, but the ability of exogenous glucagon to raise plasma glucose levels were lower in mice given a low protein diet.

13. Conclusion

Since their introduction in the terminology of scientific medicine, the terms environment, stress and microorganisms were probably never been so important in mind of mankind for the development, health and welfare of men and animals. Although the roles of stress and stress-dependent disruptions of the intestinal microbiota both in developments and in promotion of the symptoms of various diseases and disorders including those of gastrointestinal system in men and animals are well accepted, there is still a lack of information about many aspects including which strains play really a role in the etiopathogenesis of a given condition, and which mechanisms are effective in such cases [24,113]. The stress-dependent dysfunctions of HPA axis can manifest itself in different ways. In many cases it may be related to high or low cortisol concentrations in blood whereas in other situations no detectable change of cortisol occurs. Further, the response given by hypothalamus and pituitary gland to the cortisol can be increased or decreased depending on the receptor numbers [10,11,14,15]. While in classic stress response sympathetic nervous system and glucocorticoids thought to be responsible for stress-dependent processes, studies within last two decades suggest that many disordered situations of the gastrointestinal system mediated by CRF. Both CRF-related peptides and CRF receptors are also expressed within the intestine, where they may activate directly the enteric, endocrine, and immune cells and may be involved in intestinal manifestations such as mucosal permeability, secretion, mast cell function, motility, mucin formation, immune function and many disorders of the gut. In other words, the peripheral changes produced by stress can be mimicked by CRF-injection and prevented by CRF-receptor antagonists [18,20,31,32,82]. Therefore, CRF have been suggested as a new target in treating stress induced functional gastrointestinal disorders.

Recently, intestinal microbiota imbalances gain growing interests both as the subject and cause of stress and stress-related diseases which are connected with not only the gastrointestinal system but also all other systems or organs of the metazoan hosts including the adipose tissue [24,113, 179, 184,185]. Basing on experimental and clinical studies, certain phyla and species are currently related with a given specific condition [180,181]. However, all these studies are looking mainly on one side of the iceberg, like for example changes in a specific member of the microbiota in respect to stress stimuli and a specific neurotransmitter in brain, as it also the case in search of the mediating regulatory pathways. Understanding the roles of stress and stress-related microbiotal changes and their mechanisms in the role of various physiopathological conditions would be helpful in improvements of the relationships of the metazoan hosts with their microenvironments including its microbiota and thus, would contribute greatly to the health state of men and animals.

Author details

Hümeyra Ünsal* and Muharrem Balkaya

Adnan Menderes University, Faculty of Veterinary Medicine, Department of Physiology, Işıklı, Aydın, Turkey

14. References

[1] Adams JD, Jr Garcia C (2005) Spirit, Mind and Body in Chumash Healing. Evid. based. complement. alternat. med. 2: 459-463.

[2] Yang Y (2009) Chinese Herbal Medicines. Comparisons and Characteristics. 2nd Editions. China. Churchill Livingstone Elsevier, pp

[3] Fornaro M, Clementi N, Fornaro P (2009) Medicine and Psychiatry in Western Culture: Ancient Greek Myths and Modern Prejudices. Ann. gen. psychiatry 8: 21.

[4] Yapijakis C (2009) Hippocrates of Kos, the Father of Clinical Medicine, and Asclepiades of Bithynia, the Father of Molecular Medicine. In vivo: 507-514.

[5] Kelly K. The History of Medicine Medicine Becomes a Science: 1840-1999. Facts on File Inc.

[6] Bernard C. (1865). Introduction à l'étude de la médecineexpérimentale. Available: http://classiques.uqac.ca/classiques/bernard_claude/intro_etude_medecine_exp/intro_m edecine_exper.pdf

[7] Selye H (1936) A Syndrome Produced by Diverse Nocuous Agents. Nature. 138: 32.

[8] Vander Sherman and Luciano's Human Physiology: The Mechanisms of Body Function. 8th Edition. The McGraw-Hill Companies, pp. 728-732

[9] Chrousos GP, Gold PW (1992) The Concepts of Stress and Stress System Disorders. Overview of Physical and Behavioral Homeostasis. JAMA. 267: 1244-1252.

[10] Charmandari E, Tsigos C, Chrousos G (2005) Endocrinology of the Stress Response. Annu. rev. physiol. 67: 259-84.

[11] Chrousos GP (2009) Stress and Disorders of Stress Systems. Nature rev. endoc. 5: 374-381.

[12] Mayer EA, Naliboff BD, Chang L, Coutinho SV (2001) Stress and Irritable Bowel Syndrome. Am. j. physiol. gastrointest. liver physiol. 280: G519-G524.

* Corresponding Author

[13] Goymann W, Wingfield JC (2004) Allostatic Load, Social Status and Stress Hormones: The Costs of Social Status Matter. Anim. beh. 67: 591-602.

[14] McEwen BS (2000) Allostasis, Allostatic Load, and the Aging Nervous System: Role of Excitatory Amino Acids and Excitotoxicity. Neurochem. res. 25: 1219-1231.

[15] Mayer EA (2000) The Neurobiology of Stress and Gastrointestinal Disease. *Gut.* 47: 861-869.

[16] Papadimitriou A, Priftis KN (2009) Regulation of the Hypothalamic-Pituitary-Adrenal Axis. Neuroimmunomodulation. 16: 265-271.

[17] Bhatia V, Tandon RK (2005) Stress and the Gastrointestinal Tract. J. gastroenterol. hepatol. 20: 332-339.

[18] Larauche M, Kiank C, Tache Y (2009) Corticotropin Releasing Factor Signaling in Colon and Ileum: Regulation by Stress and Pathophysiological Implications. J. physiol. pharmacol. 60 (Suppl 7): 33-46.

[19] Lyte M, Vulchanova L, Brown DR (2011) Stress at the Intestinal Surface: Catecholamines and Mucosa-Bacteria Interactions. Cell tissue res. 343: 23-32.

[20] Söderholm JD, Perdue MH (2001) Stress and Gastrointestinal Tract. II. Stress and Intestinal Barrier Function. Am. j. physiol. gastrointest. liver physiol. 280: G7-G13.

[21] Davies E, MacKenzie SM (2003) Extra-Adrenal Production of Corticosteroids. Clin. Exp. pharmacol. physiol. 30: 437-445.

[22] Noti M, Sidler D, Brunner T (2009) Extra-Adrenal Glucocorticoid Synthesis in the Intestinal Epithelium: More than a Drop in the Ocean? Semin. immunopathol. 31: 237-248.

[23] Ashida H, Ogawa M, Kim M, Mimuro H, Sasakawa C (2011) Bacteria and Host Interactions in the Gut Epithelial Barrier. Nat. chem. biol. 8: 36-45.

[24] Sekirov I, Russell SL, Antunes LC, Finlay BB (2010) Gut Microbiota in Health and Disease. Physiol. rev. 90: 859-904.

[25] Sudo N, Chida Y, Aiba Y, Sonoda J, Oyama N, Yu XN, Kubo C, Koga Y (2004) Postnatal Microbial Colonization Programs the Hypothalamic-Pituitary-Adrenal System for Stress Response in Mice. J. physiol. 558: 263-275.

[26] Bailey MT, Coe CL (1999) Maternal Separation Disrupts the Integrity of the Intestinal Microflora in Infant Rhesus Monkeys. Dev psychobiol. 35:146-155.

[27] Freestone PP, Haigh RD, Williams PH, Lyte M (1999) Stimulation of Bacterial Growth by Heat-Stable Norepinophrine-Induced Autoinducers. FEMS microbial. letters. 172: 53-60.

[28] Meddings JB, Swain MG (2000) Environmental Stress-Induced Gastrointestinal Permeability is Mediated by Endogenous Glucocorticoids in the Rat. Gastroenterology. 119: 1019-1028.

[29] Spitz J, Hecht G, Taveras M, Aoys E, Alverdy J (1994) The Effect of Dexamethasone Administration on Rat Intestinal Permeability: The Role of Bacterial Adherence. Gastroenterology. 106: 35-41.

[30] Spitz JC, Ghandi S, Taveras M, Aoys E, Alverdy JC (1996) Characteristics of the Intestinal Epithelial Barrier During Dietary Manipulation and Glucocorticoid Stress. Crit. care med. 24: 635-641.

[31] Estienne M, Claustre J, Clain-Gardechaux G, Paquet A, Taché Y, Fioramonti J, Plaisancié P. (2010) Maternal Deprivation Alters Epithelial Secretory Cell Lineages in Rat Duodenum: Role of CRF-Related Peptides. Gut. 59: 744-751.

[32] Taché Y, Martinez V, Million M. Wang L (2001) Stress and the Gastrointestinal Tract III. Stress-Related Alterations of Gut Motor Function: Role of Brain Corticotropin-Releasing Factor Receptors. Am. j. physiol gastrointest. liver physiol. 280: G173-G177.

[33] Tsukada F, Sugawara M, Kohno H, Ohkubo Y (2001) Evaluation of the Effects of Restraint and Footshock Stress on Small Intestinal Motility by an Improved Method Using a Radionuclide, 51 Cr, in the Rat. Biol. pharm. bull. 24:488-90.

[34] Bradesi S, Schwetz I, Ennes HS, Lamy CM, Ohning G, Fanselow M, Pothoulakis C, McRoberts JA, Mayer EA (2005) Repeated Exposure to Water Avoidance Stress in Rats: A New Model for Sustained Visceral Hyperalgesia. Am. j. physiol. gastrointest. liver physiol. 289: G42–G53.

[35] Williams CL, Villar RG, Peterson JM, Burks TF (1988) Stress-Induced Changes in Intestinal Transit in the Rat: A Model for Iirritable Bowel Syndrome. Gastroenterology. 94: 611-621.

[36] Saunders PR, Kosecka U, McKay DM, Perdue MH (1994) Acute Stressors Stimulate Ion Secretion and Increase Epithelial Permeability in Rat Intestine. Am. j. physiol. 267: G794-G799.

[37] Million M, Taché Y, Anton P (1999) Susceptibility of Lewis and Fischer Rats to Stress-Induced Worsening of TNB-Colitis: Protective Role of Brain CRF. Am. j. physiol. 276: G1027-G1036.

[38] Söderholm JD, Streutker C, Yang PC, Paterson C, Singh PK, McKay DM, Sherman PM, Croitoru K, Perdue MH (2004) Increased Epithelial Uptake of Protein Antigens in the Ileum of Crohn's Disease Mediated by Tumour Necrosis Factor Alpha. Gut. 53: 1817-1824.

[39] Vicario M., Guilarte M, Alonso C. Yang PC, Martínez C, Ramos L, Lobo B, González A, Guilà M, Pigrau M, Saperas E, Azpiroz F, Santos J (2010) Chronological Assessment of Mast Cell-Mediated Gut Dysfunction and Mucosal Inflammation in a Rat Model of Chronic Psychosocial Stress. Brain behav. immun. 24: 1166-1175.

[40] Vicario M, Alonso C, Guilarte M, Serra J, Martínez C, González-Castro AM, Lobo B, Antolín M, Andreu AL, García-Arumí E, Casellas M, Saperas E, Malagelada JR, Azpiroz F, Santos J (2012) Chronic Psychosocial Stress Induces Reversible Mitochondrial Damage and Corticotropin-Releasing Factor Receptor Type-1 Upregulation in the Rat Intestine and IBS-like Gut Dysfunction. Psychoneuroendocrinology 37: 65-77.

[41] Söderholm JD, Yates DA, Gareau MG, Yang PC, MacQueen G, Perdue MH (2002) Neonatal Maternal Separation Predisposes Adult Rats to Colonic Barrier Dysfunction in Response to Mild Stress. Am. j. physiol. gastrointest. liver physiol. 283: G1257-G1263.

[42] Söderholm JD, Yang PC, Ceponis P, VohraA, Riddell R, Sherman PM, Perdue MH (2002) Chronic Stress Induces Mast Cell-Dependent Bacterial Adherence and Initiates Mucosal Inflammation in Rat Intestine. Gastroenterology. 123: 1099-1108.

[43] Gareau MG, Jury J, Yang PC, MacQueen G, Perdue MH (2006) Neonatal Maternal Separation Causes Colonic Dysfunction in Rat Pups Including Impaired Host Resistance. *Pediatr. res.* 59: 83-88.

[44] Gareau MG, Jury J, Perdue MH (2007) Neonatal Maternal Separation of Rat Pups Results in Abnormal Cholinergic Regulation of Epithelial Permeability. Am. j. physiol. gastrointest. liver physiol. 293: G198-G203.

[45] Iwasaki A, Kelsall BL (1999) Mucosal Dendritic Cells: Their Specialized Role in Initiating T Cell Responses. Am. j. physiol. gastroenterol. liver physiol. 276: G1074-G1078.

[46] Powell DW, Mifflin RC, Valentich JD, Crowe SE, Saada JI, West AB. (1999) Myofibroblasts. I. Paracrine Cells Important in Health and Disease. Am j. physiol. 277: C1-C9.

[47] Powell DW, Mifflin RC, Valentich JD, Crowe SE, Saada JI, West AB. (1999) Myofibroblasts. II. Intestinal Subepithelial Myofibroblasts. Am. j. physiol. 277: C183-C201.

[48] Stagg AJ, Hart AL, Knight SC, Kamm MA (2003) The Dendritic Cell: Its Role in Intestinal Inflammation and Relationship with Gut Bacteria. Gut. 52: 1522-1529.

[49] Catron DM, Itano AA, Pape KA, Mueller DL, Jenkins MK (2004) Visualizing the First 50 Hr of the Primary Immune Response to a Soluble Antigen. Immunity. 21: 341-347.

[50] Macpherson AJ, Uhr T (2004) Induction of Protective IgA by Intestinal Dendritic Cells Carrying Commensal Bacteria. Science. 303: 1662-1665.

[51] Saada JI, Barrera CA, Reyes VE, Adegboyega PA, Suarez G, Tamerisa RA, Pang KF, Bland DA, Mifflin RC, DI Mari JF, Powell DW (2004) Intestinal Myofibroblasts and Immune Tolerance. Ann. n. y. acad sci. 1029: 379-381.

[52] Niess JH, Reinecker HC (2005) Lamina Propria Dendritic Cells in the Physiology and Pathology of the Gastrointestinal Tract. Curr. opin. gastroenterol. 21: 687-691.

[53] Leon F, Symythies LE, Smith PD, Kelsall BL (2006) Involvement of Dendritic Cells in the Pathogenesis of Inflammatory Bowel Diseases. Adv. exp. med. biol. 579: 117-132.

[54] Inman CF, Singha, Lewis M, Bradley B, Stokes C, Bailey M (2010) Dendritic Cells Interact with CD4 T Cells in Intestinal Mucosa. J. leukocyte biol. 88: 571-578.

[55] Manicassamy S, Reizis B, Ravindran R, Nakaya H, Salazar-Gonzalez RM, Wang YC, Pulendran B (2010) Activation of Beta-Catenin in Dendritic Cells Regulates Immunity Versus Tolerance in the Intestine. Science. 329: 849-853.

[56] Perdue MH (1999) Mucosal Immunity and Inflammation III. The Mucosal Antigen Barrier: Cross Talk with Mucosal Cytokines Am. j. physiol. gastrointest. liver physiol. 277: G1-G5.

[57] Mason KL, Huffnagle GB, Noverr MC, Kao JY (2008) Overview of Gut Immunology. In: Huffnagle GB, Noverr MC, editors. GI Microbiota and Regulation of the Immune

System: Advances in Experimental Medicine and Biology Vol 635. Landes Bioscience Springer Science+Business Media. pp: 1-10.

[58] Boudry G, Jury J, Yang PC, Perdue MH (2007) Chronic Psychological Stress Alters Epithelial Cell Turn-Over in Rat Ileum. Am. j. physiol. gastrointest. liver physiol. 292: G1228-G1232.

[59] Cameron HL, Perdue MH (2005) Stress Impairs Murine Intestinal Barrier Function: Improvement by Glucagon-Like Peptide-2. J. pharmacol. exp. ther. 314: 214-220.

[60] Kiliaan AJ, Saunders PR, Bijlsma PB, Berin MC, Taminiau JA, Groot JA, Perdue MH. (1998) Stress Stimulates Transepithelial Macromolecular Uptake in Rat Jejunum. Am. j. physiol. gastrointest. liver. physiol. 275: G1037-G1044.

[61] Santos J, Benjamin M, Yang PC, Prior T, Perdue MH (2000) Chronic Stress Impairs Rat Growth and Jejunal Epithelial Barrier Function: Role of Mast Cells. Am. j. physiol. gastrointest. liver physiol. 278: G847-G854.

[62] Hung CR. (1998) Low Susceptibility of Stress Ulcer in Diabetic Rats: Role of Cholinergic Gastric Motility. Chin. j. physiol. 41: 151-159.

[63] Babygirija R, Zheng J, Bülbül M. Ludwig K, Takahashi T (2010) Beneficial Effects of Social Attachment to Overcome Daily Stress. Brain res.1352: 43-49.

[64] Zheng J, Babygirija R, Bülbül M, Cerjak D, Ludwig K, Takahashi T (2010) Hypothalamic Oxytocin Mediates Adaptation Mechanism Against Chronic Stress in Rats. Am. j. physiol. gastrointest. liver physiol. 299: G946-G953.

[65] Wallon C, Söderholm JD (2009) Corticotropin-Releasing Hormone and Mast Cells in the Regulation of Mucosal Barrier Function in the Human Colon. Ann. n. y. acad. sci. 1165: 206-210.

[66] Suzuki K, Harasawa R, Yoshitake Y, Mitsuoka T (1983) Effects of Crowding and Heat Stress on Intestinal flora, Body Weight Gain, and Feed Efficiency of Growing Rats and Chicks. Jpn. j. vet. sci. 45:331-338.

[67] Tannock GW (1997) Modification of the Normal Microbiota by Diet, Stress, Antimicrobial Agents, and Probiotics. In: Mackie RI, White BA, Isaacson RE, editors. Gastrointestinal Microbiology. New York. Chapman & Hall, pp 434-466

[68] Bailey MT, Lubach GR, Coe CL (2004) Prenatal Stress Alters Bacterial Colonization of the Gut in Infant Monkeys. J. pediatr. gastroenterol. nutr. 38: 414-421.

[69] Lutgendorff F, Akkermans LM, Söderholm JD (2008) The Role of Microbiota and Probiotics in Stress-Induced Gastro-Intestinal Damage. Curr. mol. med. 8(4): 282-298.

[70] Mazzon E, Sturniolo GC, Puzzolo D, Frisina N, Fries W (2002) Effect of Stress on the Paracellular Barrier in the Rat Ileum. Gut. 51: 507-513.

[71] Wang F, Graham WV, Wang Y, Witkowski ED, Schwarz BT, Turner JR (2005) Interferon-Gamma and Tumor Necrosis Factor-Alpha Synergize to Induce Intestinal Epithelial Barrier Dysfunction by Up-regulating Myosin Light Chain Kinase Expression. Am. j.pathol. 166: 409-419.

[72] Graham WV, Wang F, Clayburgh DR, Cheng JX, Yoon B, Wang Y, Lin A, Turner JR. (2006) Tumor Necrosis Factor-Induced Long Myosin Light Chain Kinase Transcription

is Regulated by Differentiation-Dependent Signaling Events. Characterization of the Human Long Myosin Light Chain Kinase Promoter. J. biol. chem. 281: 26205-26215.

[73] Al-Sadi R, Ye D, Dokladny K, Ma TY (2008) Mechanism of IL-1 Beta-Induced Increase in Intestinal Epithelial Tight Junction Permeability. J. immunol. 180: 5653-5661.

[74] Ait-Belgnaoui A, Bradesi S, Fioramonti J, Theodorou V, Bueno L (2005) Acute Stress-Induced Hypersensitivity to Colonic Distension Depends upon Increase in Paracellular Permeability: Role of Myosin Light Chain Kinase. Pain. 113: 141-147.

[75] Mazzon E, Cuzzocrea S (2008) Role of TNF-Alpha in Ileum Tight Junction Alteration in Mouse Model of Restraint Stress. Am. j. physiol. gastrointest. liver physiol. 294: G1268-G1280.

[76] Matsuo K, Zhang X, Ono Y, Nagatomi R (2009) Acute Stress-Induced Colonic Tissue HSP70 Expression Requires Commensal Bacterial Components and Intrinsic Glucocorticoid. Brain behav. immune. 23: 108-115.

[77] Boivin MA, Ye D, Kennedy JC, Al-Sadi R, Shepela C, Ma TY (2007) Mechanism of Glucocorticoid Regulation of the Intestinal Tight Junction Barrier. Am. j physiol. gastrointest. liver physiol. 292: G590-G598.

[78] Barclay GR, Turnberg LA (1987) Effect of Psychological Stress on Salt and Water Transport in the Human Jejunum. Gastroenterology. 93: 91-97.

[79] Barclay GR, Turnberg LA (1988) Effect of Cold-Induced Pain on Salt and Water Transport in the Human Jejunum. Gastroenterology. 94: 994-998.

[80] Santos J, Saunders PR, Hanssen NP, Yang PC, Yates D, Groot JA, Perdue MH (1999) Corticotropin-Releasing Hormone Mimics Stress-Induced Colonic Epithelial Pathophysiology in the Rat Am. j. physiol. 277: G391-G399.

[81] Saunders PR, Santos J, Hanssen NP, Yates D, Groot JA, Perdue MH (2002) Physical and Psychological Stress in Rats Enhances Colonic Epithelial Permeability via Peripheral CRH. Dig. dis. sci. 47: 208-215.

[82] Larauche M, Gourcerol G, Wang L, Pambukchian K, Brunnhuber S, Adelson DW, Rivier J, Million M, Taché Y (2009) A Cortagine CRF1 Agonist, Induces Stresslike Alterations of Colonic Function and Visceral Hypersensitivity in Rodents Primarily Through Peripheral Pathways. Am. j. physiol. gastrointest. liver physiol. 297: G215-G227.

[83] Charney AN, Kinsey MD, Myers L, Gainnella RA, Gots RE (1975) Na+-K+-Activated Adenosine Triphosphatase and Intestinal Electrolyte Transport. Effect of Adrenal Steroids. J. clin invest. 56: 653-660.

[84] Marnane WG, Tai YH, Decker RA, Boedeker EC, Charney AN, Donowitz M (1981) Methylprednisolone Stimulation of Guanylate Cyclase Activity in Rat Small Intestinal Mucosa: Possible Role in Electrolyte Transport. Gastroenterology.81: 90-100.

[85] Tai YH, Decker RA, Marnane WG, Charney AN, Donowitz M (1981) Effects of Methylprednisolone on Electrolyte Transport by In Vitro Rat Ileum. Am. j. physiol. 240: G365-G370.

[86] Yates DA, Santos J, Söderholm JD, Perdue MH (2001) Adaptation of stress-induced mucosal pathophysiology in rat colon involves opioid pathways. Am. j. physiol. gastrointest. liver physiol. 281: G124-G128.

[87] Santos J, Saperas E, Nogueiras C, Mourelle M, Antoli´n M, Cadahia A, Malagelada JR (1998) Release of Mast Cell Mediators into the Jejunum by Cold Pain Stress in Humans. Gastroenterology 114: 640-648.

[88] Gerova VA, Stoynov SG, Katsarov DS, Svinarov DA (2011) Increased Intestinal Permeability in Inflammatory Bowel Diseases Assessed by Iohexol Test. World j. gastroenterol. 17: 2211-2215.

[89] Gecse K, Róka R, Séra T, Rosztóczy A, Annaházi A, Izbéki F, Nagy F, Molnár T, Szepes Z, Pávics L, Bueno L, Wittmann T (2012) Leaky Gut in Patients with Diarrhea-Predominant Irritable Bowel Syndrome and Inactive Ulcerative Colitis. Digestion. 85: 40-46.

[90] Bagchi D, Carryl OR, Tran MX, Bagchi M, Garg A, Milnes MM, Williams CB, Balmoori J, Bagchi DJ, Mitra S, Stohs SJ (1999) Acute and Chronic Stress-Induced Oxidative Gastrointestinal Mucosal Injury in Rats and Protection by Bismuth Subsalicylate. Mol. cell biochem. 196: 109-116.

[91] Barreau F, Ferrier L, Fioramonti J, Bueno L (2004) Neonatal Maternal Deprivation Triggers Long Term Alterations in Colonic Epithelial Barrier and Mucosal Immunity in Rats. Gut. 53: 501-506.

[92] Zhang ZW, Lv ZH, Li JL, Li S, Xu SW, Wang XL (2011) Effects of Cold Stress on Nitric Oxide in Duodenum of Chicks. Poult. sci. 90: 1555-1561.

[93] Witthöft T, Eckmann L, Kim JM, Kagnoff MF (1998) Enteroinvasive Bacteria Directly Activate Expression of INOS and NO Production in Human Colon Epithelial Cells. Am. j. physiol. 275: G564-G571.

[94] Santos J, Yang PC, Soderholm JD, Benjamin M, Perdue MH (2001) Role of Mast Cells in Chronic Stress Induced Colonic Epithelial Barrier Dysfunction in the Rat. Gut 48: 630-636.

[95] Perdue MH, McKay DM (1994) Integrative Immunophysiology in the Intestinal Mucosa. Am. j. physiol. 267: G151-G165.

[96] Castagliuolo I, Wershil BK, Karalis K, Pasha A, Nikulasson ST, Pothoulakis C (1998) Colonic Mucin Release in Response to Immobilization Stress is Mast Cell Dependent. Am. j. physiol. gastrointest. liver physiol. 274: G1094-G1100.

[97] Kim DH, Cho YJ, Kim JH, Kim YB, Lee KJ (2010) Stress-Induced Alterations in Mast Cell Numbers and Proteinase-Activated Receptor-2 Expression of the Colon: Role of Corticotrophin-Releasing Factor. J. korean med. sci. 25: 1330-1335.

[98] Róka R, Ait-Belgnaoui A, Salvador-Cartier C, Garcia-Villar R, Fioramonti J, Eutamène H, Bueno L (2007) Dexamethasone Prevents Visceral Hyperalgesia but not Colonic Permeability Increase Induced by Luminal Protease-Activated Receptor-2 Agonist in Rats. Gut. 56: 1072-1078.

[99] Wilson LM, Baldwin AL (1999) Environmental Stress Causes Mast Cell Degranulation, Endothelial and Epithelial Changes, and Edema in the Rat Intestinal Mucosa. Microcirculation. 6: 189-198.

[100] Jorge E, Fernández JA, Torres R, Vergara P, Martin MT (2010) Functional Changes Induced by Psychological Stress are not Enough to Cause Intestinal Inflammation in Sprague-Dawley Rats. Neurogastroenterol. motil. 22: e241-e250.

[101] Godot V, Garcia G, Capel F, Arock M, Durant-Gasselin I, Asselin-Labat ML, Emilie D, Humbert M (2006) Dexamethasone and IL-10 Stimulate Glucocorticoid-Induced Leucine Zipper Synthesis by Human Mast Cells. Allergy 61: 886-890.

[102] Rijnierse A, Koster AS, Nijkamp FP, Kraneveld AD (2006) TNF-Alpha is Crucial for the Development of Mast Cell-Dependent Colitis in Mice. Am. j. physiol. gastrointest. liver physiol. 291: G969-G976.

[103] Eutamene H, Theodorou V, Fioramonti J, Bueno L (2003) Acute Stress Modulates the Histamine Content of Mast Cells in the Gastrointestinal Tract Through Interleukin-1 and Corticotropin-Releasing Factor Release in Rats. J. physiol. 553: 959-966.

[104] Wallon C, Yang PC, Keita AV, Ericson AC, McKay DM, Sherman PM, Perdue MH, Söderholm JD (2008) Corticotropin-Releasing Hormone (CRH) Regulates Macromolecular Permeability via Mast Cells in Normal Human Colonic Biopsies In Vitro. Gut. 57: 50-58.

[105] Maloy KJ, Powrie F (2011) Intestinal Homeostasis and Its Breakdown in Inflammatory Bowel Disease. Nature. 474: 298-306.

[106] McGuckin MA, Lindén SK, Sutton P, Florin TH. (2011) Mucin Dynamics and Enteric Pathogens. Nat. rev microbiol. 9: 265-278.

[107] Dharmani P, Srivastava V, Kissoon-Singh V, Chadee K (2009) Role of Intestinal Mucins in Innate Host Defense Mechanisms Against Pathogens. J. innate immun. 1: 123-135.

[108] Castagliuolo I, Lamont JT, Qiu B, Fleming SM, Bhaskar KR, Nikulasson ST, Kornetsky C, Pothoulakis C (1996) Acute Stress Causes Mucin Release From Rat Colon: Role of Corticotropin Releasing Factor and Mast Cells. Am. j. physiol. 271: G884-G892.

[109] O'Malley D, Julio-Pieper M, Gibney SM, Dinan TG, Cryan JF (2010) Distinct Alterations in Colonic Morphology and Physiology in Two Rat Models of Enhanced Stress-Induced Anxiety and Depression-like Behaviour. Stress. 13(2): 114-122.

[110] Finnie IA, Campbell BJ, Taylor BA, Milton JD, Sadek SK, Yu LG, Rhodes JM (1996) Stimulation of Colonic Mucin Synthesis by Corticosteroids and Nicotine. Clin. sci. (Lond) 91: 359-364.

[111] Tsukamoto K, Nakade Y, Mantyh C, Ludwig K, Pappas TN, Takahashi T (2006) Peripherally Administered CRF Stimulates Colonic Motility via Central CRF Receptors and Vagal Pathways in Conscious Rats. Am. j. physiol. regul. integr. comp. physiol. 290: R1537-R1541.

[112] Michelsen KS, Arditi M (2007) Toll-like Receptors and Innate Immunity in Gut Homeostasis and Pathology. Curr. opin. hematol. 14: 48-54.

[113] Grenham S, Clarke G, Cryan JF, Dinan TG (2011) Brain-Gut-Microbe Communication in Health and Disease. Front. physiol. 2: 1-14.

[114] Shibolet O, Podolsky DK (2007) TLRs in the Gut. IV. Negative Regulation of Toll-like Receptors and Intestinal Homeostasis: Addition by Subtraction Am. j. physiol. gastrointest. liver physiol. 292: G1469-G1473.

[115] Jarillo-Luna A, Rivera-Aguilar V, Martìnez-Carrillo BE, Barbosa-Cabrera E, Garfias HR, Campos-Rodríguez R (2008) Effect of Restraint Stress on the Population of Intestinal Intraepithelial Lymphocytes in Mice. Brain behav. immun. 22: 265-275.

[116] McKernan DP, Nolan A, Brint EK, O'Mahony SM, Hyland NP, Cryan JF, Dinan TG (2009) Toll-Like Receptor mRNA Expression is Selectively Increased in the Colonic Mucosa of Two Animal Models Relevant to Irritable Bowel Syndrome. PLoS ONE 4(12): e8226. Available: http://www.plosone.org/article/info%3adoi%2fF10.1371%2Fjournal.pone.0008226.

[117] Zhang Y, Woodruff M, Zhang Y, Miao J, Hanley G, Stuart C, Zeng X, Sprabhajar S, Moorman J, Zhao B, Yin D (2008) Toll-like Receptor 4 Mediates Chronic Restraint Stress-Induced Immune Suppression. J. neuroimmunol. 194:115–122.

[118] Bailey MT, Engler H, Powell ND, Padgett DA, Sheridan JF (2007) Repeated Social Defeat Increases the Bactericidal Activity of Splenic Macrophages Through a Toll-like Receptor-Dependent Pathway. Am. j. physiol. regul. integr. comp. physiol. 293: R1180-R1190.

[119] Powell ND, Bailey MT, Mays JW, Stiner-Jones LM, Hanke ML, Padgett DA, Sheridan JF (2009) Repeated Social Defeat Activates Dendritic Cells and Enhances Toll-like Receptor Dependent Cytokine Secretion. *Brain behav. immun.* 23: 225-231.

[120] McKernan DP, Gaszner G, Quigley EM, Cryan JF, Dinan TG (2011) Altered Peripheral Toll-like Receptor Responses in the Irritable Bowel Syndrome. Aliment. pharmacol. ther. 33: 1045-1052.

[121] Yang PC, Jury J, Söderholm JD, Sherman PM, Mckay DM, Perdue MH (2006) Chronic Psychological Stress in Rats Induces Intestinal Sensitization to Luminal Antigens. Am. j. pathol. 168: 104-114.

[122] Velin AK, Ericson AC, Braaf Y, Wallon C, Söderholm JD (2004) Increased Antigen and Bacterial Uptake in Follicle Associated Epithelium Induced by Chronic Psychological Stress in Rats. Gut. 53: 494-500.

[123] Keita AV, Salim SY, Jiang T, Yang PC, Franzén L, Söderkvist P, Magnusson KE, Söderholm JD (2008) Increased Uptake of Non-pathogenic E. Coli via the Follicle-Associated Epithelium in Longstanding Ileal Crohn's Disease. J. pathol. 215: 135-144.

[124] Keita AV, Söderholm JD, Ericson AC (2010) Stress-Induced Barrier Disruption of Rat Follicle-Associated Epithelium Involves Corticotropin-Releasing Hormone, Acetylcholine, Substance P, and Mast Cells. Neurogastroenterol. motil. 22: 770-778.

[125] Zheng PY, Feng BS, Oluwole C, Struiksma S, Chen X, Li P, Tang SG. Yang PC (2009) Psychological Stress Induces Eosinophils to Produce Corticotrophin Releasing Hormone in the Intestine. Gut. 58:1473-1479.

[126] Koslowski M J, Beisner J, Stange EF, Wehkamp J (2010) Innate Antimicrobial Host Defense in Small Intestinal Crohn's Disease. Int. j. med. microbiol. 300: 34-40.

[127] Cash HL, Whitham CV, Behrendt CL, Hooper LV (2006) Symbiotic Bacteria Direct Expression of an Intestinal Bactericidal Lectin. Science. 313: 1126-1130.

[128] Ayabe T, Satchell DP, Wilson CL, Parks WC, Selsted ME, Ouellette AJ (2000) Secretion of Microbicidal Alpha-Defensins by Intestinal Paneth Cells in Response to Bacteria. Nat. immunol. 1: 99-100.

[129] Macpherson AJ, Slack E (2007) The Functional Interactions of Commensal Bacteria with Intestinal Secretory IgA. Curr. opin. gastroenterol. 23: 673-8.

[130] Kelly P, Feakins R, Domizio P, Murphy J, Bevins C, Wilson J, McPhail P, Poulsom R, Dhaliwal W (2004) Paneth Cell Granule Depletion in Human Small Intestine under Infective and Nutritional Stress. Clin. exp. immunol. 135: 303-309.

[131] Alonso C, Guilarte M, Vicario M, Ramos L, Ramadan Z, Antolín M, Martínez C, Rezzi S, Saperas E, Kochhar S, Santos J, Malagelada JR (2008) Maladaptive Intestinal Epithelial Responses to Life Stress may Predispose Healthy Women to Gut Mucosal Inflammation. Gastroenterology. 135: 163-172.

[132] Murosaki S, Inagaki-Ohara K, Kusaka H, Ikeda H, Yoshikai Y (1997) Apoptosis of Intestinal Intraepithelial Lymphocytes Induced by Exogenous and Endogenous Glucocorticoids. Microbiol. immunol. 41: 139-148.

[133] Fukuzuka K, Edwards CK 3rd, Clare-Salzer M, Copeland EM 3rd, Moldawer LL, Mozingo DW (2000) Glucocorticoid and Fas Ligand Induced Mucosal Lymphocyte Apoptosis After Burn Injury. J. trauma. 49: 710-716.

[134] Reber SO, Peters S, Slattery DA, Hofmann C, Schölmerich J, Neumann ID, Obermeier F (2011) Mucosal Immunosuppression and Epithelial Barrier Defects are Key Events in Murine Psychosocial Stress-Induced Colitis. Brain behav. immun. 25: 1153-1161.

[135] Motyka B, Bhogal HS, Reynolds JD (1995) Apoptosis of Ileal Peyer's Patch B Cells is Increased by Glucocorticoids or Anti-immunoglobulin Antibodies. Eur. j. immunol. 25: 1865-1871.

[136] Ruiz-Santana S, Lopez A, Torres S, Rey A, Losada A, Latasa L, Manzano JL, Diaz-Chico BN, (2001) Prevention of Dexamethasone Induced Lymphocytic Apoptosis in the Intestine and in Peyer Patches by Enteral Nutrition. J. parenter. enteral nutr. 25: 338-345.

[137] Vaughn J (1961) Experimental Eosinophilia: Local Tissue Reactions to Ascaris Extracts. J. allergy. 32: 501-513.

[138] Browaeys J, Wallon D (1958) Éosinophilies tissulaires du rat a l'état normal et dans les éosinopénies sanguine. Le sang 29: 686-695.

[139] Elftman MD, Norbury CC, Bonneau RH, Truckenmiller ME (2007) Corticosterone Impairs Dendritic Cell Maturation and Function. Immunology. 122: 279-290.

[140] McEwen BS, Biron CA, Brunson KW, Bulloch K, Chambers WH, Dhabhar FS, Goldfarb RH, Kitson RP, Miller AH, Spencer RL, Weiss JM (1997) The Role of Adrenocorticoids

as Modulators of Immune Function in Health and Disease: Neural, Endocrine and Immune Interactions. Brain res. rev. 23: 79-133.

[141] Toft P, Lillevang ST, Tønnesen E, Svendsen P, Höhndorf K (1993) Redistribution of Lymphocytes Following E. Coli Sepsis. Scand. j. immunol. 38: 541-545.

[142] Toft P, Svendsen P, Tønnesen E, Rasmussen JW, Christensen NJ (1993) Redistribution of Lymphocytes after Major Surgical Stress. Acta anaesthesiol. scand. 37: 245-249.

[143] Tlaskalová-Hogenová H, Stepánková R, Hudcovic T, Tucková L, Cukrowska B, Lodinová-Zádníková R, Kozáková H, Rossmann P, Bártová J, Sokol D, Funda DP, Borovská D, Reháková Z, Sinkora J, Hofman J, Drastich P, Kokesová A (2004) Commensal Bacteria (Normal Microflora), Mucosal Immunity and Chronic Inflammatory and Autoimmune Diseases. Immunol. lett. 93: 97-108.

[144] Eckburg PB, Bik EM, Bernstein CN, Purdom E, Dethlefsen L, Sergent M, Gill SR, Nelson KE, Relman DA (2005) Diversity of Human Intestinal Microbial Flora. Science. 308: 1635-1638.

[145] Ley RE, Peterson DA, Gordon JI (2006) Ecological and Evolutionary Forces Shaping Microbial Diversity in the Human Intestine. Cell. 124: 837-848.

[146] O'Hara AM, Shanahan EM (2006) The gut flora as a forgotten organ. EMBO rep. 7: 688-693.

[147] Holzapfel WH, Haberer P, Snel J, Schillinger U, Jos HJ, Huis in't Veld. (1998) Overview of Gut Flora and Probiotics. Int. j. food microbiol. 41: 85-101.

[148] Mackie RI, Sghir A, Gaskins HR (1999) Developmental Microbial Ecology of the Neonatal Gastrointestinal Tract. Am. j. clin. nutr. 69(suppl.): 1035-1045.

[149] Guerrero R, Berlenga M (2006) Life's Unity and Flexibility: The Ecological Link. Int. microbiol. 9: 225-235.

[150] Savage DC (1999) Mucosal Microbiota. In: Ogra PL, Mestecky J, Lamm ME, Strober W, Bienenstock J, McGhee J, editors. Mucosal immunology. New York: Academic Press. 19-30 pp.

[151] Gill SR, Pop M, Deboy RT, Eckburg PB, Turnbaugh PJ, Samuel BS, Gordon JI, Relman DA, Fraser-Liggett CM, Nelson KE (2006) Meta Genomic Analysis of the Human Distal Gut Microbiome. Science. 312:1355-1359.

[152] Hooper LV, Gordon JI (2001) Commensal Host-Bacterial Relationships in the Gut. Science. 292: 1115-1118.

[153] Turnbaugh PJ, Ley RE, Hamady M, Fraser-Liggett CM, Knight R, Gordon JI (2007) The Human Microbiome Project. Nature. 449: 804-810.

[154] Berg RD (1996) The Indigenous Gastrointestinal Microflora. Trends microbial. 4: 430-435.

[155] Claesson MJ, Cusack S, O'Sullivan O, Greene-Diniz R, DeWeerd H, Flannery E, Marchesi R, Falush D, Dinan T, Fitzgerald G, Stanton C, VanSinderen D, O'Connor M, Harnedy N, O'Connor K, Henry C, O'Mahony D, Fitzgerald AP, Shanahan F, Twomey C, Hill C, Ross RP, O'Toole PW (2011) Composition, Variability, and Temporal Stability of the Intestinal Microbiota of the Elderly. Proc. natl. acad. sci. 108(S1): 4586-4591.

[156] Palmer C, Bik EM, DiGiulio DB, Relman DA, Brown PO (2007) Development of the Human Infant Intestinal Microbiota. PLoS Biol 5(7): e177. doi: 10.1371/journal.pbio.0050177.

[157] Andersson AF, Linberg M, Jakobsson H, Bäkhed F, Nyrén P, Engstrand L (2008) Comparative Analysis of Human Gut Microbiota by Barcoded Pyrosequencing. PLoS One. 3(7): Article ID e2836.

[158] Frank DN, Pace NR (2008) Gastrointestinal Microbiology Enters the Metagenomics Era. Curr. opin. gastroent. 24: 4-10.

[159] Miller TL, Wolin MJ (1983) Stability of Methanobrevibacter Smithii Populations in the Microbial Flora Excreted from the Human Large Bowel. Appl. environ. microbiol. 45: 317-318.

[160] Simon GL, Gorbach SL (1984) Intestinal Flora in Health and Disease. Gastroenterology 86: 174-193.

[161] Dubos R, Schaedler RW, Costello R, Hoet P (1965) Indigenous, Normal, and Autochthonous Flora of the Gastrointestinal Tract. J. exp. med. 122: 67-76.

[162] Khoury KA, Floch MH, Hersh T (1969) Small Intestinal Mucosal Cell Proliferation and Bacterial Flora in the Conventionalization of the Germfree Mouse. J. exp. med. 130: 659-670.

[163] Guarner F, Malagelada JR (2003) Gut Flora in Health and Disease. Lancet 361: 512-519.

[164] Wotsmann BS, Kardoss EB, Knight PL (1968) Cecal Enlargement, Cardiac Output and O_2 Consumption in Germfree Rats. Proc. soc. exp. biol. med. 128: 137-140.

[165] Hooper, LV, Macpherson, AJ (2010) Immune Adaptations that Maintain Homeostasis with the Intestinal Microbiota. Nat. rev. immunol. 10: 159-169.

[166] Gilmore MS, Ferretti JJ (2003) Microbiology. The Thin Line Between Gut Commensal and Pathogen. Science. 299: 1999-2002.

[167] Tannock GW (2005) New Perceptions of the Gut Microbiota: Implications for Future Research. Gastroenterol. clin. north am. 34: 361-382.

[168] Martin FP, Sprenger N, Montoliu I, Rezzi S, Kochhar S, Nicholson JK (2010) Dietary Modulation of Gut Functional Ecology Studied by Fecal Metabonomics. J. proteome res. 9: 5284-5295.

[169] Heath P, Claus SP (2011) Assessing hepatic metabolic changes during progressive colonization of germ-free mouse by 1H NMR spectroscopy. J. vis exp. (58) pii: 3642. doi: 10.3791/3642.

[170] Claus SP, Tsang TM, Wang Y, Cloarec O, Skordi E, Martin FP, Rezzi S, Ross A, Kochhar S, Holmes E, Nicholson JK (2008) Systemic Multicompartmental Effects of the Gut Microbiome on Mouse Metabolic Phenotypes. Mol. syst. biol. 4: 219.

[171] Zheng X, Xie G, Zhao A, Zhao L, Yao C, Chiu NH, Zhou Z, Bao Y, Jia W, Nicholson JK, Jia W (2011) The Footprints of Gut Microbial-Mammalian Co-metabolism. J. proteome res. 10: 5512-5522.

[172] Keeney KM, Finlay BB (2011) Enteric Pathogen Exploitation of the Microbiota-Generated Nutrient Environment of the Gut. Curr. opin. microbiol. 14: 92-98.

[173] Bouskra D, Brezillon C, Berard M, Werts C, Varona R, Boneca IG, Eberl G (2008) Lymphoid Tissue Genesis Induced by Commensals Through NOD1 Regulates Intestinal Homeostasis. Nature. 456: 507- 510.

[174] Macpherson AJ, Harris NL (2004) Interactions Between Commensal Intestinal Bacteria and the Immune System. Nat. rev. immunol. 4: 478-485.

[175] Vijay-Kumar M, Aitken JD, Carvalho FA, Cullender TC, Mwangi S, Srinivasan S, Sitaraman SV, Knight R, Ley RE, Gewirtz AT (2010) Metabolic Syndrome and Altered Gut Microbiota in Mice Lacking Toll-like Receptor 5. Science. 328: 228-231.

[176] Atarashi K, Nishimura J, Shima T, Umesaki Y, Yamamoto M, Onoue M, Yagita H, Ishii N, Evans R, Honda K, et al (2008). ATP Drives Lamina Propria T(H)17 Cell Differentiation. Nature. 455: 808-312.

[177] Chow J, Mazmanian SK (2009) Getting the Bugs out of the Immune System: Do Bacterial Microbiota "Fix" Intestinal T Cell Responses? Cell host microbe. 5: 8-12.

[178] Fetissov and Déchelotte (2011) The New Link Between Gut-Brain Axis and Neuropsychiatric Disorders. Curr. opin. clin. nutr. metab. care. 14: 477-482.

[179] Hooper LV, Wong MH, Thelin A, Hansson L, Falk PG, Gordon JI (2001) Molecular Analysis of Commensal Host-Microbial Relationships in the Intestine. Science 2: 881-884.

[180] Mozeš S, Bujňáková D, Šefčiková Z, Kmeť V (2008) Developmental Changes of Gut Microflora and Enzyme Activity in Rat Pups Exposed to Fat-Rich Diet. Obesity 16: 2610-2615.

[181] Turnbaugh PJ, Hamady M, Yatsunenko T, Cantarel BL, Duncan A, Ley RE, Sogin ML, Jones WJ, Roe BA, Affourtit JP, Egholm M, Henrissat B, Heath AC, Knight R, Gordon JI (2009) A Core Gut Microbiome in Obese and Lean Twins. Nature. 457: 480-484.

[182] Šefčiková Z, Kmeť V, Bujňáková D, Raček L', Mozeš Š (2010) Development of Gut Microflora in Obese and Lean Rats. Folia microbiol. 55: 373-375.

[183] Manco M, Putignani L, Bottazzo GF (2010) Gut Microbiota, Lipopolysaccharides, and Innate Immunity in the Pathogenesis of Obesity and Cardiovascular Risk. Endocr. rev. 31: 817-844.

[184] Turnbaugh P, Ley RE, Mahowald MA, Magrini V, Mardis ER, Gordon JI (2006) An Obesity-Associated Gut Microbiome with Increased Capacity for Energy Harvest. Nature 444: 1027-1031.

[185] Bäckhed F, Ding H, Wang T, Hooper LV, Koh GY, Nagy A, Semenkovich CF, Gordon JI (2004) The Gut Microbiota as An Environmental Factor that Regulates Fat Storage. Proc. natl. acad. sci. 2: 15718-15723.

[186] Prins A (2011) The Brain-Gut Interaction: The Conversation and the Implications. S. afr. j. clin. nutr. 24: 8-14.

[187] O'Mahony SM, Hyland NP, Dinan TG, Cryan JF. (2011) Maternal Separation as A Model of Brain-Gut Axis Dysfunction. Psychopharmacology 214: 71-88.

[188] Sudo N (2006) Stress and Gut Microbiota: Does Postnatal Microbial Colonization Programs the Hypothalamic-Pituitary-Adrenal System for Stress Response? International Congress Series 1287: 350-354.

[189] Bravo JA, Forsythe P, Chew MV, Escaravage E, Savignac HM, Dinan TG, Bienenstock J, Cryan JF (2011) Ingestion of Lactobacillus Strain Regulates Emotional Behavior and Central GABA Receptor Expression in a Mouse Via the Vagus Nerve. Proc. natl. acad. sci. 108: 16050-16055.

[190] Forsythe P, Sudo N, Dinan T, Taylor VH, Bienenstock J (2010) Mood and Gut Feelings. Brain behav. immun. 24(1): 9-16.

[191] Bailey MT, Dowd SE, Parry NM, Galley JD, Schauer DB, Lyte M (2010) Stressor Exposure Disrupts Commensal Microbial Populations in the Intestines and Leads to Increased Colonization by Citrobacter Rodentium. Infect. immun. 78: 1509-1519.

[192] Tannock GW, Savage DC (1974) Influences of Dietary and Environmental Stress on Microbial Populations in the Murine Gastrointestinal Tract. Infect, immun. 9: 591-598.

[193] Bıyık H. Balkaya M, Ünsal H, Ünsal C. (2005) The Effects of Qualitative and Quantitative Protein Malnutrition on Cecal Microbiota in Wistar Rats with or without Neutrophil Suppression. Turk. j. vet. anim. sci. 29: 767-773.

[194] Ünsal H, Balkaya M, Bıyık H, Ünsal C, Basbulbul G, Poyrazoglu E, Kozacı LD (2009) Time-dependent Effects of Dietary Qualitative and Quantitative Protein Malnutrition on Some Members of the Cecal Microbiota in Male Wistar Rats. Microb. ecol. health dis. 21: 44-449.

[195] Ünsal H, Çötelioglu Ü. (2007) The Effects of Food Restriction on Some Biochemical Parameters and Certain Bacterial Groups in the Cecum in Sprague Dawley Rats. Microb. ecol. health dis. 19: 17-24.

[196] Lyte M, Ernst S (1992) Catecholamine Induced Growth of Gram Negative Bacteria. Life sci. 50: 302-312.

[197] Bailey MT, Dowd SE, Galley JD, Hufnagle AR, Allen RG, Lyte M (2011) Exposure to a Social Stressor Alters the Structure of the Intestinal Microbiota: Implications for Stressor-Induced Immunomodulation. Brain behave. immun. 25: 397-407.

[198] O'Mahony SM, Marchesi JR, Scully P, Codling C, Ceolho AM, Quigley EM, Cryan JF, Dinan TG (2009) Early Life Stress Alters Behavior, Immunity, and Microbiota in Rats: Implications for Irritable Bowel Syndrome and Psychiatric Illnesses. *Biol. psychiatr.* 65: 263-267.

[199] Knowles SR, Nelson EA, Palombo EA (2008) Investigating the Role of Perceived Stress on Bacterial Flora Activity and Salivary Cortisol Secretion: A Possible Mechanism Underlying Susceptibility to Illness. Biol. psychol. 77: 132-137.

[200] Ünsal H, Balkaya M, Ünsal C, Bıyık H, Başbülbül G, Poyrazoğlu E (2008). The Short-term Effects of Different Doses of Dexamethasone on the Numbers of Some Bacteria in the Ileum. Dig. dis. sci. 53, 1842-1845.

[201] Kirimlioglu V, Kirimlioglu H, Yilmaz S, Piskin T, Tekerekoglu S, Bayindir Y (2006) Effect of Steroid on Mitochondrial Oxidative Stress Enzymes, Intestinal Microflora, and

Bacterial Translocation in Rats Subjected to Temporary Liver Inflow Occlusion. Transplant. proc. 38: 378-381.

[202] Lyte M (1993) The Role of Microbial Endocrinology in Infectious Disease. J. endocrinol. 137: 343-345.

[203] Freestone PP, Sandrini SM, Haigh RD, Lyte M (2008) Microbial Endocrinology: How Stress Influences Susceptibility to Infection. Trends microbiol. 16: 55-64.

[204] Freestone PP, Lyte M, Neal CP, Maggs AF, Haigh RD,Williams PH (2000) The Mammalian Neuroendocrine Hormone Norepinephrine Supplies Iron for Bacterial Growth in the Presence of Transferrin or Lactoferrin. J. bacteriol. 182: 6091-6098.

[205] Kinney KS, Austin CE, Morton DS, Sonnenfeld G (1999) Catecholamine Enhancement of Aeromonas Hydrophila Growth. Microb. pathol. 26: 85-91.

[206] Kinney KS, Austin CE, Morton DS, Sonnenfeld G (2000) Norepinephrine as a Growth Stimulating Factor in Bacteria-Mechanistic Studies. Life sci. 67: 3075-3085.

[207] Neal CP, Freestone PP, Maggs AF, Haigh RD, Williams PH, Lyte M (2001) Catecholamine Inotropes as Growth Factors for Staphylococcus Epidermidis and Other Coagulase-Negative Staphylococci. FEMS microbiol. lett. 194: 163-169.

[208] Belay T, Sonnenfeld G (2002) Differential Effects of Catecholamines on In Vitro Growth of Pathogenic Bacteria. Life sci. 71: 447-456.

[209] Belay T, Aviles H, Vance M, Fountain K, Sonnenfeld G (2003) Catecholamines and in vitro Growth of Pathogenic Bacteria: Enhancement of Growth Varies Greatly Among Bacterial Species. Life sci 73: 1527-1535.

[210] Lyte M, Arulanandam BP, Frank CD (1996) Production of Shigela-Like Toxins by Escherichia Coli O157:H7 can be Influenced by the Neuroendocrine Hormone Norepinephrine. J. lab. Clin. Med. 128: 392-398.

[211] Green BT, Lyte M, Chen C, Xie Y, Casey MA, Kulkarni-Narla A, Vulchanova L, Brown DR (2004) Adrenergic Modulation of Escherichia Coli O157:H7 Adherence to the Colonic Mucosa. Am. j. physiol. gastrointest. liver physiol. 287: G1238-G1246.

[212] Chen C, Brown DR, Xie Y, Green BT, Lyte M (2003) Catecholamines Modulate Escherichia Coli O157:H7 Adherence to Murine Cecal Mucosa. Shock. 20: 183-188.

[213] Chen C, Lyte M, Stevens MP, Vulchanova L, Brown DR (2006) Mucosally-Directed Adrenergic Nerves and Sympathomimetic Drugs Enhance Non-Intimate Adherence of Escherichia Coli O157:H7 to Porcine Cecum and Colon. Eur. j. pharmacol. 539: 116-124.

[214] Green BT, Lyte M, Kulkarni-Narla A, Brown DR (2003) Neuromodulation of Enteropathogen Internalization in Peyer's Patches from Porcine Jejunum. J. neuroimmunol. 141: 74-82.

[215] Brown DR, Price LD (2008) Catecholamines and Sympathomimetic Drugs Decrease Early Salmonella Typhimurium Uptake into Porcine Peyer's Patches. FEMS immunol. med. microbiol. 52: 29-35.

[216] Kakuno Y, Honda M, Takakura K (1997) Colonization Types of Escherichia Coli in Experimental Urinary Tract Infection in Compromised Mice Treated with Hydrocortisone. Kansenshogaku zasshi. 71: 652-658.

[217] Schreiber KL, Brown DR (2005) Adrenocorticotrophic Hormone Modulates Escherichia Coli O157: H7 Adherence to Porcine Colonic Mucosa. Stress. 8: 185-190.

[218] Sands BE (2007) Inflammatory Bowel Disease: Past, Present, and Future. J. gastroenterol. 42(1): 16-25.

[219] Foligné B, Nutten S, Steidler L, Dennin V, Goudercourt D, Mercenier A, Pot B. (2006) Recommendations for Improved Use of The Murine TNBS-Induced Colitis Model in Evaluating Anti-İnflammatory Properties of Lactic Acid Bacteria: Technical and Microbiological Aspects. Dig. dis. sci. 51: 390-400.

[220] Tamboli CP, Neut C, Desreumaux P, Colombel JF (2004) Dysbiosis in Inflammatory Bowel Disease Gut. 53: 1-4.

[221] Thomas LV, Ockhuizen T (2012) New Insights into the Impact of the Intestinal Microbiota on Health and Disease: A Symposium Report. Br. j. nutr. 107: (Suppl 1): 1-13.

[222] Steidler L (2001) Microbiological and Immunological Strategies for Treatment of Inflammatory Bowel Disease. Microbes infect. 3: 1157-1166.

[223] Scanlan PD, Shanahan F, O'Mahony C, Marchesi JR (2006) Culture-Independent Analyses of Temporal Variation of The Dominant Fecal Microbiota and Targeted Bacterial Subgroups in Crohn's Disease. J. clin. microbiol. 44: 3980-3988.

[224] Frank DN, St Amand AL, Feldman RA, Boedeker EC, Harpaz N, Pace NR (2007) Molecular-Phylogenetic Characterization of Microbial Community Imbalances in Human Inflammatory Bowel Diseases. Proc. natl. acad. sci. 104: 13780-13785.

[225] Alverdy J, Aoys E (1991) The Effect of Glucocorticoid Administration on Bacterial Translocation. Ann. surg. 214:719-723.

[226] Schiffrin EJ, Carter EA, Walker WA, Frieberg E, Benjamin J, Israel EJ (1993) Influence of Prenatal Corticosteroids on Bacterial Colonization in the Newborn Rat. J. Pediatr. Gastroenterol. nutr. 17: 271-275.

[227] Deitch EA, Winterton J, Berg R (1987) Effect of Starvation, Malnutrition and Trauma on the Gastrointestinal Tract Flora and Bacterial Translocation. Arch. Surg. 122: 1019-1024.

[228] Gorbach SL, Goldin BR (1992) Nutrition and the Gastrointestinal Microflora. Nutr. rev. 50: 378-81.

[229] Saunders DR, Wiggins HS (1981) Conservation of Mannitol, Lactulose, and Raffinose by the Human Colon. Am. j. physiol. 241: G397-G402.

[230] Roberfroid MB (2005) Introducing Inulin-Type Fructans. Br. j. nutr. 93(Suppl 1): 13-25.

[231] Drasar BS, Crowther JS, Goddard P, Hawksworth G, Hill MJ, Peach S, Williams RE, Renwick A (1973) The Relation between Diet and The Gut Microflora in Man. Proc. nutr. soc. 32: 49-52.

[232] Gracey M, Suharjono, Sunoto, Stone DE (1973) Microbial Contamination of the Gut: Another Feature of Malnutrition. Am. j. clin. nutr. 26: 1170-1174.

[233] Finegold SM, Attebery HR, Sutter VL. (1974) Effect of Diet on Human Fecal Flora: Comparison of Japanese and American Diets. Am. j. clin. nutr. 27(12): 1456-1469.

[234] Deitch EA, Winterton J, Li M, Berg R (1987) The Gut as a Portal of Entry for Bacteremia. Role of Protein Malnutrition. Ann. surg. 205: 681-692.

[235] Mallett AK, Bearne CA, Young PJ, Rowland IR, Berry C (1988) Influence of Starches of Low Digestibility on the Rat Caecal Microflora. Br. j. nutr. 60: 597-604.

[236] Deitch EA, Ma WJ, Ma L, Berg RD, Specian RD (1990) Protein Malnutrition Predisposes to Inflammatory-Induced Gut-Origin Septic States. Ann. surg. 211: 560-568.

[237] Hinton A Jr, Buhr RJ, Ingram KD (2000) Physical, Chemical, and Microbiological Changes in the Crop of Broiler Chickens Subjected to Incremental Feed Withdrawal. Poult. sci. 79: 212-218.

[238] Munro HN, Crim MC (1988) The Proteins and Amino Acids. In: Shils ME, Young VR editors. Modern nutrition in health and disease. Philadelphia: Lea & Febiger. pp. 1-37.

[239] Viteri FE, Schenider RE (1974) Gastrointestinal Alterations in Protein-Calorie Malnutrition. Med. clin. n. am. 58. 1487-1505.

[240] Heyworth B, Brown J (1975) Jejunal Microflora in Malnourished Gambian Children. Arch. dis. child. 50: 27-33.

[241] Omoike IU, Abiodun PO (1989) Upper Small Intestinal Microflora in Diarrhea and Malnutrition in Nigerian Children. J. pediatr. gastroenterol. Nutr. 9: 314-321.

[242] Jirillo E, Pasquetto N, Marcuccio L, Monno R, De Rinaldis P, Fumarola D. (1975) Endotoxemia Detected by Limulus Assay in Severe Malnourished Children. Plasma Effects on Leucocyte Migration: Preliminary Investigations. G. batteriol. virol. immunol. 68: 174-178.

[243] McCowen KC, Ling PR, Ciccarone A, Mao Y, Chow JC, Bistrian BR, Smith RJ (2001) Sustained Endotoxemia Leads to Marked Down-Regulation of Early Steps in the Insulin-Signaling Cascade. Crit. care med. 29: 839-846.

[244] Schreiber RA, Walker WA (1988) The Gastrointestinal Barrier: Antigen Uptake and Perinatal Immunity. Ann. allergy. 61: 3-12.

[245] Sanderson IR, Walker WA (1993) Uptake and Transport of Macromolecules by the Intestine: Possible Role in Clinical Disorders (an Update). Gastroenterology 104: 622-639.

[246] Stanghellini V, Barbara G, Cremon C, Cogliandro R, Antonucci A, Gabusi V, Frisoni C, De Giorgio R, Grasso V, Serra M. Corinaldesi R (2010) Gut Microbiota and Related Diseases: Clinical Features. Intern. emerg. med. 5 (Suppl 1): 57-63.

[247] Katayama M, Xu D, Specian RD, Deitch EA (1997) Role of Bacterial Adherence and the Mucus Barrier on Bacterial Translocation: Effects of Protein Malnutrition and Endotoxin in Rats. Ann Surg. 225: 317-326.

[248] Aschkenasy A (1957) On the Pathogenesis of Anemias and Leukopenias Induced by Dietary Protein Deficiency. Am. j. clin. nutr. 5: 14-25.

[249] Torun B, Viteri FE (1989) Nutrition and Function, with Emphasis on Physical Activity. In: Nutritional Problems of Children in the Developing World. M. Kretchmer M, Viteri FE, Falkner F, editors.

[250] Marroquí L, Batista TM, Gonzalez A, Vieira E, Rafacho A, Colleta SJ, Taboga SR, Boschero AC, Nadal A, Carneiro EM, Quesada I (2012) Functional and Structural Adaptations in the Pancreatic α-Cell and Changes in Glucagon Signaling During Protein Malnutrition. Endocrinology. 153:1663-1672.

Chapter 6

Extra-Adrenal Glucocorticoid Synthesis in Mucosal Tissues and Its Implication in Mucosal Immune Homeostasis and Tumor Development

Feodora I. Kostadinova. Nina Hostettler,
Pamela Bianchi and Thomas Brunner

Additional information is available at the end of the chapter

1. Introduction

While glucocorticoids (GC) exert broad effects on metabolism, behavior and immunity, local production of even small amounts of GC, which may act in a paracrine or even autocrine manner, enable a specific site of the body to regulate their exposure to GC according to their specific needs. Mucosal tissues, for example, are at the borderline to the outside world, and are therefore in constant contact with either harmless foreign particles or potentially pathogenic microorganisms, which might provoke devastating inflammatory disorders due to chronic stimulation of the mucosal immune system. Increasing the local concentration of immunoregulatory GC by extra-adrenal de novo GC synthesis or local reactivation of inactive serum metabolites provides a protective mechanism to either restore homeostasis after clearance of infection or to regulate the critical balance between immunity and tolerance.

2. Adrenal versus extra-adrenal GC synthesis

Production of GC in the adrenal glands is regulated by hypothalamic-pituitary-adrenal (HPA) axis and follows under normal conditions the circadian rhythm. However, GC are also a major humoral response to various types of stress. [1]. Immunological stress by excessive activation of immune cells rapidly results in elevated plasma levels of tumor necrosis factor alpha (TNFα), interleukin (IL) -1 and IL-6, which then stimulate the HPA axis and lead to an increase of systemic GC [2]. These and similar signals stimulate also the local GC synthesis in mucosal tissues, as will be discussed later (Table 1).

Local GC synthesis	Cellular source	Special features	Described functions	References
Thymus	Epithelial cells in cortex	Mutual antagonism	Thymic selection	[3-7]
Skin Hair follicle	Keratinocytes, melanocytes, fibroblasts etc.	Autonomous HPA-axis	Integrity and growth; response to stress factors	[8-19]
Cardiovascular system	Vessel walls, Heart	Together with mineralocorticoids	Vascular contractility and remodeling	[20-29]
Central Nervous system	Neurons, glia	Various neurosteroids	Sensitizing GABA and other receptors; feed-back on HPA-axis; cognitive functions	[30-45]
Intestine	Crypt cells	Regulation via LRH-1	Immune regulation	[46-53]
Lung	unknown	Reactivation by 11β-HSD	Immune regulation	[54]
Colon carcinoma	Tumor cells	Regulation via LRH-1	Immunosuppression	[55]

Table 1. Extra-adrenal GC sources and their functions.

Because most data published so far on local GC synthesis has been generated in animal models a brief overview of steroidogenic processes in rodents compared to humans must be made (Figure 1). A major difference is the implication of the enzyme 17α-hydroxylase in the GC synthesis in humans, but not in rodents. Pregnenolone is transformed directly into progesterone in most rodents, and in other mammalians and humans it is first hydroxylated and then metabolized into 17-OH-progesterone [56]. 11β-hydroxylase (P450C11) is an enzyme expressed in the zonae fasciculata et reticularis and is a product of the gene CYP11B1. Thus, in rodents this enzyme uses 11-deoxycorticosterone as a substrate and turns it into corticosterone, which is the active GC in these species. In humans 11β-hydroxylase metabolizes mainly 11-deoxycortisol into cortisol and to a lesser degree 11-deoxycorticosterone into corticosterone. Hence, cortisol is the major active GC in the human. 11-Deoxyorticosterone and corticosterone are important metabolites in both species, which can be hydroxylised and oxidised in the zona glomerulosa of the adrenals, subsequently leading to the mineralcorticosteroid aldosterone [57].

It is well established that the adrenal glands are the major source of systemic GC. Surgical removal of the adrenal glands results in a rapid drop of serum GC levels, which after a couple of days become undetectable, illustrating that the adrenals are primarily responsible for the GC levels detected in the circulation [46, 58]. However, in recent years there has been accumulating evidence that several other tissues are capable of producing GC and thereby regulate local processes in an adrenal-independent manner [7, 59].

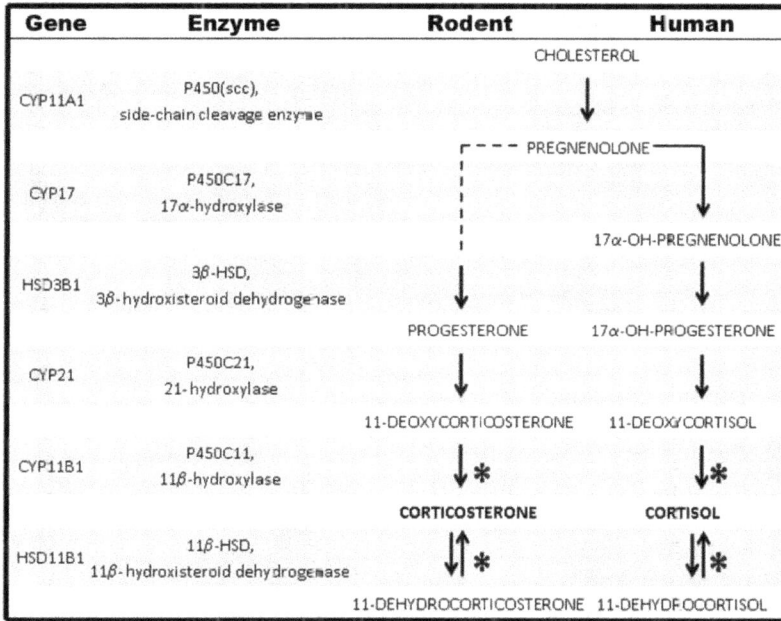

Gene	Enzyme	Rodent	Human
		CHOLESTEROL	
CYP11A1	P450(scc), side-chain cleavage enzyme	↓	
		PREGNENOLONE	
CYP17	P450C17, 17α-hydroxylase		17α-OH-PREGNENOLONE
HSD3B1	3β-HSD, 3β-hydroxisteroid dehydrogenase	↓	↓
		PROGESTERONE	17α-OH-PROGESTERONE
CYP21	P450C21, 21-hydroxylase	↓	↓
		11-DEOXYCORTICOSTERONE	11-DEOXYCORTISOL
CYP11B1	P450C11, 11β-hydroxylase	↓*	↓*
		CORTICOSTERONE	CORTISOL
HSD11B1	11β-HSD, 11β-hydroxisteroid dehydrogenase	⇵*	⇵*
		11-DEHYDROCORTICOSTERONE	11-DEHYDROCORTISOL

Legend: ☐ enzymes; ☐ metabolites: → metabolic pathway; - - - absent in rodents; * inhibitory effect of metyrapone.

Figure 1. Differences in the GC synthesis pathway in rodents and humans.

3. Extra-adrenal sources of GC synthesis

3.1. Thymus

The Thymus plays a central role in the development of the immune system. Thymocyte development and differentiation is shaped and regulated by the interaction with the thymic epithelial cells and the factors secreted by them [60, 61].

Initial characterizations of extra-adrenal GC synthesis started in the thymus. In the mid to late 90ties of the last century it was described that the non-immune cells in the thymic cortex are capable of producing various steroid metabolites. Accordingly, the expression of various enzymes of the corticosteroid synthesis pathway has been demonstrated in thymic epithelial cells [3-5]. While the function of thymic GC has been a matter of scientific debate for some time [62, 63], particularly the work of Ashwell and co-workers illustrated that GC production in the thymus has an important role in the regulation of thymocyte development and selection. Interestingly, while thymocytes are exquisitely sensitive to GC and rapidly die by apoptosis, the in situ produced corticosterone seems to oppose the signals induced by the T cell receptor and thereby lower T cell receptor-induced apoptosis (negative selection). On the other hand T cell receptor activation also inhibits the apoptosis-inducing activity of GC in thymocytes [64]. Thus, the "mutual antagonism" between T cell receptor and glucocorticoid receptor (GR) signaling seems overall to enhance survival and thereby positive selection of thymocytes by increasing the threshold of T cell receptor signals leading to negative selection [3]. The thymus in mice produces the highest amounts of GC during fetal development and in the first weeks after birth. This is the time of the most extensive lymphocyte development and differentiation, and it occurs at a time when the steroidogenesis in the adrenals is not fully active. Thus, the thymus seems to depend largely on its own by providing the necessary GC. Whether thymic epithelial cells constitutively produce GC or whether this is dependent on the interaction with activated thymocytes or soluble factors, is presently unknown. The presence or absence of factors regulating thymic GC synthesis may, however, affect positive and negative selection of thymocytes, and thereby also affect the levels of potentially autoreactive T cells in the periphery. [6, 7].

3.2. Skin

The skin is an organ with a complex structure and its purpose is to protect the inner organism from the environmental factors, infections, dehydration, thermal deregulations etc. The outer cover of the skin, the epidermis, maintains its integrity through intense self-renewing by the proliferating keratinocytes in the basal layer and the dividing cells in the hair follicles. As such skin is an important component of the defense mechanisms providing not only a reliable mechanical barrier and producing antimicrobial enzymes and other substances, but also being populated with many specialized immune cells, e.g. dendritic cells (Langerhans cells) within the epidermis, as well as resident macrophages, dendritic cells and lymphocytes in the derma [65]. The skin also displays active metabolic and endocrine functions. Along with the synthesis of vitamin D, the skin was shown to produce various hormones and regulatory factors, like parathyroid-related protein, melanocyte-stimulating hormone (MSH), β-endorphin peptides, urocortin, neurotransmitters and others (for review [10, 11]). With regard of this chapter's topic of interest is the ability of the skin to produce all components of the HPA axis. A great contribution to the understanding of GC metabolism and regulation in the skin has been made by the extensive research of Slominski and co-workers [10]. In human keratinocytes and cells of the hair follicles expression of corticotropin-releasing factor (CRF) has been demonstrated at the mRNA and protein level, whereas in mice the local synthesis of CRF has not been proven yet. The observed local increased concentration of CRF in the skin could be possibly explained by its release from neuronal cells and its active transport into the skin along the local nerve endings [12, 15]. Many cell types found in the skin, e.g. keratinocytes [66], melanocytes [13], dermal fibroblasts [67], immune cells and endothelial cells in the derma, as well as hair follicles [16] and skin tissue cultures, are able to respond to CRF stimulation and to produce proopiomelanocortin, which can be further processed into adrenocorticotropic hormone (ACTH), MSH and β -endorphin. Moreover, GC-synthesizing enzymes and active GC have been demonstrated in human and rodent skin. Metabolic assays demonstrated that ex vivo cultured normal rat skin could transform progesterone into deoxycorticosterone and corticosterone, and further to 11-dehydrocorticosterone [9]. Human skin has been demonstrated to respond to ACTH, to express various steroidogenic enzymes, and to be capable of synthesizing cortisol [8, 18]. Local steroidogenesis was demonstrated in human keratinocytes [19], sebaceous cells [13], fibroblasts [14], and melanocytes [13]. Hair follicles, also known as pilosebaceus units, appear to function as fully autonomous peripheral equivalents of the HPA axis. The CRF/ACTH-induced cortisol production appears to provide also a negative feedback on the local CRF synthesis and thereby terminate local steroidogenesis [15]. It has been suggested that this local HPA axis is implemented in the regulation of hair growth, pigmentation and modulation of local immune response [17]. Components of the HPA axis, mainly CRF, are proposed to affect the epithelial cell proliferation, apoptosis and differentiation [15]. Recent findings describe the role of local cortisol synthesis in a model of tissue injury. Up-regulation of CYP11B1 and subsequent enhanced production of cortisol was induced by the proinflammatory cytokine IL-1β and depressed by insulin-like growth factor 1 (IGF-1) [19]. In the same study elevation of cortisol synthesis was observed approximately 48 hours after acute injury and maintained the proper wound healing.

In conclusion, the skin possesses an autonomous HPA axis, regulating the normal integrity and growth, and is able to respond to stress factors. At the same time the GC-synthesizing machinery of the skin can be stimulated by inflammatory mediators in order to provide an adequate local self-limitation of immune responses.

3.3. Central nervous system

The term neurosteroids was defined after the discovery that various steroid metabolites can be detected in the brain of simultaneously adrenalectomized and gonadectomized rats [30]. Among the locally synthesized and active steroids are pregnenolone and pregnenolone sulphate, progesterone, allopregnanolone, dehydroepiandrosterone and dehydroepiandrosterone sulphate. These steroids can exert their effects in neurogenesis, development, myelinization, memory, reactions to stress through engaging nuclear receptors and modulating transcription, as well as affecting neurotransmission by modifying the activity of gamma-aminobutiric acid (GABAA), N-methyl-D-aspartic acid (NMDA), and sigma receptors (for review [31, 32, 68]). Low levels of transcripts for CYP11A1, CYP11B1 and the other enzymes of corticosterone synthesis were detected in normal rat brain, in cerebral cortex and cerebellum [33], and 11β-hydroxylase protein expression was later demonstrated in the Purkinje cells and other cells of the hippocampus [35]. In vitro conversion of precursors into corticosterone has also been demonstrated in rat fetal hippocampal neurons [34]. The extremely low levels of CYP21 transcripts and enzyme (deoxycorticosterone synthetase, P450C21) detected [36] gave raise to many doubts whether complete GC synthesis can be sustained in the brain. Nevertheless, the activity of brain tissue to convert progesterone to 11-deoxycorticosterone (resp. 17α-OH-progesterone to 11-deoxycortisol) pointed out that steroid metabolism in the brain exists. Recently, the expression of isoforms of CYP2D4 and CYP2D6 in rat and human brains, respectively, as well as demonstration of their 21-hydroxylation activity confirmed the capacity of rodent and human brain to produce GC locally [37, 69], though suggesting a slightly different enzymatic pathway compared to that of the adrenals. Nonetheless, CRF and ACTH, likely released by the hypothalamus, resp. pituitary gland, seem to regulate GC synthesis in the brain in a similar manner as in the adrenals. Interestingly, adrenalectomy even increases the expression of CYP11B1 in the rat brain [70].

Peripheral reactivation of 11-dehydrocorticosterone to corticosterone, resp. cortisone to cortisol via 11β-hydroxysteroid dehydrogenase type 1 (11β-HSD1) activity contributes considerably not only to the local concentrations and effects of GC, but also to the plasma level of GC, as shown by an almost 30% increase in corticosterone levels in the portal vein compared to the incoming arterial circulation [38, 39, 71]. In the brain 11β-HSD1 expression was found in various areas. Local levels of corticosterone in the cerebral cortex, hippocampus, hypothalamus and pituitary gland modulate the activity of the HPA axis. This effect is particularly apparent in 11β-HSD1 knockout mice. The lack of 11β-HSD1 activity in the brain of these mice leads to considerably reduced local levels of corticosterone. Hence, the HPA axis is hyperactivated and higher amounts of ACTH are produced, which in turn causes adrenal hypertrophy. Normal or even elevated systemic GC fail to transmit proper feedback responses to the hypothalamus [40-42]. Other curious effects of the local levels of GC attributed to the activity of 11β-HSD1 in the hippocampus are cognitive disorders during aging. Experiments in 11β-HSD1-deficient mice showed that these animals are protected from the decline of the learning abilities [43, 72]. 11β-HSD1 is expressed in the human prefrontal cortex, cerebellum and hippocampus, and its expression, as well as local GC levels, has also been correlated to the cognitive decline in elderly patients [44, 45], [42]. Furthermore, some clinical studies showed an improvement in verbal fluency and memory in patients treated with the specific 11β-HSD1 inhibitor carbenoxolone [44].

3.4. Cardiovascular system

The impact of mineralocorticoids and glucocorticoids on the heart and blood vessels is well known and described. Yet, the capacity of these structures to sustain their own supplies is not understood in detail. Data obtained mainly in rats indicate that vascular tissue expresses steroidogenic factors, such as StAR, CYP11A1, CYP11B1 and CYP11B2 [20, 21, 73]. Ex vivo cultured rat blood vessels were able to produce corticosterone and aldosterone [23, 73]. Expression of various steroidogenic enzymes has been shown also in the human heart and blood vessels [26, 27]. However, CYP11B1 and CYP11B2 expression was only demonstrated in patients with myocardial infarction and heart failure [28], but barely under steady state conditions or in cultured endothelial cells [29], suggesting that local GC synthesis may be triggered during pathological conditions. Presence of CYP11B2 (aldosterone synthetase) and the fact that steroidogenesis in the cardiovascular system is triggered by the angiotensin signaling system [24] points out that local steroidogensis in the vascular systems is connected to the renin-angiotensin-aldosterone regulatory mechanisms [25]. Local reactivation of 11-dehydrocorticosterone was also observed in the smooth muscle cells in arteries, where it may contribute to vascular contractility and remodeling [74], [75]. Despite a clear demonstration of steroidogenesis in the vasculature detailed studies on the anti-inflammatory role of local GC synthesis in blood vessels are still missing.

In addition to the different tissues described above local GC synthesis was also reported in the placenta [76], the ovaries [77], the testis [78], the uterus [79], and the mammary gland [80].

4. GC synthesis in mucosal tissues

Mucosal surfaces in the gastrointestinal, respiratory and urinal tract represent important contact zones between the body and the outside world. They exert important functions in the exchange of nutrients, gases and other substances between the organism and the surrounding world. They comprise an enormous interactive surface and are thereby also constantly exposed to various antigens and microorganisms. Though, most of them are harmless, and thus the body has developed mechanisms to tolerate these harmless antigens. Yet, dangerous infections of the lung and the intestine occur, in which case the local defense machinery must be engaged to protect the host from invasion. The barrier between inside and outside is primarily formed of a simple one-layered epithelium with the respective specialized functions. Beneath the epithelial layer in the lamina propria of the intestine or in the interstitium of the lung resides a large number of immune cells. Clearly the huge mucosal surface must be protected from invading pathogens, and thus these epithelial tissues are home of the largest immune system in our body. Inappropriate activation of these local immune cells by environmental antigens, though, can result in uncontrolled inflammation and associated tissue destruction. Several lines of evidence discussed in detail below indicate that locally produced GC significantly contribute to the regulation of local immune responses and the maintenance of immune homeostasis in these epithelial tissues.

4.1. GC synthesis in the intestinal epithelium

In the intestinal mucosa two super-systems collide. The intestinal lumen hosts ten times more bacteria than cells in our body are found. At the same time, the intestinal epithelium and lamina propria are also home of the largest number of B and T cells, and are also densely populated by macrophages and dendritic cells. Accidental and uncontrolled activation of these cells and/or other infiltrating immune cells by harmless commensal bacteria or food antigens is the underlying cause of a variety of inflammatory disorders, such as inflammatory bowel disease and food allergies [81]

There is accumulating evidence that local production of immunoregulatory GC significantly contributes to the control of intestinal immune homeostasis and prevents a clash between immune cells and commensal bacteria. The notion that the intestinal mucosa could be a steroidogenic organ has been already suggested some time ago, when it was found that genetic deletion of the nuclear receptor SF-1 (steroidogenic factor-1, NR5a1), largely responsible for the transcriptional control of the adrenal development and GC synthesis, could not abrogate intestinal CYP11A1 expression in the mouse embryonic gut [82]. At the same time remaining GC levels were observed in the circulation of prenatal mice, indicating that an extra-adrenal source of GC synthesis must exist [83]. Our own research started to explicitly investigate the possibility that the intestinal mucosa is an important source of immunoregulatory GC some ten years ago. Investigating the function of so-called intraepithelial lymphocytes, T cells that reside within the intestinal epithelial layer, it was found that these cells rapidly died upon isolation and ex vivo culture, but could be partially rescued when the GR was blocked by the receptor antagonist RU-486 [84]. This observation suggested that these intestinal T cells were constantly exposed to GC, and that removal of survival signals, e.g. by detachment from the epithelial layer, would promote GR-dependent apoptosis.

Subsequent studies revealed that the intestinal mucosa is home of a complex steroidogenic system, likely adapted to cope with the specialized environment of the gut. Many of the steroidogenic enzymes required for the synthesis of corticosterone from cholesterol or the reactivation of corticosterone from dehydrocorticosterone are constitutively expressed in the intestinal epithelium, whereas other enzymes become strongly induced upon immunological stress [46, 52, 53]. The ability of the intestinal tissue to synthesize corticosterone in mice [46] and humans [55] indicates that the intestinal mucosa expresses the complete and functional enzymatic machinery. This steroidogenic capacity is further confirmed by the use of metyrapone, a potent 11β-hydroxylase inhibitor with some inhibitory effects also on P450scc and 11β-HSD1, which efficiently blocks ex vivo GC synthesis in intestinal organ cultures [46, 55], confirming that GC measured were produced locally in the tissue.

While in most experiments and ex vivo organ cultures basal GC levels are detected, a significant induction is usually observed, when mice are stressed by immune cell-activating agents. Administration of T cell-activating anti-CD3ε antibody, macrophage-activating lipopolysaccharides, or TNFα, infection of mice with viruses or chemically induced intestinal inflammation promotes the expression of certain steroidogenic enzymes, e.g. CYP11A1 and CYP11B1, and strongly stimulates the synthesis of intestinal GC. In some of these in vivo experiments a role of intestinal GC synthesis in the control of intestinal immune cells could also be confirmed. Most pronounced are the effects reported on viral infection and experimental colitis. Infection of mice with the lymphocytic choriomeningitis virus (LCMV) leads to a rapid expansion of the virus, which infects various target organs, including the intestine [46, 85, 86]. The virus promotes a massive expansion of virus-specific cytotoxic T cells, which in turn control the viral expansion by killing virus-infected cells. Employing this experimental system it has been shown that intestinal T cells from mice with deregulated intestinal GC synthesis (using the pharmacological inhibitor of GC synthesis metyrapone) became more profoundly activated by the virus, and expressed activation markers and inflammatory cytokines at much higher levels [46]. Similarly, in experimental models of colitis defective intestinal GC synthesis resulted in a more rapid and more pronounced induction of intestinal inflammation, as monitored by immune cell infiltration, epithelial layer damage, weight loss, etc. [49, 53].

4.2. Regulation of intestinal GC synthesis

The regulation of adrenal GC synthesis has been well documented over many decades of research (reviewed in [87]). The connection between physical, emotional and immunological stress, and the activation of the HPA axis has been well established. Similarly, the role of the hormone ACTH in stimulating adrenal GC synthesis, and the nuclear receptor SF-1 in the transcriptional control of adrenal steroidogenesis is widely accepted [88]. In agreement with this critical role of SF-1 in the induction of steroidogenic enzymes in the adrenal glands is the observation that mice deficient for SF-1 have no detectable corticosterone in the serum. In fact, SF-1-deficient mice even lack adrenal glands, as SF-1 is also required for the embryonic development of the adrenal glands. As discussed above, mice lacking SF-1 expression still express the steroidgenic enzyme gene CYP11A1 in the primitive gut of embryonic mice, supporting the notion that in the intestine steroidogensis is differentially controlled. Along these lines, it was found that SF-1 expression is basically absent in the intestine, but functionally replaced by its close homolog LRH-1 (liver receptor homolog-1, NR5a2). LRH-1 has strong sequence homology with SF-1, and regulates gene expression by binding to identical transcription factor response elements in the promoter of their target genes [47]. In general, SF-1 and LRH-1 have a mutually exclusive expression pattern, with very low LRH-1 expression in the adrenals, but very high expression in epithelial cells from the liver, pancreas, intestine and ovaries [89].

The role of LRH-1 in the regulation of extra-adrenal GC synthesis in the intestine has been investigated in intestinal epithelial cell lines in vitro as well as in vivo models [47, 49]. Overexpression of LRH-1 in intestinal epithelial cells induces the expression of the steroidogenic enzymes CYP11A1 and CYP11B1, and mutation of corresponding response elements in their promoter abrogates their LRH-1- and SF-1-induced activation [47]. Similarly, inhibition of LRH-1 expression or function leads to reduced expression of these steroidogenic enzymes in intestinal epithelial cells. Overexpression of LRH-1 in turn directly promotes detectable levels of corticosterone in the supernatant of intestinal epithelial cell cultures. In vivo the role of LRH-1 has been investigated by the use of LRH-1 haplodeficient as well as conditional LRH-1 knockout mice [48, 49]. LRH-1 haplodeficient mice showed a largely reduced induction of steroidogenic enzymes after anti-CD3ε injection and a complete block in intestinal GC synthesis induction, confirming an important role of LRH-1 in the regulation of intestinal GC synthesis. While induction of DSS (dextran sodium sulfate)- or TNBS (trinitrobenzen sulfonic acid)-mediated colitis stimulates the expression of steroidogenic enzmymes and a transient intestinal GC synthesis [51], deletion of LRH-1 in intestinal epithelial cells largely abrogates intestinal steroidogenesis [49]. More importantly, absence of LRH-1 and associated intestinal GC synthesis also leads to a more pronounced and accelerated colitis, confirming an important role of LRH-1 and intestinal GC synthesis in the regulation of local immune responses. LRH-1 likely regulates intestinal GC synthesis not only via the induction of certain steroidogenic enzymes. Steroid acute regulator (StAR) has an important role in transporting cholesterol within the cell, and thus supplying the steroid synthesizing machinery with the substrate for GC synthesis. As LRH-1 also transcriptionally regulates StAR expression [90], LRH-1 seems to control intestinal GC synthesis at many levels.

Interestingly, LRH-1 appears to have various modes of activation. Though initially defined as orphan nuclear receptor due the lack of known ligands, the crystallization of

LRH-1 and subsequent structural analysis revealed a ligand binding to the ligand-binding domain of LRH-1. This ligand was identified as phosphatidylinositol, however, it is very likely that a larger variety of natural and synthetic ligands may bind to this ligand-binding domain and transactivate LRH-1. Of interest are recent reports demonstrating LRH-1 activation by testosterone [91], the herbizide atrazin [92] as well as several synthetic ligands with selective activities for LRH-1 over SF-1 [93]. However, ligand binding may not be an absolute requirement for LRH-1 activation. In particular, mouse LRH-1 can be activated in a ligand-independent manner, as mutation of the ligand-binding domain does not affect its activity [94].

In marked contrast, phosphorylation by upstream kinases may selectively activate both, human and mouse LRH-1. Two serine residues in the hinge region of LRH-1 have been identified as phosphorylation targets of the MAP kinase ERK1/2, and mutation of these two serine residues strongly affects LRH-1 activity [95]. In line with this idea of LRH-1 activation via the MAP kinase pathway is the observation that the MEK1 inhibitor U0126 also blocks LRH-1 activity ([95]; Bianchi, Brunner, unpublished). Next to ERK1/2 also other yet to be identified kinases may be involved in LRH-1 phosphorylation and activation.

As many other nuclear receptors LRH-1 is also efficiently regulated by cofactors and repressors. For example, SRC-1 (steroid receptor coactivator-1) binds to LRH-1 and enhances its transcriptional activity. On the other hand, various inhibitors of LRH-1, such as DAX-1 (dosage-sensitive sex reversal, adrenal hypoplasia critical region, on chromosome X, gene 1), SHP (small heterodimer partner) and Prox-1 (Prospero homeobox protein 1) have been shown to interact with LRH-1 and inhibit its activity [89, 96, 97]. Of interest is the fact that SHP is a major transcriptional target of LRH-1, and SHP induction likely represents a negative feedback loop terminating the transcriptional activity of LRH-1.

Thus far intestinal GC synthesis has been always described in the context of immunological stress and inflammation. Clearly, factors released by activated immune cells must be able to trigger steroidogenesis in intestinal epithelial cells, likely via the activation of LRH-1. Of major interest in this regard are factors that also promote adrenal GC synthesis. Surprisingly, ACTH or ACTH receptor signaling pathways, such as an increase in cellular cyclic AMP, fail to promote intestinal GC synthesis and rather inhibit it [47] indicating that next to the preferential use of SF-1 and LRH-1 there are other elements in the regulation of adrenal versus intestinal GC synthesis that are different. The pro-inflammatory cytokines IL-6 and TNFα are known as potent triggers of adrenal GC synthesis. While no evidence could be found for a role of IL-6 in the immune cell-mediated induction of intestinal steroid synthesis, TNFα appears to represent a critical mediator of intestinal GC synthesis. TNFα alone promotes the expression of steroidogenic enzymes in intestinal epithelial cells in vitro and in vivo, and stimulates the synthesis of corticosterone. More importantly, induction of intestinal GC synthesis by injection of anti-CD3ε, LPS as well as experimental colitis largely depends on the signaling via TNF receptors [53]. Surprisingly, deletion of either one of the two TNF receptors abrogates immune cell-induced intestinal GC synthesis [52], indicating that simultaneous signaling via both receptors is required.

The important role of TNFα in the induction of intestinal GC synthesis is particularly
evident when analyzing different models of experimentally induced colitis. While DSS and
the hapten TNBS promote intestinal steroidogenesis, the hapten oxazolone fails to do so,
despite very comparable induction of inflammation [53]. Clearly, inflammation alone is
insufficient to initiate intestinal steroidogensis, but the type of inflammation may be critical.
DSS and TNBS stimulate an immune response with Th1 cytokine predominance, abundant
TNFα and IFNγ, whereas oxazolone promotes a Th2 type cytokine response with no TNFα,
but IL-4 and IL-5. Supporting the important role of TNFα in these processes, it was found
that oxazolone does not trigger intestinal GC synthesis, however injection of recombinant
TNFα can restore the expression of steroidogenic enzymes and GC synthesis, and thereby
ameliorate intestinal inflammation induced by oxazolone. Thus, TNFα seems to be an
important sensor of immunological stress in the intestine and responsible for initiating
negative feedback mechanisms via the induction of intestinal GC synthesis. This is
inasmuch surprising as TNFα is an important therapeutic target in the pathogenesis of
inflammatory bowel disease (IBD), such as Crohn's disease and ulcerative colitis [98-100].
TNFα is an important disease promoting and initiating factor during IBD, and its
neutralization inhibits inflammatory processes right from the start. Its role in the regulation
of intestinal GC synthesis, however, point also out a thus far unrecognized anti-
inflammatory role of TNFα (reviewed in [51]).

4.3. GC synthesis in the lung

The intestinal and the lung epithelium have much in common. Their main function is the
absorption of nutrients and gases, respectively, and due to their enormous surface to cope
with this task they are also constantly exposed to a plethora of antigens, microbes and
potential pathogens. Thus, much alike the intestinal mucosa the lung harbors a large
number of resident immune cells, mostly macrophages and dendritic cells, and is rapidly
populated by infiltrating immune cells upon infection or stimulation with antigens.
Similarly, uncontrolled immune responses in the lung may lead to chronic disorders, such
as allergen-induced asthma and chronic obstructive pulmonary disorder (COPD). This
illustrates on one hand the need for an efficient immune response in the lung in order to
defend this vast epithelial surface from infection and invasion by pathogens, but also points
out that local immune responses must be tightly regulated to avoid chronic inflammation,
tissue damage and resulting loss of function of the absorptive epithelium.

All these thoughts suggest that similar regulatory mechanisms exist in the lung as in the
intestinal mucosa, and local GC synthesis may represent such a homeostatic control
mechanism. Indeed, it has been described that genes involved in the GC synthesis pathway
are transiently expressed in the developing mouse lung [101]. More recently, our own
research has investigated the capacity of the adult lung to express steroidogenic enzymes
and to synthesize GC in response to immunological stress [54]. Unlike the intestinal
epithelium, the entire enzymatic machinery appears to be constitutively expressed in the
adult lung tissue, and only CYP11A1, encoding P450scc, is induced upon immunological
stress initiated by injection of T cell-activating anti-CD3ε antibody or macrophage-activating

LPS. Furthermore, particularly CYP11B1, although detectable by quantitative PCR, seems to be expressed at very low levels and not to be induced as in the intestine. When analyzing corticosterone synthesis in ex vivo lung cultures two observations are compelling. The lung tissue constitutively synthesizes considerable amounts of corticosterone in unchallenged mice, and the induced GC levels upon immunological stress are much higher when compared to equal amounts of tissue in the intestine [54]. Importantly, also in the lung ex vivo GC synthesis is efficiently blocked by the pharmacological inhibitor metyrapone, supporting the idea that GC measured are de novo synthesized in the lung tissue, though here its effect may not be via the inhibition of 11β-hydroxylase. This indicates that the lung tissue may be an even more potent extra-adrenal source of immunoregulatory GC than the intestinal epithelium.

Thus far, the cellular source of lung GC synthesis has not been identified yet. Very likely, though, lung epithelial cells, either type I or type II epithelial cells, may be the relevant source of lung GC. In support of this hypothesis is the observation that lung epithelial cell lines express steroidogenic enzymes and are capable of metabolizing steroid precursors to corticosterone (Hostettler, Brunner, unpublished observations). Despite the many similarities between the intestinal and the lung epithelium in terms of response to inflammatory triggers and the synthesis of GC, there are also many differences in the induction of intestinal versus lung GC synthesis. While systemic activation of immune cells by anti-CD3 or LPS injection triggers both, intestinal and lung GC synthesis [52, 54], the response to local inflammation seems to be regulated somewhat differently. A typical model of allergic airway inflammation is the sensitization of mice with the model antigen ovalbumin in the context of alum as adjuvant, and the challenge with the antigen via aerosol. This leads to a T helper 2 type inflammatory response with a major eosinophilic and neutrophilic granulocyte infiltration of the lung tissue and lung lumen within 24 hours. Despite the massive inflammation and infiltration with immune cells only a minimal and not significant transient increase in local GC synthesis is observed, not comparable to the high concentrations measured after stimulation with anti-CD3 or LPS [54]. Given the fact that ovalbumin airway hypersensitivity and oxazolone-induced colitis are both T helper 2-driven immune responses, the idea that lack of TNFα secretion could be the missing stimulator of lung GC synthesis appears very attractive. Indeed, only minimal TNFα levels are measured in the serum and the bronchoalveolar lavage (BAL) after ovalbumin challenge [54]. Similarly, when TNFα is injected into mice local GC synthesis in the lung can be efficiently induced. However, experiments in TNF receptor-deficient mice using anti-CD3 as a trigger clearly showed that TNFα signaling is not required for immune cell-stimulated local GC synthesis in the lung tissue. Thus, very likely other cytokines and/or factors, yet to be identified, may be substituting TNFα as a sensor of immune cell activation and trigger of local GC synthesis. It is feasible to believe that such a sensor of immunological stress is not induced during allergic inflammation of the lung, e.g. asthma, but present during contact with pathogens, such as influenza infection, thereby helping to reestablish local immune homeostasis via the secretion of GC. The identification of this or these critical inducers of local GC synthesis may lead to interesting targets for therapeutic intervention of chronic inflammation of the lung via the induction of local GC synthesis.

Extra-Adrenal Glucocorticoid Synthesis in Mucosal Tissues and Its Implication in Mucosal
Immune Homeostasis and Tumor Development

139

4.4. Regulation of lung GC synthesis

Presently, not much is know regarding the molecular mechanisms of lung GC synthesis, and more detailed analysis of the regulatory pathways leading to the induction and activation of steroidogenic enzymes in the lung tissue will be needed. While the presence of all steroidogenic enzymes required for the synthesis of corticosterone from cholesterol suggests identical synthesis pathways in the lung, adrenals and intestine, metabolic assays indicate major differences between the tissues. Interestingly, ex vivo cultured lung tissue failed to convert radioactively labeled deoxycorticosterone into corticosterone, suggesting that the expression levels of CYP11B1/11β-hydroxylase are insufficient to promote this pathway of GC synthesis. In contrast, dehydrocorticosterone is efficiently metabolized by the lung tissue into corticosterone, supporting the idea that reactivation of inactive serum dehydrocorticosterone via an 11β-HDS1-dependent pathway is the primary corticosterone synthesis pathway in the lung. Along these lines is the observation that the lung expresses very low levels of CYP11B1 but very high levels of HSD11B1, and that adrenalectomy completely abolishes lung GC synthesis [54]. Though metyrapone has been reported to be selective for 11β-hydroxylase, inhibition of 11β-HSD1 has also been noted [102], explaining why ex vivo GC synthesis in lung tissue is efficiently blocked by metyrapone. A dominant role for an 11β-HSD1-dependent corticosterone synthesis pathway is also supported by the lack of evidence for a role of LRH-1 in the regulation of lung GC synthesis. While anti-CD3-induced intestinal GC synthesis was significantly reduced in LRH-1 haplodeficient mice [48], lung GC synthesis was found to be normal [54], indicating that other nuclear receptors or transcription factors are involved in the regulation of steroidogenesis in the lung tissue.

5. GC synthesis in colorectal tumors

The role of tumor immunology in the surveillance of transformed cells and the control of tumor development is a highly controversial issue. While tumor-specific immune responses and even tumor-specific T cells can be demonstrated in certain types of tumors, stimulation of tumor-specific T cells by immunization has thus far not been too successful in the prevention or treatment of tumors. A major exception is the vaccination against human papilloma virus, which strongly reduces the incidence of cervical cancer [103, 104]. Despite relatively disappointing results of such immunization protocols, clinical and histological studies support the notion that tumor-infiltrating leukocytes (TIL) are indeed capable of limiting the growth and development of certain types of cancer. An extensive study in patients with colorectal cancer revealed that those patients that had a pronounced infiltration of the tumor with lymphocytes, and in particular with memory T cells, showed a significantly prolonged survival compared to patients with little or no immune cell infiltrate [105]. Though an indirect proof, these studies demonstrate a strong correlation between anti-tumor immune responses, tumor development and patient survival. These findings, however, also suggest that tumors capable of escaping or suppressing immune responses by any means may have a major advantage and kill the patient more rapidly.

Various immune escape mechanisms have been described in different tumors. Tumor cells secrete suppressive cytokines, such as TGFβ and IL-10, express pro-apoptotic ligands (Fas ligand and TRAIL), which kill TIL, or simply reduce their immunogenicity by downregulating MHC molecules and associated antigen presentation on their surface. In this paragraph we will also discuss the proposed role of extra-adrenal GC synthesis in colorectal tumors as a mechanism of immune escape. Though various types of tumors have been shown to be active sources of steroid hormones, most of these tumors derive from steroidogenic tissues, such as the adrenal glands, ovaries or testis. For example, adrenal hyperplasia and tumors often lead to a massive release of GC, resulting in Cushing syndrome [106]. In addition, small cell bronchogenic carcinoma, carcinoids of thymus, pancreas, ovary, as well as medullary carcinoma of thyroid gland etc. have been shown to release ACTH or in rare cases CRH, and thereby to stimulate indirectly the release of systemic GC from the adrenals with subsequent suppression of the immune system [107, 108]. Yet, thus far no direct GC synthesis in tumors from non-steroidogenic tissues has been described.

As discussed in detail above, LRH-1 has a prominent role in the regulation of intestinal GC synthesis [48, 52]. Interestingly, however, LRH-1 has also been implicated in other aspects of intestinal epithelial cell biology. LRH-1 is primarily expressed in the pluripotent and proliferating cells of the intestinal crypts where it regulates the expression of cyclin D1. Furthermore, in collaboration with the Wnt signaling pathway and β-catenin it also controls the expression of cyclin E1 and c-Myc, and thereby the proliferation of crypt cells and the renewal of the intestinal epithelial layer (reviewed in [109, 110]). Not surprisingly, this mitogenic role of LRH-1 appears to be also involved in the development of intestinal tumors. Mice with a mutation in the APC gene (APC[min/+] mice) spontaneously develop adenomas in both small and large bowel. Interestingly tumor development is significantly reduced in mice with LRH-1 deficiency [111]. Thus, LRH-1 appears to be a proto-oncogene in the development of intestinal tumors. In line with this idea is the observation that different tumors derived from endoderm tissue show LRH-1 overexpression. For example, LRH-1 is overexpressed in colorectal [55] and in pancreatic tumors [112], where it also regulates cell cycle progression.

Given the important role of LRH-1 in cell cycle regulation as well as intestinal GC synthesis LRH-1-mediated synthesis of immunoregulatory GC in colorectal tumors as a mechanism to control anti-tumor immune responses appears to be an attractive idea. Indeed, considerable synthesis of cortisol can be measured in colorectal cancer cell lines as well as primary colorectal tumors using radioimmuno assay, bioassay as well as metabolic assays [55]. In line with this steroidogenic potential of colorectal tumor cells is the widely distributed expression of LRH-1 and steroidogenic enzymes. Furthermore, overexpression of LRH-1 further boost the expression of steroidogenic enyzmes and the synthesis of cortisol, whereas inhibition of LRH-1 expression downregulates these processes. Interestingly, GC synthesis in colorectal tumor cell lines as well as ex vivo cultured primary tumors seems to be constitutive, whereas in normal colonic tissue it is inducible by phorbol ester, likely via the ERK1/2-mediated activation of LRH-1. This suggests that in colorectal tumors LRH-1 may be constitutively active, and suggests that signal transduction pathways leading to tumor

development and proliferation also govern the activation of LRH-1 and associated GC
synthesis. Of interest in this regard is that LRH-1 not only controls cell cycle progression,
but that its activity is also controlled by the cell cycle [50]. Various mitogenic signals
controlling tumor cell proliferation may therefore also promote the activation of LRH-1. In
line with this idea is the observation that many colorectal tumors have activating mutations
of the epidermal growth factor receptor pathway [113] and that epidermal growth factor can
stimulate LRH-1 activation in an ERK1/2-dependent manner in Hela cells [95]. However,
more detailed analysis of the signaling pathways leading to LRH-1 activation and GC
synthesis in colorectal tumors will be required to confirm whether mitogenic stimuli are
indeed important triggers of extra-adrenal GC synthesis in tumor cells.

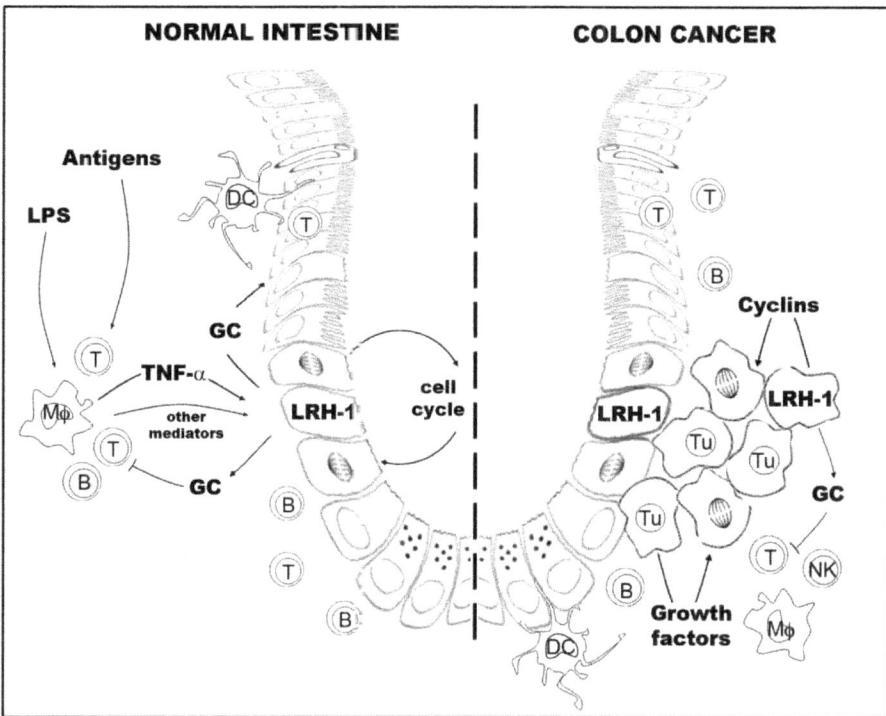

Abbreviations: B – B-Lymphocytes; DC – dendritic cells; LPS – lipopolysaccharides; Mφ – macrophages; NK – natural
killer cells; T – T-Lymphocytes; Tu – tumor cells.

Figure 2. Proposed role of intestinal GC synthesis in maintaining immune homeostasis in normal gut
mucosa and promoting immune escape in colon cancer.

While the immunoregulatory role of GC synthesis in normal intestinal tissue is quite well
established [46, 49, 52, 53], the evidence in colorectal tumors is yet relatively indirect. The
supernatant of colorectal tumor cell lines and primary tumors has been found to contain a
suppressive activity, which inhibits the activation of primary T cells, as measured by the

induction of activation marker CD69 [55]. Similarly, tumor-derived supernatant was able to promote apoptosis in GC sensitive immune cells. Importantly, these suppressive or pro-apoptotic activities were blocked by either interfering with the GC synthesis pathway in tumor cells by metyrapone, or by blocking the GR in immune cells [55]. While colorectal tumor cells may also secrete other immunoregulatory factors, such as TGFβ, these finding demonstrate that GC are present in the supernatant of tumor cells and that their concentration is high enough to promote biological responses and immunosuppression. The secretion of immunoregulatory GC by colorectal tumors may thus represent a novel mechanism how tumor cells escape from destruction by the immune system. Similar mechanisms may also exist in tumors from tissues capable of secreting bioactive GC, e.g. lung cancer.

6. Conclusion

In summary, the extremely potent GC synthesizing activity of the adrenal glands has obscured for a long time the fact that various other extra-adrenal tissues are important sources of immunoregulatory GC. This chapter has highlighted in particular the role of the pulmonary and intestinal mucosa, and its associated tumors, as potent sources of extra-adrenal GC synthesis. Their more recent identification has lead to new interpretations of how locally produced GC may be involved in the maintenance of tissue homeostasis, regulation of inflammatory processes and tumor development. Finally, the detailed analysis of the differential signal transduction pathways controlling GC synthesis in the adrenals versus extra-adrenal tissues may offer novel opportunities for the development of therapeutic interventions.

Author details

Feodora I. Kostadinova and Thomas Brunner*
Division of Biochemical Pharmacology, Department of Biology, University of Konstanz, Germany

Nina Hostettler and Pamela Bianchi
Division of Experimental Pathology, Institute of Pathology, University of Bern, Switzerland

Acknowledgement

The authors thank previous and present members of the Brunner lab, especially Igor Cima, Mathias Müller, Mario Noti, Daniel Sidler and Nadia Corazza, for their contributions to the investigation of extra-adrenal GC synthesis, Kristina Schoonjans and Johan Auwerx for fruitful collaborations and many reagents, and the Swiss National Science Foundation, Swiss Cancer League, the Bangerter Foundation, the Crohn's and Colitis Foundation of America and the German Research Foundation for continuous support of this research area.

* Corresponding Author

7. References

[1]   Sapolsky RM, Romero LM, Munck AU (2000) How Do Glucocorticoids Influence Stress Responses? Integrating Permissive, Suppressive, Stimulatory, and Preparative Actions. Endocr Rev. 21: 55-89.

[2]   Chrousos GP (1995) The Hypothalamic-Pituitary-Adrenal Axis and Immune-Mediated Inflammation. N Engl J Med. 332: 1351-62.

[3]   Vacchio MS, Papadopoulos V, Ashwell JD (1994) Steroid Production in the Thymus: Implications for Thymocyte Selection. J Exp Med. 179: 1835-46.

[4]   Lechner O, Wiegers GJ, Oliveira-Dos-Santos AJ, Dietrich H, Recheis H, et al. (2000) Glucocorticoid Production in the Murine Thymus. European journal of immunology. 30: 337-46.

[5]   Pazirandeh A, Xue Y, Rafter I, Sjovall J, Jondal M, et al. (1999) Paracrine Glucocorticoid Activity Produced by Mouse Thymic Epithelial Cells. FASEB journal : official publication of the Federation of American Societies for Experimental Biology. 13: 893-901.

[6]   Ashwell JD, Lu FW, Vacchio MS (2000) Glucocorticoids in T Cell Development and Function*. Annu Rev Immunol. 18: 309-45.

[7]   Taves MD, Gomez-Sanchez CE, Soma KK (2011) Extra-Adrenal Glucocorticoids and Mineralocorticoids: Evidence for Local Synthesis, Regulation, and Function. American journal of physiology. Endocrinology and metabolism. 301: E11-24.

[8]   Slominski A, Ermak G, Mihm M (1996) Acth Receptor, Cyp11a1, Cyp17 and Cyp21a2 Genes Are Expressed in Skin. J Clin Endocrinol Metab. 81: 2746-9.

[9]   Slominski A, Gomez-Sanchez CE, Foecking MF, Wortsman J (2000) Active Steroidogenesis in the Normal Rat Skin. Biochim Biophys Acta. 1474: 1-4.

[10] Slominski A, Wortsman J (2000) Neuroendocrinology of the Skin. Endocr Rev. 21: 457-87.

[11] Slominski A, Wortsman J, Paus R, Elias PM, Tobin DJ, et al. (2008) Skin as an Endocrine Organ: Implications for Its Function. Drug Discov Today Dis Mech. 5: 137-44.

[12] Slominski A, Wortsman J, Pisarchik A, Zbytek B, Linton EA, et al. (2001) Cutaneous Expression of Corticotropin-Releasing Hormone (Crh), Urocortin, and Crh Receptors. FASEB journal : official publication of the Federation of American Societies for Experimental Biology. 15: 1678-93.

[13] Slominski A, Zbytek B, Szczesniewski A, Semak I, Kaminski J, et al. (2005) Crh Stimulation of Corticosteroids Production in Melanocytes Is Mediated by Acth. American journal of physiology. Endocrinology and metabolism. 288: E701-6.

[14] Slominski A, Zjawiony J, Wortsman J, Semak I, Stewart J, et al. (2004) A Novel Pathway for Sequential Transformation of 7-Dehydrocholesterol and Expression of the P450scc System in Mammalian Skin. Eur J Biochem. 271: 4178-88.

[15] Ito N, Ito T, Kromminga A, Bettermann A, Takigawa M, et al. (2005) Human Hair Follicles Display a Functional Equivalent of the Hypothalamic-Pituitary-Adrenal Axis and Synthesize Cortisol. FASEB journal : official publication of the Federation of American Societies for Experimental Biology. 19: 1332-4.

[16] Paus R, Botchkarev VA, Botchkareva NV, Mecklenburg L, Luger T, et al. (1999) The Skin Pomc System (Sps). Leads and Lessons from the Hair Follicle. Annals of the New York Academy of Sciences. 885: 350-63.

[17] Paus R, Ito N, Takigawa M, Ito T (2003) The Hair Follicle and Immune Privilege. J Investig Dermatol Symp Proc. 8: 188-94.

[18] Thiboutot D, Jabara S, McAllister JM, Sivarajah A, Gilliland K, et al. (2003) Human Skin Is a Steroidogenic Tissue: Steroidogenic Enzymes and Cofactors Are Expressed in Epidermis, Normal Sebocytes, and an Immortalized Sebocyte Cell Line (Seb-1). J Invest Dermatol. 120: 905-14.

[19] Vukelic S, Stojadinovic O, Pastar I, Rabach M, Krzyzanowska A, et al. (2011) Cortisol Synthesis in Epidermis Is Induced by Il-1 and Tissue Injury. The Journal of biological chemistry. 286: 10265-75.

[20] Casal AJ, Silvestre JS, Delcayre C, Capponi AM (2003) Expression and Modulation of Steroidogenic Acute Regulatory Protein Messenger Ribonucleic Acid in Rat Cardiocytes and after Myocardial Infarction. Endocrinology. 144: 1861-8.

[21] Silvestre JS, Robert V, Heymes C, Aupetit-Faisant B, Mouas C, et al. (1998) Myocardial Production of Aldosterone and Corticosterone in the Rat. Physiological Regulation. The Journal of biological chemistry. 273: 4883-91.

[22] Silvestre JS, Heymes C, Oubenaissa A, Robert V, Aupetit-Faisant B, et al. (1999) Activation of Cardiac Aldosterone Production in Rat Myocardial Infarction: Effect of Angiotensin Ii Receptor Blockade and Role in Cardiac Fibrosis. Circulation. 99: 2694-701.

[23] Takeda Y, Miyamori I, Yoneda T, Iki K, Hatakeyama H, et al. (1994) Synthesis of Corticosterone in the Vascular Wall. Endocrinology. 135: 2283-6.

[24] Takeda Y, Miyamori I, Yoneda T, Hatakeyama H, Inaba S, et al. (1996) Regulation of Aldosterone Synthase in Human Vascular Endothelial Cells by Angiotensin Ii and Adrenocorticotropin. J Clin Endocrinol Metab. 81: 2797-800.

[25] Takeda Y (2005) Role of Cardiovascular Aldosterone in Hypertension. Curr Med Chem Cardiovasc Hematol Agents. 3: 261-6.

[26] Hatakeyama H, Miyamori I, Takeda Y, Yamamoto H, Mabuchi H (1996) The Expression of Steroidogenic Enzyme Genes in Human Vascular Cells. Biochem Mol Biol Int. 40: 639-45.

[27] Kayes-Wandover KM, White PC (2000) Steroidogenic Enzyme Gene Expression in the Human Heart. J Clin Endocrinol Metab. 85: 2519-25.

[28] Young MJ, Clyne CD, Cole TJ, Funder JW (2001) Cardiac Steroidogenesis in the Normal and Failing Heart. J Clin Endocrinol Metab. 86: 5121-6.

[29] Ahmad N, Romero DG, Gomez-Sanchez EP, Gomez-Sanchez CE (2004) Do Human Vascular Endothelial Cells Produce Aldosterone? Endocrinology. 145: 3626-9.

[30] Baulieu EE (1998) Neurosteroids: A Novel Function of the Brain. Psychoneuroendocrinology. 23: 963-87.

[31] Mellon SH (2007) Neurosteroid Regulation of Central Nervous System Development. Pharmacol Ther. 116: 107-24.

[32] Gunn BG, Brown AR, Lambert JJ, Belelli D (2011) Neurosteroids and Gaba(a) Receptor Interactions: A Focus on Stress. Front Neurosci. 5: 131.

[33] Stromstedt M, Waterman MR (1995) Messenger Rnas Encoding Steroidogenic Enzymes Are Expressed in Rodent Brain. Brain Res Mol Brain Res. 34: 75-88.

[34] MacKenzie SM, Clark CJ, Ingram MC, Lai M, Seckl J, et al. (2000) Corticosteroid Production by Fetal Rat Hippocampal Neurons. Endocr Res. 26: 531-5.

[35] MacKenzie SM, Clark CJ, Fraser R, Gomez-Sanchez CE, Connell JM, et al. (2000) Expression of 11beta-Hydroxylase and Aldosterone Synthase Genes in the Rat Brain. J Mol Endocrinol. 24: 321-8.

[36] Yu L, Romero DG, Gomez-Sanchez CE, Gomez-Sanchez EP (2002) Steroidogenic Enzyme Gene Expression in the Human Brain. Mol Cell Endocrinol. 190: 9-17.

[37] Higo S, Hojo Y, Ishii H, Komatsuzaki Y, Ooishi Y, et al. (2011) Endogenous Synthesis of Corticosteroids in the Hippocampus. PLoS One. 6: e21631.

[38] Basu R, Singh RJ, Basu A, Chittilapilly EG, Johnson CM, et al. (2004) Splanchnic Cortisol Production Occurs in Humans: Evidence for Conversion of Cortisone to Cortisol Via the 11-Beta Hydroxysteroid Dehydrogenase (11beta-Hsd) Type 1 Pathway. Diabetes. 53: 2051-9.

[39] Andrew R, Westerbacka J, Wahren J, Yki-Jarvinen H, Walker BR (2005) The Contribution of Visceral Adipose Tissue to Splanchnic Cortisol Production in Healthy Humans. Diabetes. 54: 1364-70.

[40] Harris HJ, Kotelevtsev Y, Mullins JJ, Seckl JR, Holmes MC (2001) Intracellular Regeneration of Glucocorticoids by 11beta-Hydroxysteroid Dehydrogenase (11beta-Hsd)-1 Plays a Key Role in Regulation of the Hypothalamic-Pituitary-Adrenal Axis: Analysis of 11beta-Hsd-1-Deficient Mice. Endocrinology. 142: 114-20.

[41] Carter RN, Paterson JM, Tworowska U, Stenvers DJ, Mullins JJ, et al. (2009) Hypothalamic-Pituitary-Adrenal Axis Abnormalities in Response to Deletion of 11beta-Hsd1 Is Strain-Dependent. J Neuroendocrinol. 21: 879-87.

[42] Wyrwoll CS, Holmes MC, Seckl JR (2011) 11beta-Hydroxysteroid Dehydrogenases and the Brain: From Zero to Hero, a Decade of Progress. Front Neuroendocrinol. 32: 265-86.

[43] Holmes MC, Carter RN, Noble J, Chitnis S, Dutia A, et al. (2010) 11beta-Hydroxysteroid Dehydrogenase Type 1 Expression Is Increased in the Aged Mouse Hippocampus and Parietal Cortex and Causes Memory Impairments. J Neurosci. 30: 6915-20.

[44] Sandeep TC, Yau JL, MacLullich AM, Noble J, Deary IJ, et al. (2004) 11beta-Hydroxysteroid Dehydrogenase Inhibition Improves Cognitive Function in Healthy Elderly Men and Type 2 Diabetics. Proceedings of the National Academy of Sciences of the United States of America. 101: 6734-9.

[45] MacLullich AM, Ferguson KJ, Reid LM, Deary IJ, Starr JM, et al. (2012) 11beta-Hydroxysteroid Dehydrogenase Type 1, Brain Atrophy and Cognitive Decline. Neurobiol Aging. 33: 207 e1-8.

[46] Cima I, Corazza N, Dick B, Fuhrer A, Herren S, et al. (2004) Intestinal Epithelial Cells Synthesize Glucocorticoids and Regulate T Cell Activation. The Journal of experimental medicine. 200: 1635-46.

[47] Mueller M, Atanasov A, Cima I, Corazza N, Schoonjans K, et al. (2007) Differential Regulation of Glucocorticoid Synthesis in Murine Intestinal Epithelial Versus Adrenocortical Cell Lines. Endocrinology. 148: 1445-53.

[48] Mueller M, Cima I, Noti M, Fuhrer A, Jakob S, et al. (2006) The Nuclear Receptor Lrh-1 Critically Regulates Extra-Adrenal Glucocorticoid Synthesis in the Intestine. The Journal of experimental medicine. 203: 2057-62.

[49] Coste A, Dubuquoy L, Barnouin R, Annicotte JS, Magnier B, et al. (2007) Lrh-1-Mediated Glucocorticoid Synthesis in Enterocytes Protects against Inflammatory Bowel Disease. Proc Natl Acad Sci U S A. 104: 13098-103.

[50] Atanasov AG, Leiser D, Roesselet C, Noti M, Corazza N, et al. (2008) Cell Cycle-Dependent Regulation of Extra-Adrenal Glucocorticoid Synthesis in Murine Intestinal Epithelial Cells. FASEB journal : official publication of the Federation of American Societies for Experimental Biology. 22: 4117-25.

[51] Noti M, Sidler D, Brunner T (2009) Extra-Adrenal Glucocorticoid Synthesis in the Intestinal Epithelium: More Than a Drop in the Ocean? Semin Immunopathol. 31: 237-48.

[52] Noti M, Corazza N, Tuffin G, Schoonjans K, Brunner T (2010) Lipopolysaccharide Induces Intestinal Glucocorticoid Synthesis in a Tnfalpha-Dependent Manner. FASEB journal : official publication of the Federation of American Societies for Experimental Biology. 24: 1340-6.

[53] Noti M, Corazza N, Mueller C, Berger B, Brunner T (2010) Tnf Suppresses Acute Intestinal Inflammation by Inducing Local Glucocorticoid Synthesis. The Journal of experimental medicine. 207: 1057-66.

[54] Hostettler N, Bianchi P, Gennari-Moser C, Kassahn D, Schoonjans K, et al. (2012) Local Glucocorticoid Production in the Mouse Lung Is Induced by Immune Cell Stimulation. Allergy. 67: 227-34.

[55] Sidler D, Renzulli P, Schnoz C, Berger B, Schneider-Jakob S, et al. (2011) Colon Cancer Cells Produce Immunoregulatory Glucocorticoids. Oncogene. 30: 2411-9.

[56] Keeney DS, Jenkins CM, Waterman MR (1995) Developmentally Regulated Expression of Adrenal 17 Alpha-Hydroxylase Cytochrome P450 in the Mouse Embryo. Endocrinology. 136: 4872-9.

[57] Okamoto M, Nonaka Y, Takemori H, Doi J (2005) Molecular Identity and Gene Expression of Aldosterone Synthase Cytochrome P450. Biochem Biophys Res Commun. 338: 325-30.

[58] Laurent V, Kimble A, Peng B, Zhu P, Pintar JE, et al. (2002) Mortality in 7b2 Null Mice Can Be Rescued by Adrenalectomy: Involvement of Dopamine in Acth Hypersecretion. Proceedings of the National Academy of Sciences of the United States of America. 99: 3087-92.

[59] Davies E, MacKenzie SM (2003) Extra-Adrenal Production of Corticosteroids. Clin Exp Pharmacol Physiol. 30: 437-45.

[60] Blackburn CC, Manley NR (2004) Developing a New Paradigm for Thymus Organogenesis. Nat Rev Immunol. 4: 278-89.

Extra-Adrenal Glucocorticoid Synthesis in Mucosal Tissues and Its Implication in Mucosal
Immune Homeostasis and Tumor Development

147

[61] Spits H (2002) Development of Alphabeta T Cells in the Human Thymus. Nat Rev Immunol. 2: 760-72.

[62] Ashwell JD, Vacchio MS, Galon J (2000) Do Glucocorticoids Participate in Thymocyte Development? Immunol Today. 21: 644-6.

[63] Godfrey DI, Purton JF, Boyd RL, Cole TJ (2000) Stress-Free T-Cell Development: Glucocorticoids Are Not Obligatory. Immunol Today. 21: 606-11.

[64] Zacharchuk CM, Mercep M, Chakraborti PK, Simons SS, Jr., Ashwell JD (1990) Programmed T Lymphocyte Death. Cell Activation- and Steroid-Induced Pathways Are Mutually Antagonistic. Journal of immunology. 145: 4037-45.

[65] Kupper TS, Fuhlbrigge RC (2004) Immune Surveillance in the Skin: Mechanisms and Clinical Consequences. Nat Rev Immunol. 4: 211-22.

[66] Rousseau K, Kauser S, Pritchard LE, Warhurst A, Oliver RL, et al. (2007) Proopiomelanocortin (Pomc), the Acth/Melanocortin Precursor, Is Secreted by Human Epidermal Keratinocytes and Melanocytes and Stimulates Melanogenesis. FASEB journal : official publication of the Federation of American Societies for Experimental Biology. 21: 1844-56.

[67] Slominski A, Zbytek B, Semak I, Sweatman T, Wortsman J (2005) Crh Stimulates Pomc Activity and Corticosterone Production in Dermal Fibroblasts. J Neuroimmunol. 162: 97-102.

[68] Mellon SH, Griffin LD (2002) Neurosteroids: Biochemistry and Clinical Significance. Trends Endocrinol Metab. 13: 35-43.

[69] Kishimoto W, Hiroi T, Shiraishi M, Osada M, Imaoka S, et al. (2004) Cytochrome P450 2d Catalyze Steroid 21-Hydroxylation in the Brain. Endocrinology. 145: 699-705.

[70] Ye P, Kenyon CJ, Mackenzie SM, Nichol K, Seckl JR, et al. (2008) Effects of Acth, Dexamethasone, and Adrenalectomy on 11beta-Hydroxylase (Cyp11b1) and Aldosterone Synthase (Cyp11b2) Gene Expression in the Rat Central Nervous System. J Endocrinol. 196: 305-11.

[71] Walker BR, Andrew R (2006) Tissue Production of Cortisol by 11beta-Hydroxysteroid Dehydrogenase Type 1 and Metabolic Disease. Annals of the New York Academy of Sciences. 1083: 165-84.

[72] Yau JL, McNair KM, Noble J, Brownstein D, Hibberd C, et al. (2007) Enhanced Hippocampal Long-Term Potentiation and Spatial Learning in Aged 11beta-Hydroxysteroid Dehydrogenase Type 1 Knock-out Mice. J Neurosci. 27: 10487-96.

[73] Takeda Y, Miyamori I, Yoneda T, Iki K, Hatakeyama H, et al. (1995) Production of Aldosterone in Isolated Rat Blood Vessels. Hypertension. 25: 170-3.

[74] Christy C, Hadoke PW, Paterson JM, Mullins JJ, Seckl JR, et al. (2003) 11beta-Hydroxysteroid Dehydrogenase Type 2 in Mouse Aorta: Localization and Influence on Response to Glucocorticoids. Hypertension. 42: 580-7.

[75] Hadoke PW, Macdonald L, Logie JJ, Small GR, Dover AR, et al. (2006) Intra-Vascular Glucocorticoid Metabolism as a Modulator of Vascular Structure and Function. Cellular and molecular life sciences : CMLS. 63: 565-78.

[76] Goodyer CG, Branchaud CL (1981) Regulation of Hormone Production in the Human Feto-Placental Unit. Ciba Found Symp. 86: 89-123.

[77] Yong PY, Thong KJ, Andrew R, Walker BR, Hillier SG (2000) Development-Related Increase in Cortisol Biosynthesis by Human Granulosa Cells. J Clin Endocrinol Metab. 85: 4728-33.

[78] Wang GM, Ge RS, Latif SA, Morris DJ, Hardy MP (2002) Expression of 11beta-Hydroxylase in Rat Leydig Cells. Endocrinology. 143: 621-6.

[79] Burton PJ, Krozowski ZS, Waddell BJ (1998) Immunolocalization of 11beta-Hydroxysteroid Dehydrogenase Types 1 and 2 in Rat Uterus: Variation across the Estrous Cycle and Regulation by Estrogen and Progesterone. Endocrinology. 139: 376-82.

[80] Quirk SJ, Slattery J, Funder JW (1990) 11 Beta-Hydroxysteroid Dehydrogenase Activity in the Mammary Gland. J Steroid Biochem. 35: 623-5.

[81] Brunner T (2009) Living on the Edge: Immune Cells and Immunopathology in the Intestinal Mucosa. Seminars in immunopathology. 31: 143-4.

[82] Keeney DS, Ikeda Y, Waterman MR, Parker KL (1995) Cholesterol Side-Chain Cleavage Cytochrome P450 Gene Expression in the Primitive Gut of the Mouse Embryo Does Not Require Steroidogenic Factor 1. Mol Endocrinol. 9: 1091-8.

[83] Sadovsky Y, Crawford PA, Woodson KG, Polish JA, Clements MA, et al. (1995) Mice Deficient in the Orphan Receptor Steroidogenic Factor 1 Lack Adrenal Glands and Gonads but Express P450 Side-Chain-Cleavage Enzyme in the Placenta and Have Normal Embryonic Serum Levels of Corticosteroids. Proceedings of the National Academy of Sciences of the United States of America. 92: 10939-43.

[84] Brunner T, Arnold D, Wasem C, Herren S, Frutschi C (2001) Regulation of Cell Death and Survival in Intestinal Intraepithelial Lymphocytes. Cell death and differentiation. 8: 706-14.

[85] Wasem C, Arnold D, Saurer L, Corazza N, Jakob S, et al. (2003) Sensitizing Antigen-Specific Cd8+ T Cells for Accelerated Suicide Causes Immune Incompetence. The Journal of clinical investigation. 111: 1191-9.

[86] Corazza N, Muller S, Brunner T, Kagi D, Mueller C (2000) Differential Contribution of Fas- and Perforin-Mediated Mechanisms to the Cell-Mediated Cytotoxic Activity of Naive and in Vivo-Primed Intestinal Intraepithelial Lymphocytes. Journal of immunology. 164: 398-403.

[87] Parker KL, Rice DA, Lala DS, Ikeda Y, Luo X, et al. (2002) Steroidogenic Factor 1: An Essential Mediator of Endocrine Development. Recent Prog Horm Res. 57: 19-36.

[88] Parker KL (1998) The Roles of Steroidogenic Factor 1 in Endocrine Development and Function. Mol Cell Endocrinol. 145: 15-20.

[89] Fayard E, Auwerx J, Schoonjans K (2004) Lrh-1: An Orphan Nuclear Receptor Involved in Development, Metabolism and Steroidogenesis. Trends Cell Biol. 14: 250-60.

[90] Sirianni R, Seely JB, Attia G, Stocco DM, Carr BR, et al. (2002) Liver Receptor Homologue-1 Is Expressed in Human Steroidogenic Tissues and Activates Transcription of Genes Encoding Steroidogenic Enzymes. J Endocrinol. 174: R13-7.

[91] Wu YG, Bennett J, Talla D, Stocco C (2011) Testosterone, Not 5alpha-Dihydrotestosterone, Stimulates Lrh-1 Leading to Fsh-Independent Expression of Cyp19 and P450scc in Granulosa Cells. Mol Endocrinol. 25: 656-68.

[92] Suzawa M, Ingraham HA (2008) The Herbicide Atrazine Activates Endocrine Gene Networks Via Non-Steroidal Nr5a Nuclear Receptors in Fish and Mammalian Cells. PLoS One. 3: e2117.

[93] Whitby RJ, Stec J, Blind RD, Dixon S, Leesnitzer LM, et al. (2011) Small Molecule Agonists of the Orphan Nuclear Receptors Steroidogenic Factor-1 (Sf-1, Nr5a1) and Liver Receptor Homologue-1 (Lrh-1, Nr5a2). J Med Chem. 54: 2266-81.

[94] Sablin EP, Krylova IN, Fletterick RJ, Ingraham HA (2003) Structural Basis for Ligand-Independent Activation of the Orphan Nuclear Receptor Lrh-1. Molecular cell. 11: 1575-85.

[95] Lee YK, Choi YH, Chua S, Park YJ, Moore DD (2006) Phosphorylation of the Hinge Domain of the Nuclear Hormone Receptor Lrh-1 Stimulates Transactivation. The Journal of biological chemistry. 281: 7850-5.

[96] Sablin EP, Woods A, Krylova IN, Hwang P, Ingraham HA, et al. (2008) The Structure of Corepressor Dax-1 Bound to Its Target Nuclear Receptor Lrh-1. Proceedings of the National Academy of Sciences of the United States of America. 105: 18390-5.

[97] Lee YK, Moore DD (2002) Dual Mechanisms for Repression of the Monomeric Orphan Receptor Liver Receptor Homologous Protein-1 by the Orphan Small Heterodimer Partner. The Journal of biological chemistry. 277: 2463-7.

[98] Reimund JM, Wittersheim C, Dumont S, Muller CD, Baumann R, et al. (1996) Mucosal Inflammatory Cytokine Production by Intestinal Biopsies in Patients with Ulcerative Colitis and Crohn's Disease. J Clin Immunol. 16: 144-50.

[99] Rutgeerts PJ (1999) Review Article: Efficacy of Infliximab in Crohn's Disease--Induction and Maintenance of Remission. Aliment Pharmacol Ther. 13 Suppl 4: 9-15; discussion 38.

[100] Ford AC, Sandborn WJ, Khan KJ, Hanauer SB, Talley NJ, et al. (2011) Efficacy of Biological Therapies in Inflammatory Bowel Disease: Systematic Review and Meta-Analysis. Am J Gastroenterol. 106: 644-59, quiz 60.

[101] Provost PR, Tremblay Y (2005) Genes Involved in the Adrenal Pathway of Glucocorticoid Synthesis Are Transiently Expressed in the Developing Lung. Endocrinology. 146: 2239-45.

[102] Sampath-Kumar R, Yu M, Khalil MW, Yang K (1997) Metyrapone Is a Competitive Inhibitor of 11beta-Hydroxysteroid Dehydrogenase Type 1 Reductase. J Steroid Biochem Mol Biol. 62: 195-9.

[103] Roteli-Martins C, Naud P, De Borba P, Teixeira J, De Carvalho N, et al. (2012) Sustained Immunogenicity and Efficacy of the Hpv-16/18 As04-Adjuvanted Vaccine: Up to 8.4 Years of Follow-Up. Hum Vaccin Immunother. 8.

[104] Lehtinen M, Paavonen J, Wheeler CM, Jaisamrarn U, Garland SM, et al. (2012) Overall Efficacy of Hpv-16/18 As04-Adjuvanted Vaccine against Grade 3 or Greater Cervical Intraepithelial Neoplasia: 4-Year End-of-Study Analysis of the Randomised, Double-Blind Patricia Trial. Lancet Oncol. 13: 89-99.

[105] Galon J, Costes A, Sanchez-Cabo F, Kirilovsky A, Mlecnik B, et al. (2006) Type, Density, and Location of Immune Cells within Human Colorectal Tumors Predict Clinical Outcome. Science. 313: 1960-4.

[106] Newell-Price J, Bertagna X, Grossman AB, Nieman LK (2006) Cushing's Syndrome. Lancet. 367: 1605-17.

[107] Isidori AM, Kaltsas GA, Pozza C, Frajese V, Newell-Price J, et al. (2006) The Ectopic Adrenocorticotropin Syndrome: Clinical Features, Diagnosis, Management, and Long-Term Follow-Up. J Clin Endocrinol Metab. 91: 371-7.

[108] Shahani S, Nudelman RJ, Nalini R, Kim HS, Samson SL (2010) Ectopic Corticotropin-Releasing Hormone (Crh) Syndrome from Metastatic Small Cell Carcinoma: A Case Report and Review of the Literature. Diagn Pathol. 5: 56.

[109] Botrugno OA, Fayard E, Annicotte JS, Haby C, Brennan T, et al. (2004) Synergy between Lrh-1 and Beta-Catenin Induces G1 Cyclin-Mediated Cell Proliferation. Molecular cell. 15: 499-509.

[110] Fernandez-Marcos PJ, Auwerx J, Schoonjans K (2011) Emerging Actions of the Nuclear Receptor Lrh-1 in the Gut. Biochim Biophys Acta. 1812: 947-55.

[111] Schoonjans K, Dubuquoy L, Mebis J, Fayard E, Wendling O, et al. (2005) Liver Receptor Homolog 1 Contributes to Intestinal Tumor Formation through Effects on Cell Cycle and Inflammation. Proceedings of the National Academy of Sciences of the United States of America. 102: 2058-62.

[112] Benod C, Vinogradova MV, Jouravel N, Kim GE, Fletterick RJ, et al. (2011) Nuclear Receptor Liver Receptor Homologue 1 (Lrh-1) Regulates Pancreatic Cancer Cell Growth and Proliferation. Proceedings of the National Academy of Sciences of the United States of America. 108: 16927-31.

[113] Normanno N, Tejpar S, Morgillo F, De Luca A, Van Cutsem E, et al. (2009) Implications for Kras Status and Egfr-Targeted Therapies in Metastatic Crc. Nat Rev Clin Oncol. 6: 519-27.

Chapter 7

Molecular Mechanisms Conferring Resistance/Sensitivity to Glucocorticoid-Induced Apoptosis

Ilhem Berrou, Marija Krstic-Demonacos and Constantinos Demonacos

Additional information is available at the end of the chapter

1. Introduction

1.1. Glucocorticoids therapeutic effects

Synthetic glucocorticoids (GCs) as effective anti-inflammatory therapeutics are the most widely prescribed drugs in the clinic for the treatment of various conditions including asthma, ulcerative colitis, rheumatoid arthritis and hay fever [1-4]. Glucocorticoids in some cases exert effective anti-neoplastic effects in cancers of blood origin such as acute lymphocytic leukaemia (ALL) as a result of the ability of these hormones to induce cell death in blood cells [1-3]. Resistance to glucocorticoid mediated cell death remains one of the main reasons for inefficient therapy [1] and usually occurs upon prolonged glucocorticoid treatment [2] compromising significantly the success of therapy [3]. The molecular mechanisms mediating glucocorticoid dependent initiation of programmed cell death have been extensively investigated but there are several aspects of these pathways that have not yet been clearly defined. Since understanding of these mechanisms would be beneficial towards improving the glucocorticoids therapeutic efficacy further research exemplifying resistance to glucocrticoid treatment is necessary.

Glucocorticoids (GCs) exert their anti-inflammatory and immunosuppressive effects through either genomic or non-genomic mechanisms. Non-genomic early effects of glucocorticoids are induced in tissues bearing high concentrations of this hormone by interfering with the physicochemical properties of plasma and mitochondrial membranes [4]. In particular, glucocorticoids intercalate into these membranes altering lipid peroxidation and membrane permeability [5]. In addition, non-genomic effects of glucocorticoids include early suppression of the mitogen-activated protein kinase (MAPK) and hence inflammatory signal transduction cascades such as calcium influx, phagocytosis, neutrophil degranulation and cellular adhesion [6, 7, 8, 9, 10, 11]. The non genomic effects of GCs are very important in delivering short-term therapeutic benefits to asthma and rheumatoid arthritis which are diseases characterized by high inflammatory state [12].

2. Mechanisms of GC-mediated cell death

At the molecular level GCs exert their function by interacting with their intracellular GC receptor (GR), which is a hormone responsive transcription factor that modulates gene expression of its target genes [13]. Glucocorticoids activate the cellular death machinery through transcriptional and non-transcriptional pathways by means of either the extrinsic or intrinsic pathway of apoptosis [3, 14, 15, 16].

The extrinsic pathway is induced upon activation of the membrane death receptors such as the tumour necrosis factor (TNF) receptor superfamily, member 6, Fas-Ligand (Fas-L) [17]. The binding of Fas-L leads to the activation of effector caspases (caspases 3, 6 and 7) via the activation of inducer caspases, particularly caspase 8 [18]. Evidence that glucocorticoids are involved in the regulation of the extrinsic pathway of apoptosis has been provided by observations suggesting that glucocorticoids inhibit the induction of Fas-L (but not Fas) signalling in T-cell hybridomas [19, 20]. On the contrary inhibition of the extrinsic pathway using the caspase 8 inhibitor cytokine response modifier A (crmA) in pre-B leukemic cells treated with glucocorticoids indicated that GR does not initiate apoptosis in these cells through the extrinsic pathway [21, 22]. The involvement of the intrinsic pathway, on the other hand, in the glucocorticoid mediated cell death and in particular the regulation of the balance between pro- and anti-apoptotic members of the bcl-2 family has been shown in hepatocytes, small cell lung cancer, primary ALL lymphoblasts and animal systems [23, 24].

The intrinsic pathway of cell death is stimulated in response to intracellular signals, and involves mitochondria releasing pro-apoptotic molecules, formation of the apoptosome and activation of the effector caspases via the initiator caspase 9 [25]. The balance between pro- and anti-apoptotic members of the B cell leukaemia/ lymphoma 2-like (Bcl-2) family plays a crucial role in the execution of apoptosis by glucocorticoids through the intrinsic pathway [18]. In particular, glucocorticoids regulate the expression of various genes involved in the initiation of apoptosis, including the pro-apoptotic Bcl-2 family member BCL2-like 11 (Bim) [22, 26, 27, 28]. Transactivation of Bim results in the activation of the Bcl-2–associated X protein (Bax) and the Bcl2-antagonist/killer 1 (Bak), which mediate the disruption of mitochondrial membrane potential and the release of cytochrome c into the cytosol [29]. Cytochrome c then binds to its adaptor apoptotic protease activating factor (Apaf-1), thereby activating caspase 9 and several effector caspases [30]. Furthermore, mitochondria mediate the generation of reactive oxygen species (ROS), which may potentially have an add-on effect on glucocorticoid-induced apoptosis [31].

In some cases glucocorticoids induce apoptosis by using both the intrinsic and the extrinsic pathways. This is mediated by the cleaved caspase-8 which subsequently leads to activation of the pro-apoptotic member of the Bcl-2 family, Bcl-2 homology 3 (BH3) interacting domain death agonist (Bid) [32]. The C-terminal truncated Bid (t-Bid) activates caspase 9 and the effector caspases 3, 6 and 7 [33]. The intrinsic and extrinsic pathways through which glucocorticoids induce apoptosis in cells responsive to these hormones are illustrated in Figure 1.

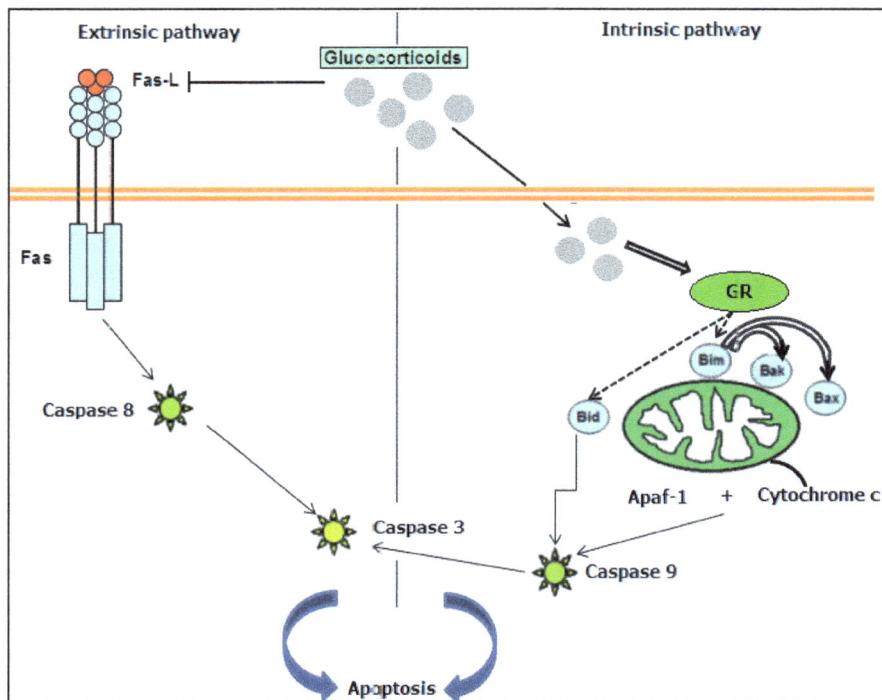

Figure 1. Schematic diagram indicating the extrinsic and intrinsic pathways through which glucocorticoids regulate apoptosis.

Several mechanisms have been proposed to explain the evasion of glucocorticoid mediated apoptosis in resistant cells [34]. These include alterations in the activity of the glucocorticoid receptor [35, 36] either due to changes in GR protein levels, presence of multiple GR variants, or post-translational modifications. GR induces apoptosis by directly modulating the expression of genes involved in cell survival/apoptosis [18, 37], or affecting gene networks involved in stress signalling resulting in an apoptotic stimulus [36, 38].

3. GR transcriptional activity is necessary for its pro-apoptotic function

Glucocorticoid induced apoptosis depends on the presence of adequate amounts of transcriptionally active GR [34, 39, 40. 41, 42]. It has also been shown that the presence of specific GR splicing variants is necessary for the stimulation of GCs dependent apoptosis [3]. Alternative hGR splicing produces two receptor variants called GRα and GRβ, which are highly homologous differing by 50 additional amino acids present in the carboxy terminal region of GRα [43]. GRα is mainly cytoplasmic, and exhibits the typical glucocorticoid receptor function in terms of ligand-dependent transcriptional regulation and as such it is the major functional GR isoform therefore its expression is crucial for cellular sensitivity to GCs [3]. GRβ on the other hand, does not bind ligands, and exerts a dominant negative effect on GRα transcriptional activity [43, 44, 45]. In clinical studies reduced GRα protein levels correlate with resistance to GCs induced apoptosis and disadvantageous prognosis in ALL [3]. Additional indication that GR transcriptional activity is necessary for the initiation of the GCs mediated apoptosis has been provided by the observation that various mutations affecting GR transcriptional activity have been detected in patients exhibiting resistance to glucocorticoids treatment [2, 46]. Furthermore, prolonged glucocorticoid treatment significantly reduces GRα expression [47], whereas GRβ expression is not affected [48].

4. GR dependent regulation of the balance between pro- and anti-apoptotic Bcl-2 family members

B cell leukaemia/ lymphoma 2-like (Bcl-2) family members are categorised into pro- and anti-apoptotic and the balance between the levels of these two types of proteins determines the cellular fate (survival or death) [23]. The involvement of the Bcl-2 family members in the glucocorticoid-induced apoptosis has been shown in cellular and animal studies [49]. For example, the expression of the anti-apoptotic Bcl-2 family member in glucocorticoid-sensitive thymocytes is lower compared to that in glucocorticoid-resistant ones [2], and overexpression of the anti-apoptotic Bcl-2 and B-cell lymphoma-extra large (Bcl-xL) in human ALL prevents glucocorticoids induced apoptosis [50, 51, 52, 53] whereas knock down of the pro-apoptotic member Bim confers resistance to dexamethasone mediated apoptosis [54]. Furthermore, over-expression of the pro-apoptotic Bax [55] and knock down of the myeloid cell leukemia sequence 1 (Mcl-1) sensitises ALL cells to glucocorticoid treatment [56]. We have shown recently that the balance between Mcl-1 and phorbol-12-myristate-13-acetate-induced protein 1 (Noxa) is a determinant of resistance / sensitivity of ALL cells to glucocorticoid-induced apoptosis [57, 58]. Several studies have shown that the pro-apoptotic Bcl-2 family member Bim plays crucial role in the glucocorticoid-induced apoptosis but further investigation is required to define the detailed molecular mechanisms of this process. Up-regulated Bim has been observed in various cell lines upon glucocorticoid treatment including ALL cells [59], primary chronic lymphocytic leukaemia (CLL) cells [27], and some patients with ALL [60]. Moreover knockout of Bim, p53 up-regulated modulator of apoptosis (Puma) or Noxa, or double knockouts of Bax and Bak confer resistance to glucocorticoid-mediated apoptosis in thymocytes [61, 62, 63]. Overall the balance of the levels between pro- and anti-apoptotic Bcl-2 family members has been recognised as a crucial factor in the determination of lymphocytes survival or death and induction of the glucocorticoid dependent programmed cell death.

Gene	Protein	Function	Role in glucocorticoid-induced apoptosis
Bcl2	B-cell Lymphoma 2 (Bcl-2)	Anti-apoptotic	Over-expression of Bcl-2 in human ALL cells prevents glucocorticoids induced apoptosis [41, 64]
BCL-xL	B-cell lymphoma-extra large (Bcl-xL)	Anti-apoptotic	Over-expression of Bcl-xL in human ALL cells prevents glucocorticoids induced apoptosis [23]
BCL2L11	BCL2 Like 11 (Bim)	Pro-apoptotic	Knock down of Bim confers resistance of ALL cells to glucocorticoid-induced apoptosis [65]. Upregulation of Bim sensitizes cells to glucocorticoid-induced apoptosis [27, 66].
Mcl1	Myeloid cell leukemia 1 (Mcl-1)	Anti-apoptotic	Knock down of Mcl-1 sensitises ALL cells to glucocorticoids apoptotic effect [56].
Phorbol-12-myristate-13-acetate-induced protein 1	Phorbol-12-myristate-13-acetate-induced protein 1 (Noxa)	Pro-apoptotic	Noxa regulates the Mcl-1 protein stability and Noxa/Mcl-1 balance determines cell survival or death [57].
p53 up-regulated modulator of apoptosis	p53 upregulated modulator of apoptosis (Puma)	Pro-apoptotic	Puma facilitates glucocorticoid-induced apoptosis of lymphocytes [62, 65].
Bax	Bcl-2–associated X (Bax)	Pro-apoptotic	Bax protein regulates glucocorticoid induced apoptosis in thymocytes [67]. Double knockouts of Bax and Bak confer resistance to glucocorticoid-induced apoptosis in thymocytes [68].
Bak	Bcl-2 homologous antagonist/killer (Bak)	Pro-apoptotic	Double knockouts of Bax and Bak confer resistance to glucocorticoid-mediated apoptosis in thymocytes [68].

Table 1. Pro- and anti-apoptotic Bcl-2 family members implicated in the glucocorticoids induced apoptosis

5. Autophagy

Autophagy is a several steps process leading to cellular degradation of unfolded or aggregated proteins and organelles in response to diverse types of stress such as starvation or metabolic stress and is an essential mechanism contributing to survival, differentiation, development, and homeostasis. Autophagy protects against chronic inflammatory conditions occurring in a variety of pathological situations such as infections, cardiovascular disease, neurodegenaration, inflammatory bowel diseases, aging and cancer [69]. Autophagy has been shown to be involved in prosurvival processes facilitating resistance of cancer cells to chemotherapy as well as under certain conditions in apoptosis [70]. Taking into account the fact that autophagy is prosurvival in addition to reports indicating that inhibitors of autophagy re-sensitise cancer cells to anticancer therapeutics [70, 71] as well as that autophagy is associated with inflammation and resistance to cancer therapy investigators were prompted to study the role of autophagy in the resistance to glucocorticoid induced apoptosis in ALL [72, 73]. These studies have indicated that dexamethasone induces autophagy before the initiation of apoptosis in ALL cells and in actual fact autophagy is a prerequisite for the efficient execution of apoptosis mediated by dexamethasone [72, 73]. More recently the molecular mechanism by which activation of autophagy overturns glucocorticoid resistance has been elucidated [74] signifying the important role of the autophagy inducer beclin-1 and the anti-apoptotic Bcl-2 family member Mcl-1 [74, 75]. Furthermore the inhibition of caspase by selective degradation of catalase and consequent generation of high concentrations of reactive oxygen species might be an alternative mechanism explaining the role of autophagy in dexamethasone induced apoptosis [76].

6. Post-translational modifications

Post-translational modifications of GR are important in regulating its transcriptional activity, protein stability, binding of GR with other transcription factors or co-modulators and subcellular localisation, and for these reasons post-translational modifications are highly relevant to glucocorticoids therapeutic efficacy [77, 78, 79, 80, 81]. GR acetylation is cell type dependent and it is suggested to suppress the receptor's transcriptional activity by reducing its ability to bind to the Glucocorticoid Responsive Elements (GREs) present in its target genes [82], or inhibit the ability of GR to translocate into the nucleus [83]. Regulation of GR transcriptional activity also takes place through ubiquitination and proteasomal degradation of the receptor upon ligand binding [84, 85]. Ubiquitination promotes interaction of GR with E2 conjugating and E3 ligase proteins causing turnover of the receptor and thus down-regulation of its transcriptional activity [85]. In support of these conclusions the proteasome inhibitor MG-132 enhances the transcriptional activity of GR [84]. Ligand-independent sumoylation has been shown to both inhibit [86, 87] as well as to stabilise and potentiate GR transcriptional activity [88]. Three sumoylation sites have been identified within the GR protein conferring GR transcriptional target selectivity [87]. We have recently reported that GR sumoylation is assisted by its phosphorylation at particular sites under certain conditions [89].

GR phosphorylation has been extensively investigated and several different kinases have been identified to induce phosphorylation of the receptor at distinct serine and threonine residues located within the N-terminal AF-1 transactivation domain of the receptor, either in the presence or in the absence of glucocorticoid hormone [90, 91, 92, 93, 94, 95]. S203 residue in human GR is targeted by cyclin/cyclin dependent kinase (CDK) complexes and is located mostly in the cytoplasm thus it is thought to be transcriptionally inactive [89, 95]. GR phosphorylated at S211 is transcriptionally active due to conformational changes which facilitate increased recruitment of the receptor to GRE-containing promoters and is a target for phosphorylation by both cyclin/CDK kinases and MAPK families depending on the cell type [91, 96]. GR phosphorylation at S226 results in inhibition of the GR function, possibly due to increased GR nuclear export and is a result of JNK activation [80, 89, 97, 98]. Finally, phosphorylation of GR at S404 attenuates GR signalling and is due to GSK3 kinase activation [99]. We have recently reported that differential GR phosphorylation in the resistant CEM-C1-15 versus sensitive CEM-C7-14 ALL cells modulates GR transcriptional activity and target selectivity resulting in diverse pro- or anti-apoptotic Bcl-2 family members' gene expression in the two cell lines [58]. In particular we have shown that GR phosphorylation at S211 is predominant in the glucocorticoid-sensitive CEM-C7-14 whereas GR phosphorylation at S226 by c-Jun N-terminal Kinase (JNK) occurs more frequently in the glucocorticoid-resistant CEM-C1-15 cells [58]. These observations lend support to the suggestion that different kinase pathways are responsible for GR phosphorylation in resistant versus sensitive cells to glucocorticoid induced apoptosis, thereby causing GR transcriptional inactivity in the resistant cell lines [58] concomitant Mcl-1 overexpression and hence resistance to GC treatment [56].

Apart from the differential expression of pro- and anti-apoptotic Bcl-2 family members [58] we have recently reported that GR isoforms localised in mitochondria are predominantly phosphorylated at serine 232 compared to serine 246 of the rat GR (corresponding to human GR Ser211 and Ser226 respectively) [95] possibly due to differential conformation of the two phosphoisoforms or diverse interaction patterns with components of the mitochondrial import machinery of the GR phosphorylated at serine 211 versus the GR phosphorylated at serine 226. These observations provide an additional potential explanation for the resistance of the CEM-C1-15 to glucocorticoids induced apoptosis in accord with recent reports indicating differential GR mitochondrial localisation in resistant compared to sensitive ALL cells to glucocorticoid induced apoptosis [93, 94, 95, 97].

7. Mitochondrial GR, glucocorticoids and cellular energy metabolism

Glucocorticoid hormones directly affect mitochondrial membranes inducing loss of mitochondrial transmembrane potential, thereby affecting vital cellular processes mediated by the function of this organelle such as ATP generation via oxidative phosphorylation, regulation of calcium flux and apoptosis [98]. In addition, glucocorticoids exert their effects on mitochondrial biogenesis through the mitochondrial GR [97, 99, 100, 101]. The intracellular trafficking of the glucocorticoid receptor has been shown to play important role in glucocorticoid-induced apoptosis [97, 102]. The glucocorticoid receptor translocates to mitochondria [97, 100, 101, 102], in various cells including rat brain and various other tissues' mitochondria [99], as well as lymphoma cells [97]. GR translocation to the nucleus occurs in both glucocorticoid-sensitive and glucocorticoid-resistant cells, whereas in contrast, GR translocation into mitochondria occurs only in the glucocorticoid-sensitive and not the resistant cells [97, 103]. The mechanisms by which GR translocates to mitochondria and its effects on the regulation of the expression of mitochondrially encoded genes have been partially elucidated [97, 100, 101, 102] and require further investigation. However, it is noteworthy that glucocorticoids modulate mitochondrial biogenesis and mitochondrial energy production pathways by regulating the transcription of the mitochondrial genome [99, 100].

The process of programmed cell death is energy dependent requiring the precise coordination of several biochemical processes including the transcriptional regulation of the expression of genes encoding enzymatic components of the energy production pathways (oxidative phosphorylation (OXPHOS) and glycolysis) [29] and mutations affecting cellular energy production lead to defects in apoptosis and tumourigenesis [104, 105, 106, 107, 108, 109]. In humans the OXPHOS pathway consists of five multi-subunit complexes whose components are encoded by genes located in both the nuclear and the mitochondrial genomes [110] supporting the notion that a transcription factor operating in both subcellular compartments could coordinate the expression of nuclear and mitochondrial genes ensuring appropriate stoichiometry and timely gene expression of the components of the respiratory chain [111]. In addition to the availability of the components encoded in the nuclear and the mitochondrial compartments an appropriate assembly mechanism of these subunits is essential for the functionality of the oxidative phosphorylation system [110]. One possible candidate transcription factor able to orchestrate nuclear and mitochondrial gene expression is the glucocorticoid receptor which mediates gene expression of both nuclear and mitochondrial encoded genes [98, 99, 100, 102, 112, 113, 114, 115, 116].

In fact, dexamethasone has been shown to affect energy metabolism and the balance between OXPHOS and glycolysis [117, 118]. Also, evidence has been recently presented indicating that changes in metabolic patterns and cellular proliferation are key aspects of resistance to GC mediated apoptosis in ALL [39]. Elevated glycolytic rate due to increased expression of genes involved in glucose metabolism are associated with resistance to glucocorticoid induced apoptosis and this resistance can be reversed by inhibitors of glycolysis in ALL [119, 120]. Moreover, glucocorticoid induced apoptosis is regulated by genes involved in cellular energy metabolism [121, 122, 123, 124] suggesting that dexamethasone contributes to the apoptosis / survival decisions in ALL cells indirectly by modulating the balance between OXPHOS and glycolysis [15, 120]. Indeed coordination of oxidative phosphorylation and glycolysis by mechanisms involving glucocorticoid receptor mediated transcriptional regulation of genes encoding enzymes implicated in both pathways has been extensively reported in the literature [99, 125, 126]. Enzymes participating in the tricarboxylic acid cycle encoded by the nuclear genome such as malate dehydrogenase 1 (Mdh1) and succinyl coenzyme A synthetase (Suclg1) are GR transcriptional target genes [127]. In addition, several mitochondrial genes encoding subunits of the OXPHOS pathway possess one or more functional glucocorticoid responsive elements [99, 100, 102, 112, 113] implying that glucocorticoids exert direct effects on mitochondrial biogenesis and respiration. Key enzymes involved in glycolysis including 6-phosphofructo-2-kinase/fructose-2, 6-bisphosphatase [126] lactate dehydrogenase B (LdhB) and aldolase A (AldoA) [128] are under GR transcriptional control [120].

To shed light on the molecular mechanisms involved in GR mediated regulation of the OXPHOS pathway bioinformatic analysis using the TRED or CCTFSP software [129, 130, 131] was performed to identify potential glucocorticoid responsive elements (GREs) in the promoters of genes encoding Surf-1, and SCO2 enzymes which are essential for the assembly of the Cytochrome c Oxidase (COX) wholoenzyme [132, 133, 134]. Similar approaches were used to detect possible existence of potential GREs in the regulatory region of the promoter of the nuclear gene encoding COX-Va. Putative GREs were identified in the regulatory regions of the promoters of Surf-1, SCO2, and COX-Va using this approach. To test whether these GREs conferred glucocorticoid responsiveness to the expression of these genes, qRT-PCR experiments were performed to quantify their mRNA levels in untreated or dexamethasone treated CEM-C1-15 (resistant to glucocorticoid induced apoptosis) and CEM-C7-14 (sensitive to glucocorticoid induced apoptosis) ALL cells [135] (Figure 2).

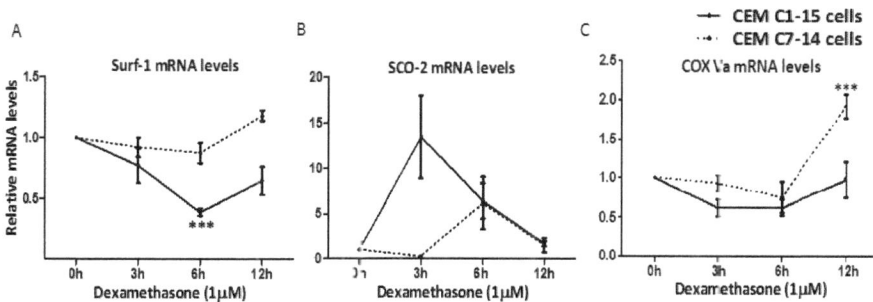

Figure 2. Relative mRNA levels of the COX assembly enzymes Surf-1 (A), SCO-2 (B), and the nuclear COX-Va (C) OXPHOS subunit were followed in the resistant CEM-C1-15 and the sensitive CEM-C7-14 to glucocorticoid induced apoptosis ALL cells treated with dexamethasone for the indicated time points by quantitative real-time PCR. Solid lines represent mRNA levels in CEM-C1-15 and dotted lines correspond to mRNA levels determined in CEM-C7-14 cells. Error bars represent standard error of the mean of five independent experiments and asterisks indicate statistical significance of $p<0.05$ compared to the untreated sample.

A marked reduction of Surf-1 mRNA levels in the resistant CEM-C1-15 cells was observed after 6 and 12 hours of dexamethasone treatment compared to the non-treated cells (Figure 2A, solid line). In contrast, in the sensitive to glucocorticoid-induced apoptosis CEM-C7-14 cells, Surf-1 mRNA levels remained constant during the first 6 hours of dexamethasone treatment and a moderate increase of Surf-1 mRNA levels was observed only 12h after the addition of the hormone (Figure 2A, dotted line). SCO-2 mRNA levels initially increased after 3h and 6h of dexamethasone treatment in CEM-C1-15 cells and later after 12h of dexamethasone treatment decreased to the level of that exhibited in the untreated cells (Figure 2B, solid line).

The fact that COX-Va expression is altered in various tumours and its association with Surf-1 in the formation of sub-complexes consisting of variable COX subunits such as

COX-I, COX-II, COX-III, and COX-IV [136] triggered our interest to investigate the regulation of the expression of the COX-Va gene. This investigation aimed to test whether differential COX-Va cellular levels in the resistant versus the sensitive CEM cells in response to glucocorticoid treatment was taking place in a similar way as that observed for Surf-1. COX-Va mRNA levels were higher in CEM-C7-14 compared to those detected in the CEM-C1-15 cells in all time points of dexamethasone treatment investigated in this study and the longer the incubation with the hormone the higher the COX-Va mRNA levels in the CEM-C7-14 cells (Figure 2C, compare dotted to solid line). Results shown in Figure 2A, 2B, and 2C support the notion that the Surf-1 and COX-Va genes encoded by the nuclear genome are under GR transcriptional control and their expression is higher in the sensitive to glucocorticoid induced apoptosis cells compared to the resistant CEM-C1-15 cells.

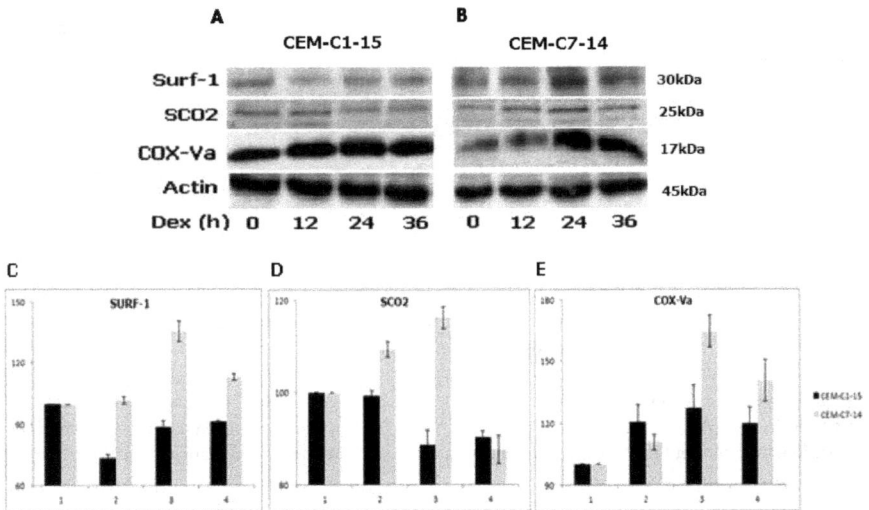

Figure 3. Western blot analysis of Surf-1, SCO-2, and COX-Va in CEM-C1-15 (A) and CEM-C7-14 (B) cells treated with dexamethasone for the indicated times. Actin was used as a loading control. Densitometric analysis of the western blots presented in A and B was carried out using Image J software. The intensity of the bands of Surf-1 (C), SCO2 (D) and COX-Va (E) at each time point was normalised to the intensity of the actin band at the respective time point and the obtained values were plotted. The intensity of the bands in the untreated cells normalised to the intensity of the actin band in the untreated cells was arbitrarily set to 100. The values representing the intensities of the bands in the treated cells were calculated as follows: Intensity of band in treated cells/intensity of actin band in treated cells x 100 / intensity of band in untreated cells/intensity of actin in untreated cells. Black bars represent the CEM-C1-15 cells and the grey bars the CEM-C7-14 cells.

The protein levels of Surf-1, SCO2 and COX-Va were also followed in CEM-C7-14 and CEM-C1-15 cells under the same conditions (Figure 3). Higher Surf-1 protein levels were observed in dexamethasone treated CEM-C7-14 cells compared to the non-treated cells for all time points tested (Figure 3A, B and C compare grey bars 2, 3 and 4 to grey bar 1). In contrast lower Surf-1 protein levels were observed in the dexamethasone treated CEM-C1-15 cells irrespectively of the length of the dexamethasone treatment compared to the untreated cells (Figure 3A, B and C compare black bars 2, 3 and 4 to black bar 1). In a similar manner to that observed for Surf-1, increasing SCO2 protein levels were observed in CEM-C7-14 cells treated with dexamethasone for 12h and 24h compared to the untreated cells (Figure 3A, B and D compare grey bars 2 and 3 to bar 1). On the contrary lower SCO2 protein levels were observed in CEM-C7-14 cells 36h after the addition of dexamethasone compared to the untreated cells (Figure 3A, B and D compare grey bar 4 to grey bar 1). On the other side the SCO2 protein levels in CEM-C1-15 cells were lower than those measured in the untreated cells for all the time points of dexamethasone treatment examined in this study (Figure 3A, B and D compare black bars 2, 3 and 4 to black bar 1). Finally the COX-Va protein levels were higher in both CEM-C1-15 and CEM-C7-14 cells treated with dexamethasone compared to the non-treated cells (Figure 3A, B and E compare black and grey bars 2, 3, and 4 to grey and black bars 1).

The expression of COX subunits and oxidative phosphorylation are affected by glucocorticoid treatment [137] possibly through the GR transcriptional activity. Given that some OXPHOS subunits are encoded by the nuclear genome, and others by the mitochondrial DNA, it was thought that glucocorticoids exert indirect effects on the regulation of transcription of mitochondrial encoded OXPHOS subunits by modulating the activity of nuclear factors involved in the gene expression of mitochondrial genes [101]. However, the identification of mitochondrial GR, and the existence of GRE-like domains in the mitochondrial genome [100, 101, 138] suggest that glucocorticoids exert direct effects on mitochondrial transcription. Taking into consideration the fact that glucocorticoid receptor potentially regulates the expression of several COX assembly factors and nuclear COX subunits (Figure 2A, 2B and 2C) it was interesting to investigate whether GR fine tunes the expression of OXPHOS genes in both nuclear and mitochondrial genomes. In order to assess this hypothesis, and in parallel, to strengthen the perception that energy metabolism is a possible pathway by which CEM cells determine resistance / sensitivity to glucocorticoid induced apoptosis we followed the mRNA levels of the mitochondrial OXPHOS subunits COX-I, COX-II and COX-III in CEM C1-15 and CEM C7-14 cells treated with dexamethasone (Figures 4A, 4B and 4C).

A similar picture to that observed for the nuclear OXPHOS components was observed for the mitochondrial OXPHOS subunits. Specifically higher cellular levels of the mitochondrial COX-I, COX-II and COX-III OXPHOS subunits were observed in CEM-C7-14 compared to CEM-C1-15 cells (Figure 4A-4C). Increased levels of COX-I mRNA in both cell lines after 12 hours of dexamethasone treatment were observed in both CEM-C1-15 and CEM-C7-14 cells (Figure 4A, compare solid with dotted line). COX-II mRNA expression initially decreased in both cell lines 3h after the addition of dexamethasone

(Figure 4B, compare solid and dotted lines 3h point) and then started to increase steadily at 6 and 12h after the treatment with the hormone but it reached higher levels in the CEM-C7-14 cells (Figure 4B, compare solid line with dotted line). COX-III gene expression remains unaffected by glucocorticoid treatment during the first 3 hours, in CEM-C1-15 cells, followed by two fold increase 6h and 12h after hormone addition (Figure 4C, solid line compare 0 time point with 6 and 12h time points). A similar pattern was evident in CEM-C7-14 cells where the induction of COX-III mRNA after 6h and 12h of dexamethasone treatment was four and five fold higher respectively compared to those detected in the untreated cells (Figure 4C, dotted line compare 0 time point with 6 and 12h time points).

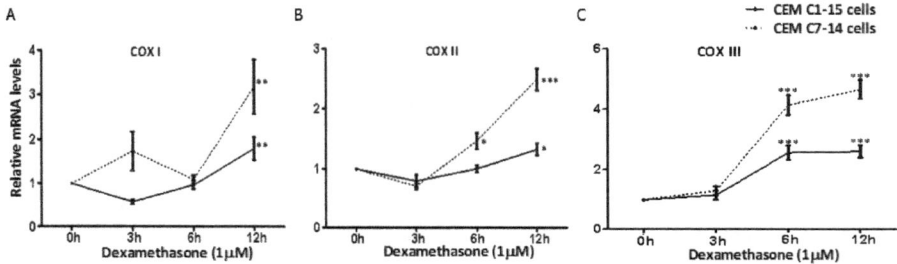

Figure 4. Relative mRNA levels of the mitochondrial OXPHOS subunits COX-I (A), COX-II (B), and COX-III (C) were followed in the resistant CEM-C1-15 and the sensitive CEM-C7-14 to glucocorticoid induced apoptosis ALL cells treated with dexamethasone for the indicated time points by quantitative real-time PCR. Solid lines represent mRNA levels in CEM-C1-15 and dotted lines correspond to mRNA levels determined in CEM-C7-14 cells. Error bars represent standard error of the mean of five independent experiments and asterisks indicate statistical significance of $p<0.05$ compared to the untreated sample.

Taken together, results presented in this manuscript endorse the hypothesis that the glucocorticoid resistance / sensitivity in CEM cells is determined by differences in the efficacy of the OXPHOS system to produce energy in the two cell lines. Support to this conclusion is lent by observations shown in Figure 2A, 2B and 2C indicating that the mRNA levels of nuclear encoded components of the OXPHOS system were higher in the sensitive CEM-C7-14 than in the resistant CEM-C1-15 cells. Higher levels of COX assembly factors in CEM-C7-14 cells imply a more efficient energy metabolism in these cells. This could be a result of distinct signalling pathways operating in the two cell lines giving rise to increased transactivation function of GR in CEM-C7-14 cells, where the receptor could be phosphorylated at S211 [58] and stimulate the expression of its potential transcription targets Surf-1 and COX-Va, whereas on the contrary, it is phosphorylated at S226 in CEM-C1-15 cells, thereby targeted to different subset of its transcriptional targets in these cells [58]. The link between altered metabolism in cancer cells and varying expression of COX subunits has been well established [139, 140, 141]. The presence of mitochondrial GR and of GRE-like domains in the mitochondrial genome [100, 102, 138, 142, 143, 144] and regulation of the mitochondrial COX subunits (COX-I, COX-II and COX-III) provide a probable mechanism explaining the dexamethasone dependent regulation of the mitochondrial COX subunits gene expression (Figure 4). In addition, differences in post translational modifications of the receptor, which in the case of CEM-C7-14 cells, allow activation [58] and possibly translocation of GR into mitochondria [96] while in CEM-C1-15 cells these events are not permissible could be an additional justification for these observations.

8. Conclusions and future perspectives

Resistance to glucocorticoid induced apoptosis in ALL has been attributed to several different processes and pathways including predominance of certain GR isoforms with reduced transcriptional activity [34, 145, 146], either due to altered binding capacity of the receptor to other transcription factors [147, 148, 149, 150] or co-regulators [81, 151], disparate expression and consequent dissimilar balance between pro- versus anti-apoptotic members of the Bcl-2 family [18], GR mitochondrial localisation [97], autophagy [72, 73, 74, 75], and post-translational modifications which affect GR transcription target selectivity and protein stability [22, 38, 89, 152, 153].

We have recently presented evidence to suggest that differential GR phosphorylation in resistant versus sensitive to glucocorticoid induced apoptosis ALL cells results in selective induction of anti-apoptotic and inhibition of pro-apoptotic Bcl-2 family members gene expression in the resistant cells [58]. Several reports have indicated the potential role of differential kinase activity in glucocorticoid resistant and sensitive cells in determining the GR subcellular localisation [96, 98, 154] and diverse effects on the induction of autophagy [72, 73, 74].

In this study we provide new evidence signifying the differential expression of OXPHOS components in glucocorticoid resistant versus sensitive ALL cells and we propose that resistant and sensitive CEM cells use different pathways to produce energy. These results are in accord with reports showing that resistance to GC in ALL is associated with increased glucose consumption [155] with concomitant induction of Mcl-1 expression and resistance to apoptosis [39]. In our anticipated model (Figure 5) in resistant lymphocytes the predominantly phosphorylated at S226 GR is possibly transcriptionally inactive and thus incapable to significantly induce OXPHOS assembly enzymes and COX subunits gene expression or translocate into mitochondria thereby exhibiting reduced oxidative phosphorylation consistent with a proliferative phenotype, and this is probably one of the mechanisms employed by the glucocorticoid-resistant CEM-C1-15 cells to survive GC treatment.

The results presented in this study endorse the hypothesis that differential GR phosphorylation affects components of cellular energy production pathways in distinct ways in resistant versus sensitive cells altering energy production and possibly ROS generation in unique ways in the two cell lines, suggesting that combination of kinase inhibitors, and glycolytic modulators together with dexamethasone could be a possible mean by which resistance to glucocorticoid induced apoptosis could be circumvented in ALL.

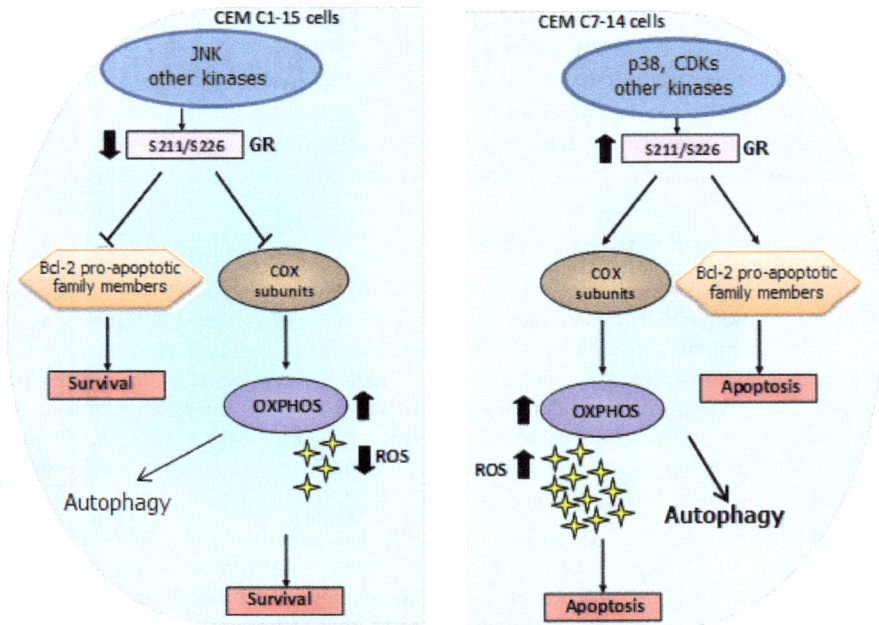

Figure 5. Model summarising the proposed mechanism determining resistance / sensitivity of CEM cells to glucocorticoid-induced apoptosis. Differential phosphorylation of GR in glucocorticoid resistant versus sensitive cells leads to the reduction of gene expression of OXPHOS subunits and pro-apoptotic Bcl-2 family members in the resistant cells (left panel) whereas the opposite is the case for the sensitive cells (right panel).

Author details

Ilhem Berrou, Marija Krstic-Demonacos, Constantinos Demonacos

University of Manchester, School of Pharmacy and Faculty of Life Sciences, Manchester, UK

9. References

[1] Buttgereit F, Saag KG, Cutolo M, da Silva JAP, Bijlsma JWJ (2005) The molecular basis for the effectiveness, toxicity, and resistance to glucocorticoids: focus on the treatment of rheumatoid arthritis. Scand J Rheumatol 34: 14-21.

[2] Sionov RV, Spokoini R, Kfir-Erenfeld S, Cohen O, Yefenof E (2008) Mechanisms regulating the susceptibility of hematopoietic malignancies to glucocorticoid-induced apoptosis. Adv Cancer Res 101: 127-248.

[3] Schmidt S, Rainer J, Ploner C, Presul E, Riml S, et al. (2004) Glucocorticoid-induced apoptosis and glucocorticoid resistance: molecular mechanisms and clinical relevance. Cell Death Differ 11 Suppl 1: S45-55.

[4]   Losel R, Wehling M (2003) Nongenomic actions of steroid hormones. Nat Rev Mol Cell Biol 4: 46-56.

[5]   Buttgereit F, Straub RH, Wehling M, Burmester GR (2004) Glucocorticoids in the treatment of rheumatic diseases: an update on the mechanisms of action. Arthritis Rheum 50: 3408-3417.

[6]   Stellato C (2004) Post-transcriptional and nongenomic effects of glucocorticoids. Proc Am Thorac Soc 1: 255-263.

[7]   Solito E, Mulla A, Morris JF, Christian HC, Flower RJ, et al. (2003) Dexamethasone induces rapid serine-phosphorylation and membrane translocation of annexin 1 in a human folliculostellate cell line via a novel nongenomic mechanism involving the glucocorticoid receptor, protein kinase C, phosphatidylinositol 3-kinase, and mitogen-activated protein kinase. Endocrinology 144: 1164-1174.

[8]   Qiu J, Wang CG, Huang XY, Chen YZ (2003) Nongenomic mechanism of glucocorticoid inhibition of bradykinin-induced calcium influx in PC12 cells: possible involvement of protein kinase C. Life Sci 72: 2533-2542.

[9]   Long F, Wang YX, Liu L, Zhou J, Cui RY, et al. (2005) Rapid nongenomic inhibitory effects of glucocorticoids on phagocytosis and superoxide anion production by macrophages. Steroids 70: 55-61.

[10] Liu L, Wang YX, Zhou J, Long F, Sun HW, et al. (2005) Rapid non-genomic inhibitory effects of glucocorticoids on human neutrophil degranulation. Inflamm Res 54: 37-41.

[11] Koukouritaki SB, Gravanis A, Stournaras C (1999) Tyrosine phosphorylation of focal adhesion kinase and paxillin regulates the signaling mechanism of the rapid nongenomic action of dexamethasone on actin cytoskeleton. Mol Med 5: 731-742.

[12] Löwenberg M, Stahn C, Hommes DW, Buttgereit F (2008) Novel insights into mechanisms of glucocorticoid action and the development of new glucocorticoid receptor ligands. Steroids 73: 1025-1029.

[13] Smith LK, Cidlowski JA (2010) Glucocorticoid-induced apoptosis of healthy and malignant lymphocytes. Prog Brain Res 182: 1-30.

[14] Frankfurt O, Rosen ST (2004) Mechanisms of glucocorticoid-induced apoptosis in hematologic malignancies: updates. Curr Opin Oncol 16: 553-563.

[15] Distelhorst CW (2002) Recent insights into the mechanism of glucocorticosteroid-induced apoptosis. Cell Death Differ 9: 6-19.

[16] Lepine S, Sulpice JC, Giraud F (2005) Signaling pathways involved in glucocorticoid-induced apoptosis of thymocytes. Crit Rev Immunol 25: 263-288.

[17] Thorburn A (2004) Death receptor-induced cell killing. Cell Signal 16: 139-144.

[18] Ploner C, Schmidt S, Presul E, Renner K, Schrocksnadel K, et al. (2005) Glucocorticoid-induced apoptosis and glucocorticoid resistance in acute lymphoblastic leukemia. J Steroid Biochem Mol Biol 93: 153-160.

[19] D'Adamio F, Zollo O, Moraca R, Ayroldi E, Bruscoli S, et al. (1997) A new dexamethasone-induced gene of the leucine zipper family protects T lymphocytes from TCR/CD3-activated cell death. Immunity 7: 803-812.

[20] Ashwell JD, Lu FW, Vacchio MS (2000) Glucocorticoids in T cell development and function. Annu Rev Immunol 18: 309-345.

[21] Planey SL, Abrams MT, Robertson NM, Litwack G (2003) Role of apical caspases and glucocorticoid-regulated genes in glucocorticoid-induced apoptosis of pre-B leukemic cells. Cancer Res 63: 172-178.

[22] Garza AS, Miller AL, Johnson BH, Thompson EB (2009) Converting cell lines representing hematological malignancies from glucocorticoid-resistant to glucocorticoid-sensitive: signaling pathway interactions. Leuk Res 33: 717-727.

[23] Almawi WY, Melemedjian OK, Jaoude MM (2004) On the link between Bcl-2 family proteins and glucocorticoid-induced apoptosis. J Leukoc Biol 76: 7-14.

[24] Bouillet P, Metcalf D, Huang DC, Tarlinton DM, Kay TW, et al. (1999) Proapoptotic Bcl-2 relative Bim required for certain apoptotic responses, leukocyte homeostasis, and to preclude autoimmunity. Science 286: 1735-1738.

[25] Shi Y (2004) Caspase activation, inhibition, and reactivation: a mechanistic view. Protein Sci 13: 1979-1987.

[26] Abrams MT, Robertson NM, Yoon K, Wickstrom E (2004) Inhibition of glucocorticoid-induced apoptosis by targeting the major splice variants of BIM mRNA with small interfering RNA and short hairpin RNA. J Biol Chem 279: 55809-55817.

[27] Iglesias-Serret D, de Frias M, Santidrian AF, Coll-Mulet L, Cosialls AM, et al. (2007) Regulation of the proapoptotic BH3-only protein BIM by glucocorticoids, survival signals and proteasome in chronic lymphocytic leukemia cells. Leukemia 21: 281-287.

[28] Wang Z, Malone MH, He H, McColl KS, Distelhorst CW (2003) Microarray analysis uncovers the induction of the proapoptotic BH3-only protein Bim in multiple models of glucocorticoid-induced apoptosis. J Biol Chem 278: 23861-23867.

[29] Elmore S (2007) Apoptosis: a review of programmed cell death. Toxicol Pathol 35: 495-516.

[30] Lauber K, Appel HA, Schlosser SF, Gregor M, Schulze-Osthoff K, et al. (2001) The adapter protein apoptotic protease-activating factor-1 (Apaf-1) is proteolytically processed during apoptosis. J Biol Chem 276: 29772-29781.

[31] Arai Y, Nakamura Y, Inoue F, Yamamoto K, Saito K, et al. (2000) Glucocorticoid-induced apoptotic pathways in eosinophils: comparison with glucocorticoid-sensitive leukemia cells. Int J Hematol 71: 340-349.

[32] Segal M, Niazi S, Simons MP, Galati SA, Zangrilli JG (2007) Bid activation during induction of extrinsic and intrinsic apoptosis in eosinophils. Immunol Cell Biol 85: 518-524.

[33] Kaufmann T, Tai L, Ekert PG, Huang DC, Norris F, et al. (2007) The BH3-only protein bid is dispensable for DNA damage- and replicative stress-induced apoptosis or cell-cycle arrest. Cell 129: 423-433.

[34] Oakley RH, Cidlowski JA (2011) Cellular processing of the glucocorticoid receptor gene and protein: new mechanisms for generating tissue-specific actions of glucocorticoids. J Biol Chem 286: 3177-3184.

[35] Evans RM (1988) The steroid and thyroid hormone receptor superfamily. Science 240: 889-895.

[36] Yamamoto KR (1985) Steroid receptor regulated transcription of specific genes and gene networks. Annu Rev Genet 19: 209-252.

[37] Ploner C, Rainer J, Niederegger H, Eduardoff M, Villunger A, et al. (2008) The BCL2 rheostat in glucocorticoid-induced apoptosis of acute lymphoblastic leukemia. Leukemia 22: 370-377.

[38] Kfir-Erenfeld S, Sionov RV, Spokoini R, Cohen O, Yefenof E (2010) Protein kinase networks regulating glucocorticoid-induced apoptosis of hematopoietic cancer cells: fundamental aspects and practical considerations. Leuk Lymphoma 51: 1968-2005.

[39] Beesley AH, Weller RE, Senanayake S, Welch M, Kees UR (2009) Receptor mutation is not a common mechanism of naturally occurring glucocorticoid resistance in leukaemia cell lines. Leuk Res 33: 321-325.

[40] Medh RD, Webb MS, Miller AL, Johnson BH, Fofanov Y, et al. (2003) Gene expression profile of human lymphoid CEM cells sensitive and resistant to glucocorticoid-evoked apoptosis. Genomics 81: 543-555.

[41] Herold MJ, McPherson KG, Reichardt HM (2006) Glucocorticoids in T cell apoptosis and function. Cell Mol Life Sci 63: 60-72.

[42] Helmberg A, Auphan N, Caelles C, Karin M (1995) Glucocorticoid-induced apoptosis of human leukemic cells is caused by the repressive function of the glucocorticoid receptor. EMBO J 14: 452-460.

[43] Zhou J, Cidlowski JA (2005) The human glucocorticoid receptor: one gene, multiple proteins and diverse responses. Steroids 70: 407-417.

[44] Oakley RH, Jewell CM, Yudt MR, Bofetiado DM, Cidlowski JA (1999) The dominant negative activity of the human glucocorticoid receptor beta isoform. Specificity and mechanisms of action. J Biol Chem 274: 27857-27866.

[45] Kino T, Liou SH, Charmandari E, Chrousos GP (2004) Glucocorticoid receptor mutants demonstrate increased motility inside the nucleus of living cells: time of fluorescence recovery after photobleaching (FRAP) is an integrated measure of receptor function. Mol Med 10: 80-88.

[46] Hillmann AG, Ramdas J, Multanen K, Norman MR, Harmon JM (2000) Glucocorticoid receptor gene mutations in leukemic cells acquired in vitro and in vivo. Cancer Res 60: 2056-2062.

[47] Zilberman Y, Zafrir E, Ovadia H, Yefenof E, Guy R, et al. (2004) The glucocorticoid receptor mediates the thymic epithelial cell-induced apoptosis of CD4+8+ thymic lymphoma cells. Cell Immunol 227: 12-23.

[48] Webster JC, Oakley RH, Jewell CM, Cidlowski JA (2001) Proinflammatory cytokines regulate human glucocorticoid receptor gene expression and lead to the accumulation of the dominant negative beta isoform: a mechanism for the generation of glucocorticoid resistance. Proc Natl Acad Sci U S A 98: 6865-6870.

[49] Youle RJ, Strasser A (2008) The BCL-2 protein family: opposing activities that mediate cell death. Nat Rev Mol Cell Biol 9: 47-59.

[50] Hartmann BL, Geley S, Loffler M, Hattmannstorfer R, Strasser-Wozak EM, et al. (1999) Bcl-2 interferes with the execution phase, but not upstream events, in glucocorticoid-induced leukemia apoptosis. Oncogene 18: 713-719.

[51] Broome HE, Yu AL, Diccianni M, Camitta BM, Monia BP, et al. (2002) Inhibition of Bcl-xL expression sensitizes T-cell acute lymphoblastic leukemia cells to chemotherapeutic drugs. Leuk Res 26: 311-316.

[52] Bailly-Maitre B, de Sousa G, Boulukos K, Gugenheim J, Rahmani R (2001) Dexamethasone inhibits spontaneous apoptosis in primary cultures of human and rat hepatocytes via Bcl-2 and Bcl-xL induction. Cell Death Differ 8: 279-288.

[53] Huang ST, Cidlowski JA (2002) Phosphorylation status modulates Bcl-2 function during glucocorticoid-induced apoptosis in T lymphocytes. FASEB J 16: 825-832.

[54] Lu J, Quearry B, Harada H (2006) p38-MAP kinase activation followed by BIM induction is essential for glucocorticoid-induced apoptosis in lymphoblastic leukemia cells. FEBS Lett 580: 3539-3544.

[55] Salomons GS, Brady HJM, Verwijs-Janssen M, Van Den Berg JD, Hart AAM, et al. (1997) The Baxα:Bcl-2 ratio modulates the response to dexamethasone in leukaemic cells and is highly variable in childhood acute leukaemia. Int J Cancer 71: 959-965.

[56] Wei G, Twomey D, Lamb J, Schlis K, Agarwal J, et al. (2006) Gene expression-based chemical genomics identifies rapamycin as a modulator of MCL1 and glucocorticoid resistance. Cancer Cell 10: 331-342.

[57] Alves NL, Derks IA, Berk E, Spijker R, van Lier RA, et al. (2006) The Noxa/Mcl-1 axis regulates susceptibility to apoptosis under glucose limitation in dividing T cells. Immunity 24: 703-716.

[58] Lynch JT, Rajendran R, Xenaki G, Berrou I, Demonacos C, et al. (2010) The role of glucocorticoid receptor phosphorylation in Mcl-1 and NOXA gene expression. Mol Cancer 9: 38.

[59] Jiang N, Koh GS, Lim JY, Kham SK, Ariffin H, et al. (2011) BIM is a prognostic biomarker for early prednisolone response in pediatric acute lymphoblastic leukemia. Exp Hematol 39: 321-329.

[60] Schmidt S, Rainer J, Riml S, Ploner C, Jesacher S, et al. (2006) Identification of glucocorticoid-response genes in children with acute lymphoblastic leukemia. Blood 107: 2061-2069.

[61] Bouillet P, Metcalf D, Huang DCS, Tarlinton DM, Kay TWH, et al. (1999) Proapoptotic Bcl-2 Relative Bim Required for Certain Apoptotic Responses, Leukocyte Homeostasis, and to Preclude Autoimmunity. Science 286: 1735-1738.

[62] Villunger A, Michalak EM, Coultas L, Mullauer F, Bock G, et al. (2003) p53- and drug-induced apoptotic responses mediated by BH3-only proteins puma and noxa. Science 302: 1036-1038.

[63] Herr I, Gassler N, Friess H, Büchler M (2007) Regulation of differential pro- and anti-apoptotic signaling by glucocorticoids. Apoptosis 12: 271-291.

[64] Memon SA, Moreno MB, Petrak D, Zacharchuk CM (1995) Bcl-2 blocks glucocorticoid-but not Fas- or activation-induced apoptosis in a T cell hybridoma. J Immunol 155: 4644-4652.

[65] Erlacher M, Michalak EM, Kelly PN, Labi V, Niederegger H, et al. (2005) BH3-only proteins Puma and Bim are rate-limiting for gamma-radiation- and glucocorticoid-induced apoptosis of lymphoid cells in vivo. Blood 106: 4131-4138.

[66] Real PJ, Tosello V, Palomero T, Castillo M, Hernando E, et al. (2009) Gamma-secretase inhibitors reverse glucocorticoid resistance in T cell acute lymphoblastic leukemia. Nat Med 15: 50-58.

[67] Hoijman E, Rocha Viegas L, Keller Sarmiento MI, Rosenstein RE, Pecci A (2004) Involvement of Bax protein in the prevention of glucocorticoid-induced thymocytes apoptosis by melatonin. Endocrinology 145: 418-425.

[68] Rathmell JC, Lindsten T, Zong WX, Cinalli RM, Thompson CB (2002) Deficiency in Bak and Bax perturbs thymic selection and lymphoid homeostasis. Nat Immunol 3: 932-939.

[69] Fésüs L, Demény MÁ, Petrovski G (2011) Autophagy shapes inflammation Antioxid Redox Signal 14: 2233-2243.

[70] Mizushima N (2007) Autophagy: process and function. Genes Dev 21: 2861-2873.

[71] Chen S, Rehman SK, Zhang W, Wan A, Yao L, et al. (2010) Autophagy is a therapeutic target in anticancer drug resistance. Biochim Biophys Acta 1806: 220-229.

[72] Grander D, Kharaziha P, Laane E, Pokrovskaja K, Panaretakis T (2009) Autophagy as the main means of cytotoxicity by glucocorticoids in hematological malignancies. Autophagy 5: 1198-1200.

[73] Laane E, Tamm KP, Buentke E, Ito K, Khahariza P, et al. (2009) Cell death induced by dexamethasone in lymphoid leukemia is mediated through initiation of autophagy. Cell Death Differ 16: 1018-1029.

[74] Bonapace L, Bornhauser BC, Schmitz M, Cario G, Ziegler U, et al. (2010) Induction of autophagy-dependent necroptosis is required for childhood acute lymphoblastic leukemia cells to overcome glucocorticoid resistance. J Clin Invest 120: 1310-1323.

[75] Heidari N, Hicks MA, Harada H (2010) GX15-070 (obatoclax) overcomes glucocorticoid resistance in acute lymphoblastic leukemia through induction of apoptosis and autophagy. Cell Death Dis 1: e76.

[76] Yu L, Wan F, Dutta S, Welsh S, Liu Z, et al. (2006) Autophagic programmed cell death by selective catalase degradation. Proc Natl Acad Sci U S A 103: 4952-4957.

[77] Luecke HF, Yamamoto KR (2005) The glucocorticoid receptor blocks P-TEFb recruitment by NFkappaB to effect promoter-specific transcriptional repression. Genes Dev 19: 1116-1127.

[78] De Bosscher K, Vanden Berghe W, Haegeman G (2000) Mechanisms of anti-inflammatory action and of immunosuppression by glucocorticoids: negative interference of activated glucocorticoid receptor with transcription factors. J Neuroimmunol 109: 16-22.

[79] Nawata H, Okabe T, Yanase T, Nomura M (2008) Mechanism of action and resistance to glucocorticoid and selective glucocorticoid receptor modulator to overcome glucocorticoid-related adverse effects. Clinical & Experimental Allergy Reviews 8: 53-56.

[80] Perissi V, Rosenfeld MG (2005) Controlling nuclear receptors: the circular logic of cofactor cycles. Nat Rev Mol Cell Biol 6: 542-554.

[81] Davies L, Paraskevopoulou E, Sadeq M, Symeou C, Pantelidou C, et al. (2011) Regulation of glucocorticoid receptor activity by a stress responsive transcriptional cofactor. Mol Endocrinol 25: 58-71.

[82] Nader N, Chrousos GP, Kino T (2009) Circadian rhythm transcription factor CLOCK regulates the transcriptional activity of the glucocorticoid receptor by acetylating its hinge region lysine cluster: potential physiological implications. FASEB J 23: 1572-1583.

[83] Matthews JG, Ito K, Barnes PJ, Adcock IM (2004) Defective glucocorticoid receptor nuclear translocation and altered histone acetylation patterns in glucocorticoid-resistant patients. J Allergy Clin Immunol 113: 1100-1108.

[84] Wallace AD, Cidlowski JA (2001) Proteasome-mediated glucocorticoid receptor degradation restricts transcriptional signaling by glucocorticoids. J Biol Chem 276: 42714-42721.

[85] Deroo BJ, Rentsch C, Sampath S, Young J, DeFranco DB, et al. (2002) Proteasomal inhibition enhances glucocorticoid receptor transactivation and alters its subnuclear trafficking. Mol Cell Biol 22: 4113-4123.

[86] Holmstrom S, Van Antwerp ME, Iniguez-Lluhi JA (2003) Direct and distinguishable inhibitory roles for SUMO isoforms in the control of transcriptional synergy. Proc Natl Acad Sci U S A 100: 15758-15763.

[87] Tian S, Poukka H, Palvimo JJ, Janne OA (2002) Small ubiquitin-related modifier-1 (SUMO-1) modification of the glucocorticoid receptor. Biochem J 367: 907-911.

[88] Le Drean Y, Mincheneau N, Le Goff P, Michel D (2002) Potentiation of glucocorticoid receptor transcriptional activity by sumoylation. Endocrinology 143: 3482-3489.

[89] Davies L, Karthikeyan N, Lynch JT, Sial EA, Gkourtsa A, et al. (2008) Cross talk of signaling pathways in the regulation of the glucocorticoid receptor function. Mol Endocrinol 22: 1331-1344.

[90] Krstic MD, Rogatsky I, Yamamoto KR, Garabedian MJ (1997) Mitogen-activated and cyclin-dependent protein kinases selectively and differentially modulate transcriptional enhancement by the glucocorticoid receptor. Mol Cell Biol 17: 3947-3954.

[91] Hoeck W, Groner B (1990) Hormone-dependent phosphorylation of the glucocorticoid receptor occurs mainly in the amino-terminal transactivation domain. J Biol Chem 265: 5403-5408.

[92] Ismaili N, Garabedian MJ (2004) Modulation of glucocorticoid receptor function via phosphorylation. Ann N Y Acad Sci 1024: 86-101.

[93] Beck IM, Vanden Berghe W, Vermeulen L, Yamamoto KR, Haegeman G, et al. (2009) Crosstalk in inflammation: the interplay of glucocorticoid receptor-based mechanisms and kinases and phosphatases. Endocr Rev 30: 830-882.

[94] Galliher-Beckley AJ, Cidlowski JA (2009) Emerging roles of glucocorticoid receptor phosphorylation in modulating glucocorticoid hormone action in health and disease. IUBMB Life 61: 979-986.

[95] Galliher-Beckley AJ, Williams JG, Cidlowski JA (2011) Ligand-independent phosphorylation of the glucocorticoid receptor integrates cellular stress pathways with nuclear receptor signaling. Mol Cell Biol 31: 4663-4675.

[96] Adzic M, Djordjevic A, Demonacos C, Krstic-Demonacos M, Radojcic MB (2009) The role of phosphorylated glucocorticoid receptor in mitochondrial functions and apoptotic signalling in brain tissue of stressed Wistar rats. Int J Biochem Cell Biol 41: 2181-2188.

[97] Sionov RV, Cohen O, Kfir S, Zilberman Y, Yefenof E (2006) Role of mitochondrial glucocorticoid receptor in glucocorticoid-induced apoptosis. J Exp Med 203: 189-201.

[98] Hock MB, Kralli A (2009) Transcriptional Control of Mitochondrial Biogenesis and Function. Ann Rev Physiol. Palo Alto: Annual Reviews. pp. 177-203.

[99] Scheller K, Sekeris CE (2003) The effects of steroid hormones on the transcription of genes encoding enzymes of oxidative phosphorylation. Exp Physiol 88: 129-140.

[100] Demonacos CV, Karayanni N, Hatzoglou E, Tsiriyiotis C, Spandidos DA, et al. (1996) Mitochondrial genes as sites of primary action of steroid hormones. Steroids 61: 226-232.

[101] Demonacos C, Tsawdaroglou NC, Djordjevic-Markovic R, Papalopoulou M, Galanopoulos V, et al. (1993) Import of the glucocorticoid receptor into rat liver mitochondria in vivo and in vitro. J Steroid Biochem Mol Biol 46: 401-413.

[102] Demonacos C, Djordjevic-Markovic R, Tsawdaroglou N, Sekeris CE (1995) The mitochondrion as a primary site of action of glucocorticoids: the interaction of the glucocorticoid receptor with mitochondrial DNA sequences showing partial similarity to the nuclear glucocorticoid responsive elements. J Steroid Biochem Mol Biol 55: 43-55.

[103] Sionov RV, Kfir S, Zafrir E, Cohen O, Zilberman Y, et al. (2006) Glucocorticoid-induced apoptosis revisited: a novel role for glucocorticoid receptor translocation to the mitochondria. Cell Cycle 5: 1017-1026.

[104] Kondoh H, Lleonart ME, Gil J, Wang J, Degan P, et al. (2005) Glycolytic enzymes can modulate cellular life span. Cancer Res 65: 177-185.

[105] Kwong JQ, Henning MS, Starkov AA, Manfredi G (2007) The mitochondrial respiratory chain is a modulator of apoptosis. J Cell Biol 179: 1163-1177.

[106] Cuezva JM, Krajewska M, de Heredia ML, Krajewski S, Santamaria G, et al. (2002) The bioenergetic signature of cancer: a marker of tumor progression. Cancer Res 62: 6674-6681.

[107] Lemarie A, Grimm S (2011) Mitochondrial respiratory chain complexes: apoptosis sensors mutated in cancer? Oncogene 30: 3985-4003.

[108] Tomiyama A, Serizawa S, Tachibana K, Sakurada K, Samejima H, et al. (2006) Critical role for mitochondrial oxidative phosphorylation in the activation of tumor suppressors Bax and Bak. J Natl Cancer Inst 98: 1462-1473.

[109] Huang G, Chen Y, Lu H, Cao X (2007) Coupling mitochondrial respiratory chain to cell death: an essential role of mitochondrial complex I in the interferon-[beta] and retinoic acid-induced cancer cell death. Cell Death Differ 14: 327-337.

[110] Coenen MJ, van den Heuvel LP, Smeitink JA (2001) Mitochondrial oxidative phosphorylation system assembly in man: recent achievements. Curr Opin Neurol 14: 777-781.

[111] Fontanesi F, Soto IC, Horn D, Barrientos A (2006) Assembly of mitochondrial cytochrome c-oxidase, a complicated and highly regulated cellular process. Am J Physiol Cell Physiol 291: C1129-C1147.

[112] Weber K, Brück P, Mikes Z, Küpper J-H, Klingenspor M, et al. (2002) Glucocorticoid hormone stimulates mitochondrial biogenesis specifically in skeletal muscle. Endocrinology 143: 177-184.

[113] Van Itallie CM (1992) Dexamethasone treatment increases mitochondrial RNA synthesis in a rat hepatoma cell line. Endocrinology 130: 567-576.

[114] Kulinsky V, Kolesnichenko L (2007) Regulation of metabolic and energetic functions of mitochondria by hormones and signal transduction systems. Biochemistry (Moscow) Supplemental Series B: Biomedical Chemistry 1: 95-113.

[115] Ritz P, Dumas JF, Ducluzeau PH, Simard G (2005) Hormonal regulation of mitochondrial energy production. Curr Opin Clin Nutr Metab Care 8: 415-418.

[116] Vijayasarathy C, Biunno I, Lenka N, Yang M, Basu A, et al. (1998) Variations in the subunit content and catalytic activity of the cytochrome c oxidase complex from different tissues and different cardiac compartments. Biochim Biophys Acta 1371: 71-82.

[117] Martens ME, Peterson PL, Lee CP (1991) In vitro effects of glucocorticoid on mitochondrial energy metabolism. Biochim Biophys Acta 1058: 152-160.

[118] Pandya JD, Agarwal NA, Katyare SS (2007) Dexamethasone treatment differentially affects the oxidative energy metabolism of rat brain mitochondria in developing and adult animals. Int J Dev Neurosci 25: 309-316.

[119] Holleman A, den Boer ML, Kazemier KM, Janka-Schaub GE, Pieters R (2003) Resistance to different classes of drugs is associated with impaired apoptosis in childhood acute lymphoblastic leukemia. Blood 102: 4541-4546.

[120] Hulleman E, Kazemier KM, Holleman A, VanderWeele DJ, Rudin CM, et al. (2009) Inhibition of glycolysis modulates prednisolone resistance in acute lymphoblastic leukemia cells. Blood 113: 2014-2021.

[121] Adebodun F (1999) Phospholipid metabolism and resistance to glucocorticoid-induced apoptosis in a human leukemic cell line: a 31P-NMR study using a phosphonium analog of choline. Cancer Lett 140: 189-194.

[122] Brown GC, Borutaite V (2008) Regulation of apoptosis by the redox state of cytochrome c. Biochim Biophys Acta 1777: 877-881.

[123] Carlet M, Janjetovic K, Rainer J, Schmidt S, Panzer-Grumayer R, et al. (2010) Expression, regulation and function of phosphofructo-kinase/fructose-biphosphatases (PFKFBs) in glucocorticoid-induced apoptosis of acute lymphoblastic leukemia cells. BMC Cancer 10: 638.

[124] Dong H, Zitt C, Auriga C, Hatzelmann A, Epstein PM (2010) Inhibition of PDE3, PDE4 and PDE7 potentiates glucocorticoid-induced apoptosis and overcomes glucocorticoid resistance in CEM T leukemic cells. Biochem Pharmacol 79: 321-329.

[125] Vander Kooi BT, Onuma H, Oeser JK, Svitek CA, Allen SR, et al. (2005) The glucose-6-phosphatase catalytic subunit gene promoter contains both positive and negative glucocorticoid response elements. Mol Endocrinol 19: 3001-3022.

[126] Lange AJ, Espinet C, Hall R, El-Maghrabi MR, Vargas AM, et al. (1992) Regulation of gene expression of rat skeletal muscle/liver 6- phosphofructo-2-kinase/fructose-2, 6-bisphosphatase: Isolation and characterization of a glucocorticoid response element in the first intron of the gene. J Biol Chem 267: 15673-15680.

[127] Datson NA, Van Der Perk J, De Kloet ER, Vreugdenhil E (2001) Identification of corticosteroid-responsive genes in rat hippocampus using serial analysis of gene expression. Eur J Neurosci 14: 675-689.

[128] Datson NA, Morsink MC, Meijer OC, de Kloet ER (2008) Central corticosteroid actions: Search for gene targets. Eur J Pharmacol 583: 272-289.

[129] Zhao F, Xuan Z, Liu L, Zhang MQ (2005) TRED: a Transcriptional Regulatory Element Database and a platform for in silico gene regulation studies. Nucleic Acids Res 33: D103-107.

[130] Marinescu VD, Kohane IS, Riva A (2005) MAPPER: a search engine for the computational identification of putative transcription factor binding sites in multiple genomes. BMC Bioinformatics 6: 79.

[131] Kolchanov NA, Merkulova TI, Ignatieva EV, Ananko EA, Oshchepkov DY, et al. (2007) Combined experimental and computational approaches to study the regulatory elements in eukaryotic genes. Brief Bioinform 8: 266-274.

[132] Yang H, Brosel S, Acin-Perez R, Slavkovich V, Nishino I, et al. (2010) Analysis of mouse models of cytochrome c oxidase deficiency owing to mutations in Sco2. Hum Mol Genet 19: 170-180.

[133] Fontanesi F, Soto IC, Horn C, Barrientos A (2006) Assembly of mitochondrial cytochrome c-oxidase, a complicated and highly regulated cellular process. Am J Physiol Cell Physiol 291: C1129-1147.

[134] Fernandez-Vizarra E, Tiranti V, Zeviani M (2009) Assembly of the oxidative phosphorylation system in humans: what we have learned by studying its defects. Biochim Biophys Acta 1793: 200-211.

[135] Harmon JM, Thompson EB (1981) Isolation and characterization of dexamethasone-resistant mutants from human lymphoid cell line CEM-C7. Mol Cell Biol 1: 512-521.

[136] Williams SL, Valnot I, Rustin P, Taanman JW (2004) Cytochrome c oxidase subassemblies in fibroblast cultures from patients carrying mutations in COX10, SCO1, or SURF1. J Biol Chem 279: 7462-7469.

[137] Rachamim N, Latter H, Malinir N, Asher C, Wald H, et al. (1995) Dexamethasone enhances expression of mitochondrial oxidative phosphorylation genes in rat distal colon. Am J Physiol 269: C1305-C1310.

[138] Sekeris CE (1990) The mitochondrial genome: a possible primary site of action of steroid hormones. In Vivo 4: 317-320.

[139] Herrmann JM, Funes S (2005) Biogenesis of cytochrome oxidase-sophisticated assembly lines in the mitochondrial inner membrane. Gene 354: 43-52.

[140] Krieg RC, Knuechel R, Schiffmann E, Liotta LA, Petricoin EF, 3rd, et al. (2004) Mitochondrial proteome: cancer-altered metabolism associated with cytochrome c oxidase subunit level variation. Proteomics 4: 2789-2795.

[141] Grandjean F, Bremaud L, Robert J, Ratinaud MH (2002) Alterations in the expression of cytochrome c oxidase subunits in doxorubicin-resistant leukemia K562 cells. Biochem Pharmacol 63: 823-831.

[142] Scheller K, Sekeris CE (2003) The effects of steroid hormones on the transcription of genes encoding enzymes of oxidative phosphorylation. Exp Physiol 88: 129-140.

[143] Chen JQ, Eshete M, Alworth WL, Yager JD (2004) Binding of MCF-7 cell mitochondrial proteins and recombinant human estrogen receptors α and β to human mitochondrial dna estrogen response elements. J Cell Biochem 93: 358-373.

[144] Chen JQ, Eshete M, Alworth WL, Yager JD (2004) Binding of MCF-7 cell mitochondrial proteins and recombinant human estrogen receptors alpha and beta to human mitochondrial DNA estrogen response elements. J Cell Biochem 93: 358-373.

[145] Pujols L, Xaubet A, Ramirez J, Mullol J, Roca-Ferrer J, et al. (2004) Expression of glucocorticoid receptors alpha and beta in steroid sensitive and steroid insensitive interstitial lung diseases. Thorax 59: 687-693.

[146] Rainer J, Lelong J, Bindreither D, Mantinger C, Ploner C, et al. (2012) Research resource: transcriptional response to glucocorticoids in childhood acute lymphoblastic leukemia. Mol Endocrinol 26: 178-193.

[147] De Bosscher K, Vanden Berghe W, Haegeman G (2003) The interplay between the glucocorticoid receptor and nuclear factor-kappaB or activator protein-1: molecular mechanisms for gene repression. Endocr Rev 24: 488-522.

[148] Ma J, Xie Y, Shi Y, Qin W, Zhao B, et al. (2008) Glucocorticoid-induced apoptosis requires FOXO3A activity. Biochem Biophys Res Commun 377: 894-898.

[149] Nicholson L, Hall AG, Redfern CP, Irving J (2010) NFkappaB modulators in a model of glucocorticoid resistant, childhood acute lymphoblastic leukemia. Leuk Res 34: 1366-1373.

[150] Tissing WJ, Meijerink JP, den Boer ML, Pieters R (2003) Molecular determinants of glucocorticoid sensitivity and resistance in acute lymphoblastic leukemia. Leukemia 17: 17-25.

[151] Sivils JC, Storer CL, Galigniana MD, Cox MB (2011) Regulation of steroid hormone receptor function by the 52-kDa FK506-binding protein (FKBP52). Curr Opin Pharmacol 11: 314-319.

[152] Chen W, Dang T, Blind RD, Wang Z, Cavasotto CN, et al. (2008) Glucocorticoid receptor phosphorylation differentially affects target gene expression. Mol Endocrinol 22: 1754-1766.

[153] Miller AL, Webb MS, Copik AJ, Wang Y, Johnson BH, et al. (2005) p38 Mitogen-activated protein kinase (MAPK) is a key mediator in glucocorticoid-induced apoptosis of lymphoid cells: correlation between p38 MAPK activation and site-specific phosphorylation of the human glucocorticoid receptor at serine 211. Mol Endocrinol 19: 1569-1583.

[154] Itoh M, Adachi M, Yasui H, Takekawa M, Tanaka H, et al. (2002) Nuclear export of glucocorticoid receptor is enhanced by c-Jun N-terminal kinase-mediated phosphorylation. Mol Endocrinol 16: 2382-2392.

[155] Bhadri VA, Trahair TN, Lock RB (2011) Glucocorticoid resistance in paediatric acute lymphoblastic leukaemia. J Paediatr Child Health.

Chapter 8

The Role of GILZ in Anti-Inflammatory and Immunosuppressive Actions of Glucocorticoids

Huapeng Fan and Eric F. Morand

Additional information is available at the end of the chapter

1. Introduction

Chronic inflammatory diseases place a social and financial burden on society. Glucocorticoids, a class of steroid hormones existing in almost every vertebrate, have been exploited for more than 60 years as a therapeutic option for the inflammatory diseases. For example, the therapeutic effects of synthetic glucocorticoids, first observed in rheumatoid arthritis (RA), led to the awarding of a Nobel prize in 1950 (Slocumb et al., 1950). Based on their rapid, profound and wide-ranging effects, glucocorticoids are a mainstay of treatment for virtually all inflammatory diseases besides RA, and now are among the most frequently prescribed of all medications (Hillier, 2007). Indeed, a community practice survey in 2000 indicated that up to 1% of the entire adult population is taking systemic glucocorticoids at any given time (van Staa et al., 2000). Glucocorticoids have widespread systemic effects, particularly on the inflammation and immune response (Barnes, 2006; Chrousos, 1995). However, glucocorticoids are associated with dose dependent side effects, including diabetes mellitus, osteoporosis, weight gain, and hypertension (Huscher et al., 2009), as well as increased risk of cardiovascular events (Davis et al., 2007). Much effort has been expended identifying glucocorticoid anti-inflammatory mechanisms of action (Barnes, 2006; Schaïcke et al., 2002). Understanding of the mechanism of action of glucocorticoids is essential in order to devise better ways to treat inflammatory disease, ideally retaining the beneficial effects of glucocorticoids but not their adverse effects.

The discovery of a glucocorticoid-induced protein that could emulate the beneficial, but not harmful, effects of glucocorticoids, would represent a landmark in inflammation translational research on a glucocorticoid alternative therapy. Glucocorticoid induced leucine zipper (GILZ) may be such a candidate molecule. GILZ was first identified in 1997 in a gene extraction library, where it was found to be dramatically induced by dexamethasone (D'Adamio et al., 1997). Subsequent studies, mostly utilizing forced over expression of GILZ have ascertained that GILZ has anti-inflammatory functions that include interactions with the NF-κB and AP-1 pathways (Di Marco *et al.*, 2007; Mittelstadt & Ashwell, 2001), which closely mimics the anti-inflammatory effects of glucocorticoids. Moreover, it has recently been shown that GILZ is also expressed in rheumatoid arthritis (RA) synovial tissues, where it exerts inhibitory effects on cytokine expression, and inhibiting the expression of GILZ results in exacerbation of disease in a mouse model of RA. As we will summarise in this Chapter, GILZ is a pivotal endogenous regulator of inflammation and immune responses, which could represent a potential new therapeutic alternate to glucocorticoids.

2. GILZ structure and expression

2.1. Molecular structure of GILZ

As shown in **Fig 1**, GILZ, also named TSC22 domain family protein 3 (TSC22D3), is a 137-amino acid protein, consisting of three major domains: the N-terminal (1-75 aa), leucine zipper (76-97 aa), and C-terminal domains (98-137 aa) (Beaulieu & Morand, 2011). To date, four isoforms of GILZ have been characterized as splice variants from the *Tsc22d* gene and named GILZ1-4 (Soundararajan *et al.*, 2007). The leucine zipper motif of GILZ is located in the central part of the protein and mainly mediates the homodimerization of GILZ required for many of its functions (Di Marco *et al.*, 2007), while the other two domains are responsible for protein-protein interactions between GILZ and transcription factors and signaling molecules. For example, the C-terminal of GILZ is a proline-rich region necessary for direct binding of GILZ to the p65 subunit of NF-κB (Di Marco *et al.*, 2007; Riccardi *et al.*, 2001). In 2001, Aryoldi and colleagues showed that the over expression of GILZ in T cells inhibits the activation of NF-κB by binding the p65 subunit of NF-κB and preventing its nuclear translocation (Ayroldi *et al.*, 2001). GILZ was co-precipitated with the p65 subunit of NF-κB in macrophages stimulated with glucocorticoids, and expression of GILZ with an NF-κB reporter inhibits reporter activity (Berrebi *et al.*, 2003). The N-terminal domain of GILZ directly binds with the upstream MAP kinase pathway activating molecule Raf-1, to inhibit its function. The interaction between GILZ and c-Fos and c-Jun (two constituents of AP-1) also occurs via the N-terminal domain of GILZ. Moreover, GILZ also binds to Ras via its tuberous sclerosis complex (TSC) box (61-75 aa), or even interacts with Ras and Raf together to form a trimer.

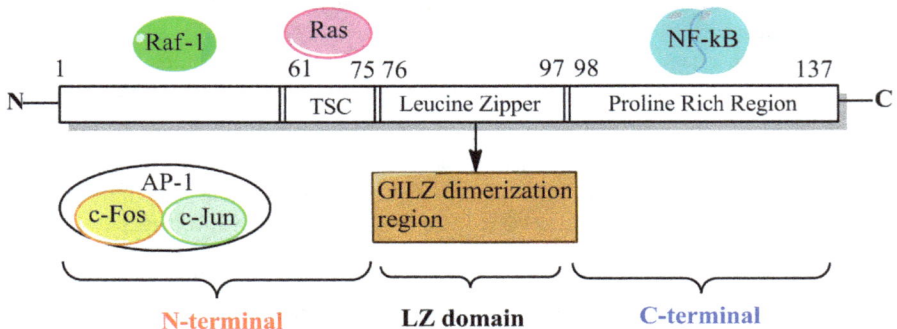

Figure 1. Functional domains of GILZ

2.2. Expression of GILZ

GILZ gene expression is exquisitely sensitive to induction by glucocorticoids. For example, in human RA synovial fibroblasts, dexamethasone (Dex), a synthetic drug derived from glucocorticoid class of steroid, induced a more than 10-fold increase in GILZ transcripts at a concentration of only 1 nM, while 100 nM dexamethasone increased GILZ mRNA by over 100-fold (Beaulieu et al., 2010a). In vivo, exogenous glucocorticoids induce GILZ expression, while blockade of endogenous glucocorticoids inhibits GILZ expression in mouse, and GILZ expression is reduced in response to reductions in circulating cortisol in humans (Beaulieu et al., 2010a; Lekva et al., 2009). The dramatic effect of glucocorticoids on GILZ is mediated via the direct binding of the glucocorticoid/glucocorticoid receptor (GR) complex to six glucocorticoid-responsive elements (GREs) located in the promoter region of the GILZ gene. The GILZ promoter also contains two functional forkhead-responsive elements (FHREs), which when bound to the transcription factor forkhead box O 3 (FoxO3) facilitate maximal GILZ expression induced by glucocorticoid receptor binding (Asselin-Labat et al., 2005b).

Although GILZ expression is mainly controlled by glucocorticoids (Beaulieu et al., 2010b; Berrebi et al., 2003; Eddleston et al., 2007a), it is also modulated by a variety of cytokines (Eddleston et al., 2007a). For example, GILZ is up-regulated by IL-10 (Berrebi et al., 2003), IL-15 and TGF-β (Ayroldi & Riccardi, 2009; Cohen et al., 2006a), whereas GILZ is down-regulated by IL-2 in some cell types IL-2 can inhibit FoxO3 transcriptional activity, thus inhibiting glucocorticoid induced GILZ expression (Asselin-Labat et al., 2005a). Some inflammatory stimuli, such as tumor necrosis factor (TNF) and lipopolysaccharide (LPS), were also found to reduce GILZ mRNA expression in fibroblast like synoviocytes (Beaulieu et al., 2010b). GILZ expression can also be regulated by other anti-inflammatory molecule such as Annexin A1. Yang et al have reported that in Annexin A1 deficient cells, dexamethasone failed to significantly induce GILZ, in contrast to wild type cells (Yang et al., 2009), which indicates a regulatory role of Annexin A1 on GILZ expression.

Interestingly, GILZ expression is also modulated by the oxygen environment. Wang and colleagues recently found that hypoxia not only remarkably upregulated the expression of GILZ, but also significantly enhanced Dex-induced expression of GILZ in macrophages and the spleen of rats (Wang et al., 2011). They also reported ERK MAP kinase activity is involved in the upregulation of GILZ induced by hypoxia.

To date, GILZ has been discovered to be expressed in a variety of tissues (**Table 1**). This information indicates a widespread distribution of GILZ in the human body and suggests it is well placed for a role as a pivotal regulator of inflammation. Moreover, growing evidence showed that GILZ is present in a wide range of cell types that are sensitive to glucocorticoids in vitro. In 1997, GILZ was first identified in T cells, in which GILZ inhibited T cell receptor (TCR)-mediated T cell activation (D'Adamio et al., 1997). Since then, GILZ has been shown to be expressed in other immune cells, including monocytes/macrophages, mast cells, and dendritic cells (Berrebi et al., 2003; Cohen et al., 2006b; Godot et al., 2006; Hamdi et al., 2007a), and to have numerous anti-inflammatory functions in these cells. These functions are outlined in the following sections. Besides immune cells, GILZ has also been shown to express in other cell types such as epithelial cells and bone-marrow-derived mesenchymal stem cells (MSCs). For example, GILZ was reported to inhibit NF-κB activation in epithelial cells and MSCs (Eddleston *et al.*, 2007b; Yang *et al.*, 2008). The studies also reported the expression of GILZ is necessary for dexamethasone-mediated inhibition of IL-8 production in respiratory epithelial cells and similarly for the dexamethasone-dependent inhibition of cyclo-oxygenase 2 expression in MSCs.

Tissue types	Expression of GILZ	Reference(s)
Lymphoid tissue	Lymphocytes mainly from thymus, spleen, and lymph nodes	(Asselin-Labat *et al.*, 2004; D'Adamio *et al.*, 1997; Riccardi *et al.*, 2001)
Brain	Ubiquitously expressed in rat brain	(van der Laan, 2008)
Renal epithelium	mammalian kidney epithelial cells	(Soundararajan *et al.*, 2009)
Collecting duct	the cortical collecting duct of the mouse kidney	(Robert-Nicoud *et al.*, 2001)
Ovaries	normal ovary and epithelial ovary cancer	(Redjimi *et al.*, 2009)
Bone tissue	fetal osteoblasts, mesenchymal stem cells, and osteoclasts	(Lekva *et al.*, 2010)
Skeletal muscle and cardiac tissue	skeletal muscle tissue and myoblasts	(Bruscoli *et al.*, 2010)

Table 1. Expression of GILZ in different tissues

3. Effects of GILZ on the immune response

3.1. Innate immunity

A variety of studies suggest that GILZ has critical inhibitory effects on the activity of the innate immune system. In a monocytic cell line (THP-1), RANTES (also known as CCL5) and MIP-1α (also known as CCL3), antigen presenting MHC class II molecules, B7 co-stimulatory molecules CD80 and CD86, and the the pathogen-associated molecular pattern (PAMP) receptor TLR2, are all modulated by GILZ, with an expected effect on reducing recruitment and activation of inflammatory cells (Berrebi *et al.*, 2003; Cohen *et al.*, 2006b). Furthermore, in liver disease, GILZ expression in Kupffer macrophages due to glucocorticoids treatment reduces the production of pro-inflammatory mediators in response to LPS (Hamdi *et al.*, 2007a). Besides macrophages and monocytes, GILZ is also expressed in human airway epithelial cells and inhibited by IL-1β, TNF and interferon (IFN)-γ, and overexpression of GILZ inhibited the activation of NF-κB by IL-1β and TLR ligands (Eddleston *et al.*, 2007b). Currently, it is known that GILZ expression is inhibited by different pro-inflammatory mediators. For example, GILZ was not produced in granulomas in Crohn disease and tuberculosis since the macrophages in the granulomas were activated with the strong expression of the RANTES gene (Berrebi *et al.*, 2003). By contrast, GILZ expression is retained in macrophages in Burkitt lymphomas, potentially contributing to the failure of the immune system to reject the tumor (Berrebi *et al.*, 2003). Taken together, these results above indicate a wide range of inhibitory effects of GILZ in a variety of innate immune responses. Clearly, immune responses, such as the expression of cytokines, chemokines and TLRs, are highly pertinent to the known pathology of inflammatory diseases such as RA. Of note, no *in vivo* studies of the role of GILZ in regulating classic innate immune responses, such as responses to endotoxin or other TLR ligands, have been reported.

3.2. Adaptive immunity

Parallel to innate immune responses, multiple critical functions of GILZ have been found which regulate the activity of antigen-presenting and effector cells of the adaptive immune response. For example, GILZ can mediate the effects of glucocorticoids on dendritic cells (DCs), whose maturation and antigen presentation are impaired in the presence of increased GILZ. Cohen *et al* demonstrated that GILZ over expression altered MHC and co-stimulatory molecule expression, resulting in reduced antigen presentation (Cohen *et al.*, 2006a), and subsequent decreased T lymphocyte activation. Moreover, the expression of GILZ is induced by glucocorticoids and transforming growth factor β (TGF-β) in immature DCs, and oral administration of glucocorticoids to patients increased the expression of GILZ in antigen-presenting cells (Cohen *et al.*, 2006b). The overexpression of GILZ is also able to drive the development of regulatory DCs, which secrete IL-10, and prevent the production of pro-inflammatory cytokines induced by CD40L. Furthermore, these GILZ-expressing regulatory DCs were found to induced CD25[hi]FoxP3[+]CTLA-4[+], IL-10 secreting T-regulatory cells from CD4[+] T-lymphocytes (Hamdi *et al.*, 2007b), resulting in inhibition of subsequent immune responses to specific antigens (Suffia *et al.*, 2006). Regulatory T cells (Tregs) that inhibit activation of other T lymphocytes are generated in response to GILZ over expressing dendritic cells (Hamdi *et al.*, 2007b), providing a further immunomodulatory effect of GILZ. This immunosuppressive effect of GILZ on DCs is extremely relevant in the context of inflammatory pathology since DCs determine whether antigen presentation will lead to an immune response or a tolerogenic response.

Additional knowledge of the effects of GILZ in adaptive immunity arises from studies of modified GILZ expression in T lymphocyte cells. For example, Cannarile and colleagues have demonstrated increased secretion of cytokines associated with a T$_H$2 response, such as IL-4, IL-10, IL-5, and IL-13, and reduced expression of cytokines associated with a T$_H$1 response such as IFN-γ in GILZ overexpressing cells compared with wild type T cells (Cannarile *et al.*, 2006a). In their study on GILZ transgenic T lymphocytes, they found there was decreased expression of T-box protein 21 (T-bet) (Cannarile *et al.*, 2006a), a transcription factor specifically associated with a T$_H$1 response, and increased expression of the transcription factors GATA-3 and STAT6. As STAT6 modulates GATA3 which is important for polarization towards a T$_H$2 phenotype (Wurster *et al.*, 2000; Zheng & Flavell, 1997), these studies indicate that the expression of GILZ promotes T lymphocyte development towards a

TH2 instead of TH1 phenotype. Moreover, mice transgenic for GILZ under the control of the CD2 promoter, that overexpresse GILZ in T cells, display a TH2-skewed phenotype, and are protected from the TH1-dependent model of dinitrobenzene sulfonic acid (DNBS)-induced colitis but exhibit an increase in the 'allergenic' TH2 Oxazolone-induced colitis (Cannarile *et al.*, 2009). Another study investigated the levels of inflammatory mediators in wild type and GILZ transgenic mice induced with DNBS, and were able to demonstrate a decrease in pro-inflammatory cytokines and NF-κB activation in GILZ transgenic mice compared to wild type. Furthermore, in T-cell specific GILZ transgenic mice, young animals do not exhibit a significant difference in thymic weight. However, there was a significant decrease in CD4+CD8+ double positive thymocytes. There was also a parallel increase in CD4-CD8- double negative and CD8+ T-cells, but no change in the CD4+ population (Delfino *et al.*, 2004). In the aged mice, the CD4+ population also increased in a significant manner, although not as dramatically as the CD8+ or the CD4-CD8- populations, signifying a disturbance in thymic maturation. The observation above is interesting since GILZ might mediate some of the glucocorticoid-triggered apoptotic effects during thymic development. Microarray studies also show that GILZ is expressed in resting B cells, and it is presumed that GILZ down-regulation facilitates B-cell activation (Glynne *et al.*, 2000).

4. Effect of GILZ on signalling pathways

4.1. NF-κB pathway

To date, much research has focused on the function of the NF-κB pathway in the anti-inflammatory effects of glucocorticoids (Auphan *et al.*, 1995; DeBosscher & Haegeman, 2009; Gossye *et al.*, 2009). Glucocorticoids are known as effective inhibitors of the NF-κB pathway, and considerable research directed at understanding the antagonistic effects of glucocorticoids on this pathway has been undertaken (De Bosscher *et al.*, 2003). As shown in **Fig 2**, GILZ, significantly up regulated in the presence of glucocorticoids, participates in the inhibition of NF-κB by glucocorticoids through a physical interaction with the NF-κB p65 subunit (Ayroldi *et al.*, 2001), preventing its nuclear translocation. The inhibition of GILZ is independent from other IκB- or Rel-related proteins, since GILZ was found to co-immunoprecipitate with NF-κB p65 subunit in the presence or absence of IκB (Ayroldi *et al.*, 2001). Subsequently, Yang *et al* demonstrated the role of GILZ in the inhibition of the inflammatory mediator COX-2 in MCSs in response to IL-1α and TNF-α, by preventing NF-κB p65 subunit nuclear transport (Yang *et al.*, 2008). Similarly, the mechanism of GILZ-NF-κB mediated inhibition of COX-2 transcription has been shown in epithelial cells (Eddleston *et al.*, 2007b). The inhibition of NF-κB by GILZ has also been demonstrated *in vivo*, in a transgenic mouse model in which GILZ expression is driven by the CD2 promoter, resulting in the overexpression of GILZ in thymocytes (Delfino *et al.*, 2006). When subjected to T-cell receptor-triggered apoptosis, the nuclear translocation and DNA binding of NF-κB were impaired in T cells from GILZ transgenic mice, whereas the translocation of transcription factors belonging to the NFAT family was not affected. All the findings above arouse interest in GILZ and its function in the pathogenesis of NF-κB–related inflammatory diseases. For example, GILZ transgenic mice demonstrated reduced NF-κB activation in spinal cord injury in comparison to wild type mice, and overexpression of GILZ protects TH1 inflammatory responses in colitis associated with inhibition of nuclear and phosphorylated p65 (Cannarile *et al.*, 2009; Esposito *et al.* 2011). Moreover, Srinivasan and colleagues have described a novel NF-κB p65-binding GILZ-derived peptide which exhibited therapeutic potential as a small molecule NF-κB inhibitor in experimental autoimmune encephalomyelitis (EAE), a model of human multiple sclerosis (Srinivasan & Janardhanam, 2011a).

4.2. AP-1 pathway

The transcription factor AP-1 is another major participant in inflammatory and immune responses (Adcock & Caramori, 2001). AP-1, as a heterodimer of the c-Fos and c-Jun proteins, can be phosphorylated to significantly increase its transcriptional activity. The direct inhibitory effects of the glucocorticoid-glucocorticoid receptor complex on AP-1 signaling are well documented (De Bosscher *et al.*, 2003). It is also known that glucocorticoids lead to the repression of mitogen-activated protein kinase (MAPK) activity and hence AP-1 activation through the expression of phosphatases that exert inhibitory interactions with various MAPK members (Aeberli *et al.*, 2006). Of interest, Mittelstadt and colleagues showed direct binding of GILZ to the AP-1 components c-Jun and c-Fos (**Fig 2**) in Jurkat cells (an immortalized line of T cells) (Mittelstadt & Ashwell, 2001). The paper also showed GILZ is critical for the regulation of FasL expression in response to glucocorticoids. FasL is a promoter containing NFAT binding elements and under regulation of the NFAT/AP-1 complex signalling. FasL promoter and its enhancer elements, early growth response factor (Erg) -2 and Erg-3 were inhibited by transient transfection of GILZ in Jurkat cells. The authors demonstrated that c-Fos and c-Jun do in fact interact with N-terminal, but not the LZ or PER domains, of GILZ. Furthermore, Ayroldi et al. confirmed the interaction of GILZ with c-Fos and c-Jun, and further showed that GILZ expression interferes with c-Fos transcription in response to anti-CD3 stimulation of IL-2, but not c-Jun, and also by negatively interfering with upstream signalling of Raf-1-ERK pathway (Ayroldi *et al.*, 2002).

4.3. MAP kinase pathways

The MAP kinase family consists of extracellular signal-regulated kinase (ERK), p38 kinase, and JNK, all of which can be activated by upstream molecules such as Ras and Raf-1 (Rincon, 2001) and all of which phosphorylate downstream proteins in the respective cascades to regulate expression of a variety of genes related to inflammation, cell proliferation, differentiation and apoptosis. GILZ has also been shown to bind to both Raf-1 (Ayroldi *et al.*, 2002) and Ras (Ayroldi *et al.*, 2007) and thereby to modulate downstream signalling (**Fig 2**). Ayroldi and colleagues reported that GILZ overexpression in anti-CD3-stimulated T cells can bind to Raf-1, which inhibits phosphorylation of Raf-1 and results in suppression of MEK and ERK1/2 phosphorylation (Ayroldi *et al.*, 2002). They also found that GILZ can bind to Raf-1 via the NH$_2$-terminal region of GILZ and Ras via the TSC box of GILZ. The interaction of GILZ with Ras or Raf-1 has been shown to be dependent on the activation of Ras, where GILZ will bind predominately to Raf-1 in the absence of active Ras. However, as Ras is activated, Raf-1 will bind to Ras to a stronger degree than it will bind to GILZ. Furthermore, the affinity of GILZ to Ras will also increase, leading to predominately GILZ-Ras complexes (Ayroldi, 2007). GILZ may also form a trimer with both Ras and Raf-1, and this is also dependent on Ras activation. All the results above suggest that GILZ inhibits cell activation and inflammation via regulation of MAPK signaling molecules.

4.4. PI3K/Akt and apoptotic signalling pathways

The inhibition by GILZ of Ras and Raf-1 also decreases the activation of another downstream signalling pathway, the PI3 kinase (PI3K)/Akt pathway, which is involved in cell survival as well as activation. Recent studies have uncovered a crucial role for FoxO3 in mediation of PI3K/Akt pathway. In the cell, non-phosphorylated FoxO3 migrates into the nucleus and up-regulates several mediators of cell cycle progression, such as G1/S-specific cyclin-D1, p27^{KIP1} (also known as cyclin-dependent kinase inhibitor 1B), Fas ligand (also known as tumor necrosis factor ligand superfamily member 6) and Bim (also known as Bcl-2-like protein 11), to inhibit cell proliferation (Schmidt *et al.*, 2002). Activation of Akt leads to the phosphorylation of FoxO3, which results in the nuclear exclusion of FoxO3 and thus leads to the inhibition of their cognate transcriptional targets. Interestingly, the gene encoding GILZ has been identified as a transcriptional target of FoxO3 (Asselin-Labat *et al.*, 2005b). Other studies have demonstrated that GILZ can inhibit its own expression through a negative feedback effect to promote nuclear exclusion of FoxO3 shown in **Fig 2** (Latre de Late et al., 2010). However, until now, the net effect of the PI3K/Akt-FoxO3–GILZ regulatory loop on cell proliferation has not yet been clearly defined.

GILZ has also been shown to modulate the expression of a variety of apoptosis pathway proteins in accordance with the observations that GILZ can prevent anti-CD3 mediated apoptosis (D'Adamio *et al.*, 1997). Asselin-Labat and colleagues showed that an increase in GILZ expression down-regulates the expression of Bim, a pro-apoptotic member of the Bcl-2 family, but has no effect on Bcl-xL protein, an anti-apoptotic Bcl-2 family protein, to prevent apoptosis. In the same study, they demonstrated that knockdown of GILZ accelerates IL-2-deprivation-mediated apoptosis in the IL-2-dependent, CTLL-2 cell line, through increased levels of Bim (Asselin-Labat *et al.*, 2004). Furthermore, they showed that GILZ acts on Bim through the transcriptional factor FoxO3. Using a Bim-promoter-luciferase construct, GILZ expression was shown to repress Bim transcription, and these effects were abrogated with the co-expression of FoxO3 (Asselin-Labat *et al.*, 2004). However, it had been previously shown in CD4$^+$CD8$^+$ double positive T cells that overexpression of GILZ leads to an increase in the spontaneous apoptosis, and an interaction with, and reduction of, Bcl-xL. Furthermore, GILZ expression was associated with an increase in the activation of extrinsic apoptotic caspases -3 and -8, but not caspase-9, involved in the mitochondrial/cytochrome C pathway (Delfino *et al.*, 2004). The authors suggested that NF-κB inhibition is the mechanism by which TCR mediated apoptosis is inhibited by GILZ in over expression models, and that NF-κB may be involved in control of Bcl-xL (Delfino *et al.*, 2006). Whilst the mechanism of GILZ in regulation of cell apoptosis has yet to be well understood, it follows the general trend of GILZ to display a dual activity in regards to apoptosis and cell survival.

4.5. Other non-inflammatory signalling pathways

In addition to mediating glucocorticoid effects in inflammation and immunity, GILZ may also play a critical role in non-immune function such as adipogenesis and osteogenesis. For example, Shi *et al* reported that GILZ directly binds to CCAAT/enhancer-binding protein (C/EBP) DNA binding sites in the *PPAR-γ2* promoter, with consequent inhibition of mesenchymal cell adipogenesis (Shi *et al.*, 2003). Previously, glucocorticoids had been shown to activate C/EBP directly, and therefore promote PPAR-γ2 expression and adipocyte differentiation (Shi *et al.*, 2003). This observation thus suggests a potential role of GILZ as a direct transcriptional repressor of gene expression in a direction opposite to the effects of Glucocorticoids. Of note, this is in contrast to the effects of GILZ binding to pro-inflammatory transcription factors where it mimics the effects of glucocorticoids. Moreover, as PPAR-γ2 is a key regulator of adipogenesis, GILZ's prevention of C/EBP action inhibits adipogenesis, and thereby promotes osteogenesis (Zhang *et al.*, 2008b), again an effect opposite to those of glucocorticoids which promote osteoporosis. The findings offer the suggestion of a possible GILZ-based therapy wherein GILZ exhibits beneficial glucocorticoid anti-inflammatory actions without the negative side effects of adiposity and osteoporosis.

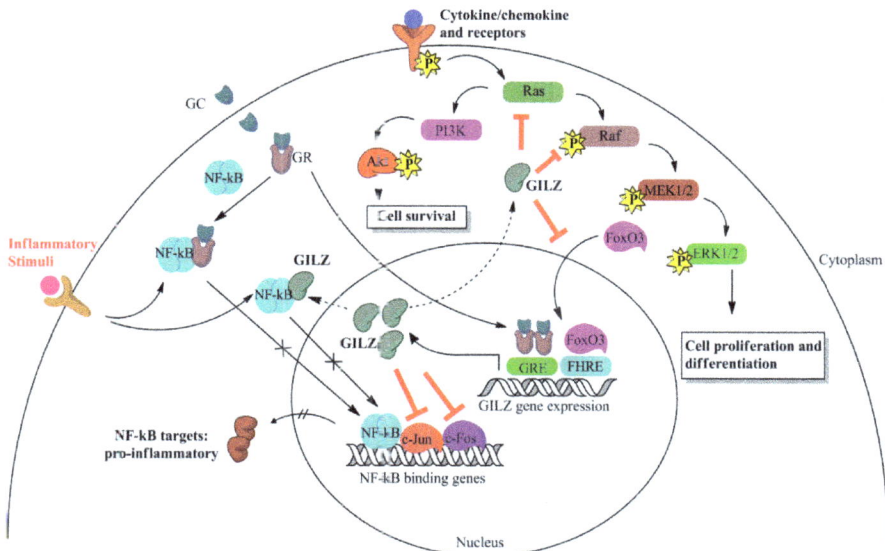

Figure 2. Roles of GILZ as a mediator in immune signaling pathways

NF-κB, activated by a variety of inflammatory stimulation, translocates into the nucleus and binds to target genes encoding pro-inflammatory factors. Glucocorticoid bound to the receptor GR can directly interact with NF-κB to prevent its nuclear translocation. In addition, the GC/GR complex can translocate into the nucleus and bind to glucocorticoid response elements on the *GILZ* gene to induce GILZ expression. GILZ in turn binds to NF-κB and prevents its nuclear translocation. GILZ can also directly bind to c-Jun and c-Fos, two constituents of AP-1, to inhibit their transcriptional activity and gene expression of pro-inflammatory molecules. The location, in the cytoplasm or nucleus, where GILZ binds to AP-1 subunits is still unknown. In the cytoplasm, GILZ also modulates cell survival by blocking Ras activation and the downstream PI3K/Akt signaling pathway. GILZ binds and inhibits Ras and Raf phosphorylation and thus inhibits downstream MEK-1/2 and ERK-1/2 activation. As part of a negative feedback loop, GILZ prevents nuclear translocation of FoxO3, which is in turn a key transcriptional factor to upregulate *GILZ* gene expression.

5. Effect of GILZ on inflammatory and autoimmune diseases

The reported actions of GILZ suggest GILZ may exert anti-inflammatory effects in immune and inflammatory diseases. Studies in animal disease models, or in human pathology, remain limited, but favour a role for GILZ as a modulator of immune-inflammatory responses. For example, Cannarile and colleagues reported GILZ effects on delayed-type hypersensitivity (DTH) responses in the GILZ transgenic mouse (Cannarile *et al.*, 2006b). In response to ovalbumin (OVA) immunization, GILZ overexpression mice exhibited significantly less swelling than wild type control, which indicates the essential role of GILZ in T cells in inhibiting T$_H$1 dependent DTH responses. The authors also investigated a murine model of colitis, in which it was shown that significant inhibition was observed in mice overexpressing GILZ in T cells (Cannarile *et al.*, 2009). In addition, studies of these T cells showed reduction of the T$_H$1 cytokine IFN-γ. Moreover, colon lysates from GILZ overexpressing mice have lower total and phosphorylated Ser536 NF-κB p65, which indicates that GILZ overexpression in T cells protects mice from T$_H$1-mediated colitis disease by inhibition of NF-κB activity.

Recently, Beaulieu and colleagues investigated the role of endogenous GILZ in RA (Beaulieu *et al.*, 2010a). GILZ was potently induced by glucocorticoids in cultured human RA synovial cells *in vitro*, and in murine arthritis *in vivo*. GILZ silencing by *in vivo* siRNA administration resulted in increased severity of the collagen-induced model of RA in mice, and in parallel GILZ overexpression inhibited chemokine and cytokine expression in human synovial cells. These results suggest GILZ as a key endogenous regulatory molecule in RA. Another study showed that GILZ was noticeably absent in granulomas in Crohn disease and tuberculosis (Berrebi *et al.*, 2003), which suggests inhibitor regulation of GILZ in the presence of chronic inflammatory disease, while human asthma patients demonstrated increased GILZ expression in response to glucocorticoid therapy (Kelly *et al.*, 2011).

GILZ is also reported to attenuate experimental autoimmune encephalomyelitis (EAE), a disease model of human multiple sclerosis. Srinivasan and colleagues demonstrated that delivery of a GILZ-derived peptide is protective against EAE in mice (Srinivasan & Janardhanam, 2011b). The GILZ fragment they isolated, containing a proline rich domain, can directly interact with p65 NF-κB, thereby inhibiting p65 translocation from activated human CD4+ T cells isolated from peripheral blood mononuclear cells (PBMCs) (Srinivasan & Janardhanam, 2011a). As T cells are a major target of glucocorticoids in EAE (Wust et al., 2008), these data provide further evidence that exogenous GILZ could exert therapeutically useful anti-inflammatory properties.

6. Perspective and expectations: GILZ as a glucocorticoid sparing target

GILZ, a molecule mainly modulated by glucocorticoids, play a pivotal role in the regulation of inflammation and immune responses. Expressed in multiple cells and tissues, GILZ inhibits the expression of a variety of inflammatory mediators and modulates the immune response. In this chapter, we have summarised GILZ structure and function, the effects of GILZ in immune responses, and its interaction with a number of key transduction pathways pivotal to the pathogenesis of inflammatory diseases. The more recent observations that GILZ exerts immunomodulatory and anti-inflammatory effects *in vivo* that mimic the inhibitory actions of glucocorticoids strongly suggests GILZ is a potential substitute for glucocorticoids in the therapy of inflammatory diseases.

As we have noted, currently a number of important anti-inflammatory molecules, such as Annexin A1 and MKP-1, are induced by glucocorticoids, and evidence that synthetic glucocorticoids lose their effectiveness in the absence of these molecules has been adduced (Furst et al., 2007; Ralph & Morand, 2008; Yang et al., 2009; Yang et al., 2004; Yang et al., 2006). Attention to the molecules that glucocorticoids amplify the expression of will permit discovery of the means to develop a surrogate for glucocorticoids' beneficial impact on immune activation without their toxicity. Importantly, the presence of GILZ exerts immune and inflammation modulatory effects in the absence of glucocorticoids. A GILZ-based therapeutic approach, therefore, could potentially offer profound glucocorticoid-like regulatory effects in autoimmune disease. Investigation of the metabolic effects of any GILZ-based therapy is required in order to ensure that the undesirable effects of glucocorticoids are not recapitulated. Early results are encouraging in this regard. In mesenchymal stem cells, differentiation towards osteogenic precursors is enhanced by GILZ, whereas silencing of GILZ reduced osteogenic differentiation (Zhang et al., 2008a), suggesting that a GILZ therapy might have protective rather than harmful effects on bone. GILZ expression was also associated with osteoblast development, and GILZ silencing increased osteoblast expression of OPG and RANKL in favour of osteoclastogenesis (Lekva et al., 2010), further suggesting that GILZ-based therapy might have a bone-protective effect. Studies of the role of GILZ in glucocorticoid-induced osteoporosis *in vivo* are eagerly awaited.

GILZ-based therapies could be based around the administration of recombinant protein or NF-κB binding peptides. As we have introduced above, Srinivasan and colleagues have described a novel NF-κB p65 binding GILZ peptide which exhibited therapeutic potential as a NF-κB inhibitor in EAE (Srinivasan & Janardhanam, 2011b). Alternatively, a gene therapy approach, which has already been successfully used *in vivo* to suppress arthritis via delivery of the anti-inflammatory cytokine IL-10 (Apparailly *et al.*, 2002), could be applied to GILZ. Inducing GILZ expression other than through the use of glucocorticoids, for example by modifying activity of the transcription factor FoxO3, could represent a further means to increase available GILZ protein, as could inhibition of the as-yet unidentified mechanisms of GILZ protein turnover. Finally, structure-function analysis of the molecules with which GILZ interacts in order to achieve its immune modifying effects could reveal targets for synthetic GILZ mimetics. Although considerable work remains, the first proof of concept studies of an *in vivo* GILZ-based therapeutic approach is under development in the authors' laboratory (unpublished observations).

In conclusion, glucocorticoids remain among the most widely used drugs in human diseases, and in particular in autoimmune disease. Their effectiveness is increasingly well understood, based on their effects on inflammatory signal transduction, but their use is constrained by toxicity, which also relates to their specific physiological actions. GILZ is a key molecule in glucocorticoid biology, which now represents a candidate mediator of glucocorticoid regulation of immune and inflammatory responses, and deserves further investigation.

Author details

Huapeng Fan and Eric F. Morand
Centre for Inflammatory Diseases, Monash University, Australia

Acknowledgement

The authors are supported by a Project Grant from the National Health and Medical Research Council of Australia.

7. References

Adcock IM, Caramori G. Cross-talk between pro-inflammatory transcription factors and glucocorticoids. *Immunol Cell Biol* 79(4):376-384, 2001.

Aeberli D, Yang Y, Mansell A, Santos L, Leech M, Morand EF. Endogenous macrophage migration inhibitory factor modulates glucocorticoid sensitivity in macrophages via effects on MAP kinase phosphatase-1 and p38 MAP kinase. *FEBS Lett* 580(3):974-981, 2006.

Apparailly F, Millet V, Noel D, Jacquet C, Sany J, Jorgensen C. Tetracycline-inducible interleukin-10 gene transfer mediated by an adeno-associated virus: application to experimental arthritis. *Hum Gene Ther* 13(10):1179-1188, 2002.

Asselin-Labat M, Biola-Vidamment A, Kerbrat S, Lombes M, Bertoglio J, Pallardy M. Fox03 Mediates Antagonistic Effects of Glucocorticoids and Interleukin-2 on Glucocorticoid-Induced Leucine Zipper Expression. *Molecular Endocrinology* 19(7):1752-1764, 2005a.

Asselin-Labat ML, Biola-Vidamment A, Kerbrat S, Lombes M, Bertoglio J, Pallardy M. FoxO3 mediates antagonistic effects of glucocorticoids and interleukin-2 on glucocorticoid-induced leucine zipper expression. *Molecular endocrinology (Baltimore, Md* 19(7):1752-1764, 2005b.

Asselin-Labat ML, David M, Biola-Vidamment A, Lecoeuche D, Zennaro MC, Bertoglio J, Pallardy M. GILZ, a new target for the transcription factor FoxO3, protects T lymphocytes from interleukin-2 withdrawal-induced apoptosis. *Blood* 104(1):215-223, 2004.

Auphan N, Didonato JA, Rosette C, Helmberg A, Karin M. Immunosuppression by Glucocorticoids: Inhibition of NF-κB Activity Through Induction of IκB Synthesis. *Science* 270(5234):286-290, 1995.

Ayroldi E. GILZ mediates the antiproliferative activity of glucocorticoids by negative regulation of Ras signaling. *J. Clin. Invest.* 117:1605-1615, 2007.

Ayroldi E, Migliorati G, Bruscoli S, Marchetti C, Zollo O, Cannarile L, D'adamio F, Riccardi C. Modulation of T-cell activation by the glucocorticoid-induced leucine zipper factor via inhibition of nuclear factor kappaB. *Blood* 98(3):743-753, 2001.

Ayroldi E, Riccardi C. Glucocorticoid-induced leucine zipper (GILZ): a new important mediator of glucocorticoid action. *FASEB Journal* 23:1-10, 2009.

Ayroldi E, Zollo O, Bastianelli A, Marchetti C, Agostini M, Di Virgilio R, Riccardi C. GILZ mediates the antiproliferative activity of glucocorticoids by negative regulation of Ras signaling. *J Clin Invest* 117(6):1605-1615, 2007.

Ayroldi E, Zollo O, Macchiarulo A, Di Marco B, Marchetti C, Riccardi C. Glucocorticoid-induced leucine zipper inhibits the Raf-extracellular signal-regulated kinase pathway by binding to Raf-1. *Molecular and cellular biology* 22(22):7929-7941, 2002.

Barnes PJ. How corticosteroids control inflammation: Quintiles Prize Lecture 2005. *British Journal of Pharmacology* 148(3):245-254, 2006.

Beaulieu E, Morand EF. Role of GILZ in immune regulation, glucocorticoid actions and rheumatoid arthritis. *Nat Rev Rheumatol* advance online publication, 2011.

Beaulieu E, Ngo D, Santos L, Smith M, Jorgensen C, Escriou V, Scherman D, Courties G, Apparailly F, Morand EF. Glucocorticoid-induced leucine zipper is an endogenous anti-inflammatory mediator in arthritis *Arthritis Rheum*, 2010a.

Beaulieu E, Ngo D, Santos L, Yang YH, Smith M, Jorgensen C, Escriou V, Scherman D, Courties G, Apparailly F, Morand E. Glucocorticoid- Induced Leucine Zipper is an Endogenous Antiinflammatory Mediator in Arthritis. *Arthritis and Rheumatism* 62(9), 2010b.

Berrebi D, Bruscoli S, Cohen N, Foussat A, Migliorati G, Bouchet-Delbos L, Maillot MC, Portier A, Couderc J, Galanaud P, Peuchmaur M, Riccardi C, Emilie D. Synthesis of glucocorticoid-induced leucine zipper (GILZ) by macrophages: an anti-inflammatory and immunosuppressive mechanism shared by glucocorticoids and IL-10. *Blood* 101(2):729-738, 2003.

Bruscoli S, Donato V, Velardi E, Di Sante M, Migliorati G, Donato R, Riccardi C. Glucocorticoid-induced leucine zipper (GILZ) and long GILZ inhibit myogenic differentiation and mediate anti-myogenic effects of glucocorticoids. *J Biol Chem* 285(14):10385-10396, 2010.

Cannarile L, Cuzzocrea S, Santucci L, Agostini M, Mazzon E, Esposito E, Muia C, Coppo M, Di Paola R, Riccardi C. Glucocorticoid-induced leucine zipper is protective in Th1-mediated models of colitis. *Gastroenterology* 136(2):530-541, 2009.

Cannarile L, Fallarino F, Agostini M, Cuzzocrea S, Mazzon E, Vacca C, Genovese T, Migliorati G, Ayroldi E, Riccardi C. Increased GILZ expression in transgenic mice up-regulates Th-2 lymphokines. *Blood* 107(3):1039-1047, 2006a.

Cannarile L, Fallarino F, Agostini M, Cuzzocrea S, Mazzon E, Vacca C, Genovese T, Migliorati G, Ayroldi E, Riccardi C. Increased GILZ expression in transgenic mice up-regulates Th-2 lymphokines. *Blood* 107(3):1039-1047, 2006b.

Chrousos G. The Hypothalamic-Pitutitary-Adrenal Axis and Immune Mediated Infalmmation. *The New England Journal of Medicine* 332(30):1351-1363, 1995.

Cohen N, Mouley E, Hamdi H, Maillot M, Pallardy M, Godot V, Capel F, Balian A, Naveau S, Galanaud P, Lemoine FM, Emilie D. GILZ expression in human dendritic cells redirects their maturation and prevents antigen-specific T lymphoctye response. *Blood* 107(5):2037-2044, 2006a.

Cohen N, Mouly E, Hamdi H, Maillot MC, Pallardy M, Godot V, Capel F, Balian A, Naveau S, Galanaud P, Lemoine FM, Emilie D. GILZ expression in human dendritic cells redirects their maturation and prevents antigen-specific T lymphocyte response. *Blood* 107(5):2037-2044, 2006b.

D'adamio F, Zollo O, Moraca R, Ayroldi E, Bruscoli S, Bartoli A, Cannarile L, Migliorati G, Riccardi C. A new dexamethasone-induced gene of the leucine zipper family protects T lymphocytes from TCR/CD3-activated cell death. *Immunity* 7(6):803-812, 1997.

Davis JM, 3rd, Maradit Kremers H, Crowson CS, Nicola PJ, Ballman KV, Therneau TM, Roger VL, Gabriel SE. Glucocorticoids and cardiovascular events in rheumatoid arthritis: a population-based cohort study. *Arthritis and rheumatism* 56(3):820-830, 2007.

De Bosscher K, Vanden Berghe W, Haegeman G. The interplay between the glucocorticoid receptor and nuclear factor-kappaB or activator protein-1: molecular mechanisms for gene repression. *Endocrine reviews* 24(4):488-522, 2003.

Debosscher K, Haegeman G. MInireview: Latest Perspectives on Antiinflammaotry Actions of GLucocorticoids. *Molecuar Endocrinology* 23(3):281-291, 2009.

Delfino DV, Agostini M, Spinicelli S, Vacca C, Riccardi C. Inhibited cell death, NF-kappaB activity and increased IL-10 in TCR-triggered thymocytes of transgenic mice overexpressing the glucocorticoid-induced protein GILZ. *International immunopharmacology* 6(7):1126-1134, 2006.

Delfino DV, Agostini M, Spinicelli S, Vito P, Riccardi C. Decrease of Bcl-xL and augmentation of thymocyte apoptosis in GILZ overexpressing transgenic mice. *Blood* 104(13):4134-4141, 2004.

Di Marco B, Massetti M, Bruscoli S. Macchiarulo A, Di Virgilio R, Velardi E, Donato V, Migliorati G, Riccardi C. Glucocorticoid-induced leucine zipper (GILZ)/NF-kappaB interaction: role of GILZ homo-dimerization and C-terminal domain. *Nucleic Acids Res* 35(2):517-528, 2007.

Eddleston J, Herschbach J, Wageliε-Steffen AL, Christiansen S, Zuraw BL. The anti-inflammatory effect of glucocorticoids is mediated by glucocorticoid-induced leucine zipper in epithelial cells. *Journal of Allergy and Clinical Immunology* 119(1):115-122, 2007a.

Eddleston J, Herschbach J, Wageliε-Steffen AL, Christiansen SC, Zuraw BL. The anti-inflammatory effect of glucocorticoids is mediated by glucocorticoid-induced leucine zipper in epithelial cells. *J Allergy Clin Immunol* 119(1):115-122, 2007b.

Esposito E, Bruscoli S, Mazzon E, Paterniti I, Coppo M, Velardi E, Cuzzocrea S, Riccardi C. Glucocorticoid-Induced Leucine Zipper (GILZ) Over-Expression in T Lymphocytes Inhibits Inflammation and Tissue Damage in Spinal Cord Injury. *Neurotherapeutics*, 2011.

Furst R, Schroeder T, Eilken HM, Bubik MF, Kiemer AK, Zahler S, Vollmar AM. MAPK phosphatase-1 represents a novel anti-inflammatory target of glucocorticoids in the human endothelium. *FASEB J* 21(1):74-80, 2007.

Glynne R, Ghandour G, Rayner J, Mack DH, Goodnow CC. B-lymphocyte quiescence, tolerance and activation as viewed by global gene expression profiling on microarrays. *Immunol Rev* 176:216-246, 2000.

Godot V, Garcia G, Capel F, Arock M, Durand-Gasselin I, Asselin-Labat ML, Emilie D, Humbert M. Dexamethasone and IL-10 stimulate glucocorticoid-induced leucine zipper synthesis by human mast cells. *Allergy* 61(7):886-890, 2006.

Gossye V, Elewaut D, Bougarne N, Bracke D, Calenbergh SV, Haegeman G, Debosscher K. Differential Mechanism of NF-B Inhibition by Two Glucocorticoid Receptor Modulators in Rheumatoid Arthritis Synovial Fibroblasts. *Arhtritis and Rheumatism* 60(11):3241-3250, 2009.

Hamdi H, Bigorgne A, Naveau S, Balian A, Bouchet-Delbos L, Cassard-Doulcier AM, Maillot MC, Durand-Gasselin I, Prevot S, Delaveaucoupet J, Emilie D, Perlemuter G. Glucocorticoid-induced leucine zipper: A key protein in the sensitization of monocytes to lipopolysaccharide in alcoholic hepatitis. *Hepatology (Baltimore, Md* 46(6):1986-1992, 2007a.

Hamdi H, Godot V, Maillot MC, Prejean MV, Cohen N, Krzysiek R, Lemoine FM, Zou W, Emilie D. Induction of antigen-specific regulatory T lymphocytes by human dendritic cells expressing the glucocorticoid-induced leucine zipper. *Blood* 110(1):211-219, 2007b.

Hillier SG. Diamonds are forever: the cortisone legacy. *The Journal of endocrinology* 195(1):1-6, 2007.

Huscher D, Thiele K, Gromnica-Ihle E, Hein G, Demary W, Dreher R, Zink A, Buttgereit F. Dose-related patterns of glucocorticoid-induced side effects. *Annals of the Rheumatic Diseases* 68(7):1119-1124, 2009.

Kelly M, King E, Rider C, Gwozd C, Holden N, Eddleston J, Zuraw B, Leigh R, O'byrne P, Newton R. Corticosteroid-induced gene expression in allergen-challenged asthmatic subjects taking inhaled budesonide. *Br J Pharmacol*, 2011.

Latre De Late P, Pepin A, Assaf-Vandecasteele H, Espinasse C, Nicolas V, Asselin-Labat ML, Bertoglio J, Pallardy M, Biola-Vidamment A. Glucocorticoid-induced leucine zipper (GILZ) promotes the nuclear exclusion of FOXO3 in a Crm1-dependent manner. *J Biol Chem* 285(8):5594-5605.

Lekva T, Bollerslev J, Kristo C, Olstad OK, Ueland T, Jemtland R. The Glucocorticoid-Induced Leucine Zipper Gene (GILZ) Expression Decreases after Successful Treatment of Patients with Endogenous Cushing's Syndrome and May Play a Role in Glucocorticoid-Induced Osteoporosis. *J Clin Endocrinol Metab*, 2009.

Lekva T, Bollerslev J, Kristo C, Olstad OK, Ueland T, Jemtland R. The glucocorticoid-induced leucine zipper gene (GILZ) expression decreases after successful treatment of patients with endogenous Cushing's syndrome and may play a role in glucocorticoid-induced osteoporosis. *J Clin Endocrinol Metab* 95(1):246-255, 2010.

Mittelstadt PR, Ashwell JD. Inhibition of AP-1 by the glucocorticoid-inducible protein GILZ. *J Biol Chem* 276(31):29603-29610, 2001.

Ralph JA, Morand EF. MAPK phosphatases as novel targets for rheumatoid arthritis. *Expert opinion on therapeutic targets* 12(7):795-808, 2008.

Redjimi N, Gaudin F, Touboul C, Emilie D, Pallardy M, Biola-Vidamment A, Fernandez H, Prevot S, Balabanian K, Machelon V. Identification of glucocorticoid-induced leucine zipper as a key regulator of tumor cell proliferation in epithelial ovarian cancer. *Mol Cancer* 8:83, 2009.

Riccardi C, Bruscoli S, Ayroldi E, Agostini M, Migliorati G. GILZ, a glucocorticoid hormone induced gene, modulates T lymphocytes activation and death through interaction with NF-[kappa]B. *Adv. Exp. Med. Biol.* 495:31-39, 2001.

Rincon M. MAP-kinase signaling pathways in T cells. *Curr Opin Immunol* 13(3):339-345, 2001.

Robert-Nicoud M, Flahaut M, Elalouf JM, Nicod M, Salinas M, Bens M, Doucet A, Wincker P, Artiguenave F, Horisberger JD, Vandewalle A, Rossier BC, Firsov D. Transcriptome of a mouse kidney cortical collecting duct cell line: effects of aldosterone and vasopressin. *Proc Natl Acad Sci U S A* 98(5):2712-2716, 2001.

Scha¨Cke H, Do¨Cke W, Asadullah* K. Mechanisms involved in the side effects of glucocorticoids. *Pharmacology and Therapeutics* 96:23-43, 2002.

Schmidt M, Fernandez De Mattos S, Van Der Horst A, Klompmaker R, Kops GJ, Lam EW, Burgering BM, Medema RH. Cell cycle inhibition by FoxO forkhead transcription factors involves downregulation of cyclin D. *Molecular and cellular biology* 22(22):7842-7852, 2002.

Shi X, Shi W, Li Q, Song B, Wan M, Bai S, Cao X. A glucocorticoid-induced leucine-zipper protein, GILZ, inhibits adipogenesis of mesenchymal cells. *EMBO Rep* 4(4):374-380, 2003.

Slocumb CH, Polley HF, Hench PS, Kendall EC. Effects of cortisone and ACTH on patients with rheumatoid arthritis. *Proc Staff Meet Mayo Clin* 25(17):476-478, 1950.

Soundararajan R, Melters D, Shih I-C, Wang J, Pearce D. Epithelial sodium channel regulated by differential composition of a signaling complex. *Proceedings of the National Academy of Sciences* 106(19):7804-7809, 2009.

Soundararajan R, Wang J, Melters D, Pearce D. Differential Activities of Glucocorticoid-induced Leucine Zipper Protein Isoforms. *The Journal of Biological Chemistry* 282(50):36303-36313, 2007.

Srinivasan M, Janardhanam S. Novel p65 binding GILZ peptide suppresses experimental autoimmune encephalomyelitis. *J Biol Chem*, 2011a.

Srinivasan M, Janardhanam S. Novel p65 binding GILZ peptide suppresses experimental autoimmune encephalomyelitis. *Journal of Biological Chemistry*, 2011b.

Suffia IJ, Reckling SK, Piccirillo CA, Goldszmid RS, Belkaid Y. Infected site-restricted Foxp3+ natural regulatory T cells are specific for microbial antigens. *The Journal of experimental medicine* 203(3):777-788, 2006.

Van Der Laan S. Chromatin immunoprecipitation scanning identifies glucocorticoid receptor binding regions in the proximal promoter of a ubiquitously expressed glucocorticoid target gene in brain. *J. Neurochem.* 106:2515-2523, 2008.

Van Staa TP, Leufkens HGM, Abenhaim L, Begaud B, Zhang B, Cooper C. Use of oral corticosteroids in the United Kingdom. *QJM* 93(2):105-111, 2000.

Wang Y, Ma Y-Y, Song X-L, Cai H-Y, Chen J-C, Song L-N, Yang R, Lu J. Upregulations of Glucocorticoid-Induced Leucine Zipper by Hypoxia and Glucocorticoid Inhibit Proinflammatory Cytokines under Hypoxic Conditions in Macrophages. *The Journal of Immunology*, 2011.

Wurster A, Tanaka T, Grusby MJ. The biology of Stat4 and Stat6. *Oncogene* 19:2577-2584, 2000.

Wust S, Van Den Brandt J, Tischner D, Kleiman A, Tuckermann JP, Gold R, Luhder F, Reichardt HM. Peripheral T cells are the therapeutic targets of glucocorticoids in experimental autoimmune encephalomyelitis. *J Immunol* 180(12):8434-8443, 2008.

Yang N, Zhang W, Shi XM. Glucocorticoid-induced leucine zipper (GILZ) mediates glucocorticoid action and inhibits inflammatory cytokine-induced COX-2 expression. *J Cell Biochem* 103(6):1760-1771, 2008.

Yang YH, Aeberli D, Dacumos A, Xue JR, Morand EF. Annexin-1 regulates macrophage IL-6 and TNF via glucocorticoid-induced leucine zipper. *J Immunol* 183(2):1435-1445, 2009.

Yang YH, Morand EF, Getting SJ, Paul-Clark M, Liu DL, Yona S, Hannon R, Buckingham JC, Perretti M, Flower RJ. Modulation of inflammation and response to dexamethasone by Annexin 1 in antigen-induced arthritis. *Arthritis and rheumatism* 50(3):976-984, 2004.

Yang YH, Toh ML, Clyne CD, Leech M, Aeberli D, Xue J, Dacumos A, Sharma L, Morand EF. Annexin 1 negatively regulates IL-6 expression via effects on p38 MAPK and MAPK phosphatase-1. *J Immunol* 177(11) 8148-8153, 2006.

Zhang W, Yang N, Shi XM. Regulation of mesenchymal stem cell osteogenic differentiation by glucocorticoid-induced leucine zipper (GILZ). *J Biol Chem* 283(8):4723-4729, 2008a.

Zhang W, Yang N, Shi XM. Regulation of MSC osteogenic differentiation by glucocorticoid-induced leucine zipper (GILZ). *J. Biol. Chem.* 283:4723-4729, 2008b.

Zheng W, Flavell R. The Transcription Factor GATA-3 Is Necessary and Sufficient for Th2 Cytokine Gene Expression in CD4 T Cells. *Cell* 9:587-596, 1997.

Glucocorticoids in Behaviour Models

Using Rodent Models to Simulate Stress of Physiologically Relevant Severity: When, Why and How

Carine Smith

Additional information is available at the end of the chapter

1. Introduction

Given the demands of modern life, it is no wonder that the concept of stress has become a household topic for discussion. Also in the academic realm the phenomenon which is stress, is topping the charts in terms of research interest. The short term costs as well as the long term maladaptive effects of stress have been a popular topic of research in especially physiology and psychology for the past few decades, ever since Hans Selye defined the term "stress" in 1956 (Selye, 1956). Stress-related chronic disease, such as cardiovascular disease, diabetes and depression, places an ever-increasing burden on society – medically, socially and financially. Therefore, if we are to limit the spread and impact of this "pandemic", it is imperative to properly manage the effects of stress on our bodies. This of course, is only possible if we have a complete understanding of the body's response to stress.

The response to stress is almost never localised and contained. Rather, a stress response is initiated in response to a local physical (e.g. contusion to skeletal muscle) or mental (e.g. the loss of a loved one) stressor, but always culminates in a wide-spread, systemic response process that affects many organs and systems. Consider for a moment a less complex research model in a different discipline. Metabolic pathways (e.g. the Krebs cycle or glycolysis) can easily be manipulated in cell culture assays using one single cell type at a time, since these pathways (including substrate supply and waste removal systems) are contained in its entirety within each cell. In contrast, with the stress response pathways this is clearly not the case.

The stress response is a complex network of events, which is directed via two interlinked pathways, one endocrine (the hypothalamic pituitary adrenal (HPA)-axis) and one neural (the locus coeruleus norepinephrine (LC-NE) or sympatho-adrenal medullary (SAM)-system). While the neural pathway is mainly activated neurally in response to stress perception, leading to the well-known "fight-or-flight" response, the endocrine pathway has many more triggers. Apart from neural activation, the HPA-axis is also activated by a large number of hormones and even chemical messengers, such as interleukin-6, a cytokine and mediator of inflammation, which is known to increase cortisol secretion. A contributing factor to the complexity of the HPA-axis is the fact that cortisol, the main end product of this stress response, has both endocrine and metabolic functions. Although cortisol is commonly known as the "stress hormone" in the context of psychological stress, its main function is actually metabolic – to maintain glucose supply to the brain. Therefore, the HPA-axis is structured not only for activation in response to perceived stress, but also to react to metabolic stimuli. Furthermore, while the stress response should be powerful and fast in an acute stress situation, the response should be controlled and relatively more limited in a situation of chronic stress, to prevent detrimental effects to the organism in the long term. One can appreciate therefore the need for relatively complex signalling networks in this regard, which serves to activate, limit or inhibit the stress response. To achieve this, numerous molecular mechanisms are in place, and react and interact in response to various stress signals. To give just one example, the glucocorticoid receptor, which is present on most cells to enable cortisol's effect on these cells, is up-regulated in response to acute stress, but down-regulated after a period of chronic stress.

Such complexities make the choice of a suitable stress research model both a difficult, and vital one. While some mechanisms, e.g. activation agents of specific adrenal or pituitary cell types, may be elucidated in cell culture, a whole-system model is required in order to assess the net effect of any stressor to these systems. This does not imply that there is no place for *ex vivo* or *in vitro* studies in the discipline of stress research, far from it! A large number of cell-based – and more recently organotypic culture-based – studies have contributed substantially to our understanding of specific mechanisms and/or partial pathways relevant to stress. The important point here is that ideally, *in vitro* work should at some point be followed up by *in vivo* investigations, in order to test the applicability of results obtained *in vitro*, to a whole system.

The importance of *in vivo* assessments, and the need for conducting them in a model specifically suitable to answer the question at hand, is clear when one considers the huge number of described animal models in the scientific literature. Apart from more conventional models using genetically "intact" rodents, recent advances in biotechnology have made possible research using non-physiological models such as gene-knock out animals. These animals may be genetically modified to erase the gene coding for a particular protein, so that the researcher may elect to produce animals completely lacking a particular protein of interest (e.g. IL-6 knockout mice), or in some cases lacking it in only one organ or system (e.g. STAT-3 knocked out or "switched off" in skeletal muscle only). These models may be used to shed light on various *in vivo* mechanisms which could previously not be properly elucidated using the conventional methods. However, these models have their limitations. For example, when doing research on inflammation, an animal in which a pro-inflammatory cytokine was knocked out, may display increased or decreased basal levels of other pro-inflammatory cytokines, or an altered anti-inflammatory cytokine profile, or even up- or down-regulated cytokine responses on activation, as a spontaneous compensatory mechanism. The resultant net effect of the genetic manipulation therefore may result in a model that is not physiologically accurate, and responses measured may not accurately reflect normal *in vivo* responses. Furthermore, these compensatory mechanisms and/or the mere absence of an important protein may also result in other – sometimes unanticipated – side-effects (such as severe constipation in IL-6 knockout mice). Apart from being a confounding factor in the intended study, in some cases these undesired outcomes may result in poor health or even shortened life expectancy of the experimental animal, so that it limits the application of such a model even further. Of course, chain-reaction compensatory responses will also limit the extent to which results obtained in such models, may be extrapolated to a (at least genetically) normal situation.

Relatively "old-fashioned", or more conventional methods, when applied optimally, therefore still have an important place in research, both in applied areas such as pharmacology and in areas of basic research. Only when a situation that is physiologically relevant is recreated or simulated, can one realistically assess either the response to a challenge, or the outcome of a remedial intervention.

Therefore, in this chapter, I would like to reflect on methods used to simulate a variety of stressors to the body, starting with a variety of models used to simulate psychological stress, ranging in severity from non-extreme (mild) psychological stress to extreme mental trauma. I will also discuss general considerations in picking the appropriate animal model to use, which may determine the difference between success and failure in your research. Details on the various models will be provided, including issues such as repeatability and standardisation. Models will also be discussed in terms of their suitability for different research approaches or objectives, as well as in terms of their limitations. Arguments for and against the use of any particular model will also be illustrated using actual research data.

2. General considerations when choosing a rodent stress model

Small rodents are an obvious choice for research models in need of a whole body system, since they are relatively small and prolifically reproducing mammals, making them relatively economical to breed and house. Although rats and mice are physiologically very similar to humans in terms of organs and systems implicated in their response to stress, there are some fundamental differences between rodents and humans that may greatly influence results obtained using such models. It is necessary to understand these differences and the impact that it may have on any particular study employing rodents, and to adapt protocols to accommodate these differences in order to maximise the validity of results obtained. Let us consider just a few general factors that have huge impact on study outcome, but which may often be ignored or overlooked.

2.1. When to stress: lights on or off?

The timing of stress exposure, interventions to relieve stress and sampling of blood or tissue for analysis is a vital consideration, with many confounders complicating the issue. Firstly, the rat is nocturnally active, while humans obviously are not naturally nocturnal. Therefore, the question arises of whether to stress the rats during their active time, at night, or during the day, when they are asleep – which would most accurately mimic the physiological responses of humans? One could argue that it would be more applicable to expose an animal to a psychological stressor while it is awake, i.e. in the darkness – after all, how can one stress a rat when it is half asleep during the day anyway? However, this seemingly logical argument is not correct, for a very simple reason. Whether the rodent is asleep or wide awake when exposed to an experimental stressor is not the determining factor – rather, the normal rhythmic changes of hormones over the course of a day hugely affects the ability to respond to stress.

A typical circadian rhythm graph for corticosterone is presented in Figure 1. The circadian rhythm illustrated is expected in experiments employing a normal light-dark cycle – convention would be a 12 hour light-dark cycle, with lights switched on at 7am, and off at 7pm. Reversal of the light cycle has significant effects on the circadian rhythms, the "pattern" of which follows the delay in timing from the conventional one. This effect of light and darkness may be partially explained by the fact that sympathetic input to the adrenal gland is photo-sensitive: in periods of darkness, a dramatic increase in basal norepinephrine secretions from sympathetic nerves occurs (Hashimoto et al., 1999), so that basal corticosterone secretion is up-regulated in periods of darkness. However, one can also see from the curve that corticosterone secretion starts to increase after the nadir at a time of day when there is still much light – this further illustrates the complexity of this regulation, pointing to the existence of additional important causative factors.

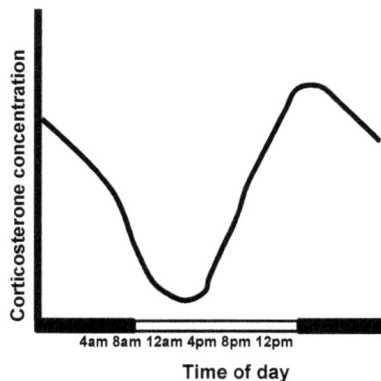

Figure 1. Expected circadian rhythm graph for corticosterone in rats. Dark bars at the bottom indicate "lights off" periods and open bar indicates the "lights on" period.

It is of importance to note that adaptation to changes in lighting conditions is not synchronised, and so does not occur within similar time frames, for all hormones. For example, while the corticosterone rhythm was shown to adapt to a 12-hour delay (phase reversal) and become constant after about 6 days, the rhythm for adrenaline only adapted after 10 days, indicating that the pituitary adrenocortical system adapts more readily to light-dark cycle shifts, while the sympatho-adrenal medullary system requires relatively more time (Miki and Sudo, 1996).

Researchers working on models using juvenile animals should also take note that the circadian rhythms for these hormone fluctuations are not fully developed at birth. The diurnal rhythm for corticosterone for example is only regular from about day 30-32 in rats (Allen and Kendall, 1967). Also, circadian rhythms are affected by many stress-related disorders – in this context, a chronic mild stress model of depression has been shown to cause fluctuations in corticosterone rhythm which only normalised after 8 weeks of chronic mild stress, and which was dependent on resilience of animals exposed to stress (Christiansen et al., 2012).

Therefore, in planning an experiment, it is most important to decide whether the stress exposure and sample collection should take place during the rising or falling phase of a hormone pulse. In the context of stress for example, one would time stress exposure and sample collection to coincide with the natural decrease of hormones expected to increase in response to stress, such as corticosterone and the catecholamines. Otherwise, if done at a time when hormone levels were increasing naturally, the circadian rhythm may effectively mask the acute response to stress. Even though these experiments should always include control samples taken from unstressed animals at the same time of day, unsynchronised sampling may still increase the variability of data, and thus decrease statistical power. This consideration is especially important in models employing physiologically relevant levels of stress, since the response seen is usually not enormous, and any potential confounders should be excluded as far as possible. Therefore, a suggestion is that all stress exposure interventions should be performed in the early morning hours, so that subsequent sample collection may to completed before noon, when the nadir for corticosterone occurs.

2.2. Metabolic rate

Another very important way in which rodents differ from humans is their much faster basal metabolic rate. Rats have a metabolic rate roughly 10 times and mice 30 times that of humans. This would obviously have huge implications for any study design with a pharmacological component. For example, when testing the potential of a stress relief medication, one would have to either increase the dose recommended by the manufacturer for human consumption, or decrease the dosage interval in rodents to ensure the maintenance of a therapeutic concentration of the drug at the level of the target tissue. Both these approaches have their drawbacks though. On the one hand, administration of a mega dose may result in intolerance reactions to the drug, most often including side effects such as gastroenteritis, with obvious confounding results given the interaction between inflammation and the glucocorticoid response. When choosing this method, parameters to monitor gut integrity, such as prostaglandin E2 levels or serum lipopolysaccharide levels, should ideally be included in the testing profile. On the other hand, decreasing the dosage interval requires more frequent handling of the experimental animals, which increases the possibility of an undesired stress response to the constant handling. This last obstacle can be partially overcome with the use of osmotic mini-pumps – these tiny pumps are implanted subcutaneously behind the neck of the rodent where it cannot reach, and releases the drug constantly at a pre-selected rate and over a pre-selected number of days. It is debatable however whether or not this method accurately reflects *in vivo* conditions for and effects of a drug that is, for example, intended to be administered orally once or twice a day, rather than continuously. A further limitation of this method is that labile substances can't be tested in this way, since the drug can only be maintained at body temperature (i.e. not cooled) for the duration of the infusion.

2.3. Social issues

A factor that should be of particular interest to researchers investigating effects of psychological stress, is the social hierarchy that exists within experimental rodent colonies. Rats in particular are a very social species, and individual housing of rats actually causes a degree of psychological stress. Therefore, standard practise is to house rats in groups of four to five, when using standard sized cages. This in itself is a limiting factor, since it is logistically not really possible to monitor appetite or food and water consumption of individual rats (which are usually done using metabolic cages in which rats are individually housed) without causing a stress response to housing conditions. Logistic factors aside, it is interesting to see that within these small groups, a social hierarchy quickly emerges, with some rats being submissive, while others are clearly dominant. Dominant rats have been shown to grow faster and to be relatively more resistant to stress interventions that submissive rats. This is both good and bad for the researcher. On the one hand, having this social hierarchy in a way simulates human situations, making the model more representative of the human population as a whole. On the other hand, the variation in the response to stress resulting from social hierarchy results in great variations in data obtained within the same experimental group, which could hide differences between experimental groups. This lowers the statistical power of any experiment, necessitating the use of larger experimental groups, which of course is more time and resource consuming. In our experience, experimental groups for the purpose of research into the psychological stress response should consist of at least 10-15 rats, on condition that all rats have been properly accustomed to the environment, handlers and protocols.

2.4. Practical tips

Apart from the factors discussed above, there are a few more general considerations to keep in mind when setting up an animal model of stress. I will touch on these just briefly. Research has shown that the mood (emotional state) of the animal handler(s) also affect the basal anxiety level of animals. Therefore some personality types may be more suited to work using animal models than others. For example, in our group we had two students conducting stress studies on sibling rats from the same litters. One student was completely at ease with the rats and handled them with natural ease, while the other student was very nervous around the rats and anxious about handling them. When assessing corticosterone levels in the control rats from the first student's study, serum concentrations were all lower than 10ng/ml. However, those from the more nervous student all had values in excess of 40ng/ml. (All samples were collected at the same time of day, so that diurnal variation did not play a role.) Of course, the fact that even unstressed animals had clearly elevated corticosterone levels, severely limits the conclusions that may be drawn from this specific experiment.

Different strains of animals have also been shown to vary substantially in their natural sensitivity to stress. This has been comprehensively reviewed elsewhere, in the context of neurobiology (Ellenbroek et al., 2005). Perhaps of specific interest for the stress researcher is the fact that these differences in stress sensitivity seems to be the effect of differences at adrenocortical level, rather than a central effect, since restraint were reported to elicit similar hippocampal and hypothalamic responses across five rat strains, although differences were quite clearly present at adrenal level (Gomez et al., 1996). An interesting fact is that some of these supposedly strain-dependent differences are more the result of nurture than nature: for example, if a spontaneously hypertensive rat (SHR) is reared by a Wistar-Kyoto rat (WKY), its hypertension is significantly less pronounced. One should therefore exercise caution in the selection of a strain to breed for the purpose of stress research. Furthermore, even within an established strain, differences occur. For example, first-time rat mothers have been shown to yield pups with relatively less resistance to stress, so that litters from first-time mothers should be avoided by the stress researcher. Also, a vital point to remember is that the experimental animal does not speak human! When conducting research in humans, it is possible – and ethically required – to explain to any volunteer the intervention that he or she will be subjected to, including expected risks. Therefore, when a human is stressed experimentally (e.g. by participating in a maths test or public speaking), although they will mount a psychological stress response, they also know that the test, or stressor, won't be permanently detrimental. A rodent on the other hand, has no way of knowing whether an acutely applied stressor will be lethal or not, so that even mild stressors are perceived as quite severe the first time. Therefore, if the requirement for research purposes is to simulate stress of a physiologically relevant severity in rodents, the stress intervention may actually seem relatively mild in comparison to what one might expect to be necessary.

From just these few considerations it is clear that the ideal *in vivo* model for psychological stress may simply not exist. However, if one is aware of potential confounders, the protocol may be optimised, and interpretation of results approached with the necessary caution, making in vivo models very valuable and realistic tools. So, how does one go about setting up the optimum model?

3. Design and setup of an animal model

Moving on to the actual setting up of a model, there are several precautions to include in the protocol, that are unique to studies on stress, especially psychological stress. For this section, I will limit myself to a discussion of rat models for stress, since this is the species of choice for this discipline, and also the species that I have most experience working with.

Putting first things first, one has to decide what situation of stress should be simulated. This is directly dependent on the research question. For example, if the question is related to the effect of a calming tablet administered to someone who has been exposed to a sudden trauma (e.g. car hi-jacking), a model where rats are subjected to a severe acute stressor is obviously the best choice. When a daily supplement is tested for stress relieving properties, or the effect of long-term occupational/stress on a specific organ is investigated, a model with multiple exposures to a relatively milder stressor would be more ideal. Sometimes, it may even be useful to combine protocols to achieve a mix of acute and chronic stress, in order to most accurately simulate actual human situations. Rats have been reported to be able to adjust to any mild stressor within a period of about 3 days (Garcia et al., 2000). Therefore, a study requiring mild stress to continue for a relatively long time, may require combination of a number of stressors in order to maintain a stressful environment.

3.1. What does a rat find stressful?

The decision of the type of stressor again depends on the situation being simulated. Stressors in real life vary from "mild irritation" to traumatic. Similar variety is therefore required in models for stress. Arguably the most popular simulation of prolonged trauma is a model known as maternal separation. Normally, pups remain with their mother throughout the first few weeks of their life until they are weaned at the age of 21-30 days, dependent on laboratory standard operating procedure. In the maternal separation model, rat pups are removed from their mother during a critical time in their development, usually during the first two or three weeks after birth, for a period of three hours per day. This traumatic separation is characterised by changes in both behavioural responses (such as anxious-like behaviour and hyperactivity in the open field test) and HPA-axis responses (such as decreased expression of glucocorticoid receptor in the hippocampus and $\approx$15% higher basal blood corticosterone concentrations) to stress, that persists into adulthood. These changes suggest an increased natural anxiety in response to chronic severe stress during early development. This technique is uniquely suited for and commonly used for investigating the development of psychiatric disorders such as anxiety and depression. Note that the endocrine responses seen in this model is relatively small in comparison to for example restraint stress models, even though it represents trauma, i.e. the most severe type of stress. One has to keep in mind though that these changes are assessed in the "rested" state, and reflects chronic changes, which are always smaller in magnitude than acute responses assessed directly after application of an acute stressor.

A somewhat milder form of stress may be simulated using restraint (sometimes called immobilisation). This technique is highly variable due to research group-specific differences in the execution of this technique. On the extreme end, animals are literally taped down on a flat board, immobilising them completely, for a period between one and two hours. Rats are fairly vocal in response to this particular protocol, so that it is advisable to conduct this particular protocol in soundproof facilities, to prevent negative effects on the rest of the animals housed in the same unit. A much milder form of restraint is to place rats in small cages that limit their movement. An example of a Perspex restraint cage (restraining up to 6 rats simultaneously) as used by our group is presented in Figure 2.

This particular cage has compartments 5cm wide x 7cm high x 18 cm long, and works best for restraint of mature Wistar rats, weighing around 300-350 g (this type of restraint is only successful when rats fit tightly into restraint compartments). Note the use of Perspex as material for the cages: this prevents the rats from having a stress response to being isolated from their group because they can still see their "neighbours". Also, body heat from peers warms the sides of the cages, creating a similar effect to when rats sleep clumped together, as they habitually do. When rats are put into these compartments, they typically turn around once or twice (invariably getting stuck halfway through the turn), and then stop trying to move. Grooming behaviour – a known self-pacifying behaviour in rats – indicates that rats are feeling claustrophobic, i.e. a psychological stress response can be expected. Rats are usually restrained for a period of 30 minutes to 2 hours once per day. During this time, they do not have access to food or water, but sufficient ventilation holes at both ends allow for normal ventilation. Keep in mind that when restraining nocturnal animals during light hours, they won't have a huge requirement to feed or drink, so that the absence of food and water is not perceived as stressful and does not impact significantly on their normal metabolism.

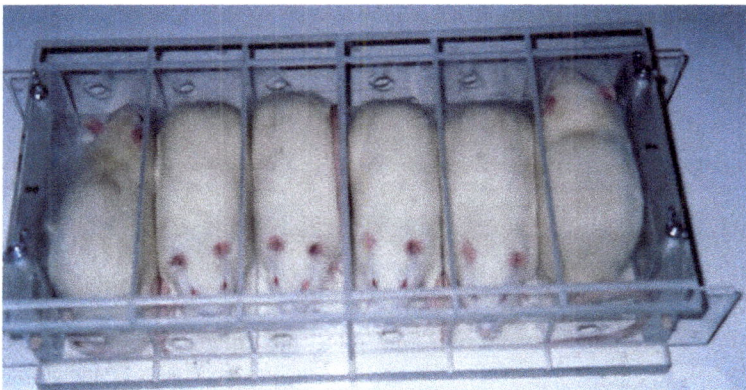

Figure 2. Restraint stress by confinement in purpose-designed Perspex cages elicits a mild form of psychological stress in rats. Adult male Wistar rats weighing more than 300g were used in this particular instance. Note the two rats on each side that were able to turn around in the cage once, but prefer not to attempt it again.

The response obtained using this model is of mild severity, and is ideal for studying normal adaptation to both acute and chronic stress. Given the wide relevance of this severity of stress to the human population, it is also a valuable model to use in the pharmacological, psychological and physiological testing of therapies, drugs and daily supplements intended to decrease stress levels or counter the side-effects of stress. This particular model is relatively easy to standardise in terms of diet, stress duration, light-dark cycle, etc. and is highly repeatable within a research group, as long as particular care is taken in selection of animal handlers and other factors already discussed. However, inter-research group differences do exist, so that care should be taken to consider changes in stress intervention protocols when comparing results reported by different laboratories. Commonly expected values with the restraint model used as an acute stress intervention lasting one hour, in our hands, are presented below (Figure 3) for changes in body mass, corticosterone, testosterone and the pro-inflammatory cytokine interleukin (IL)-1β.

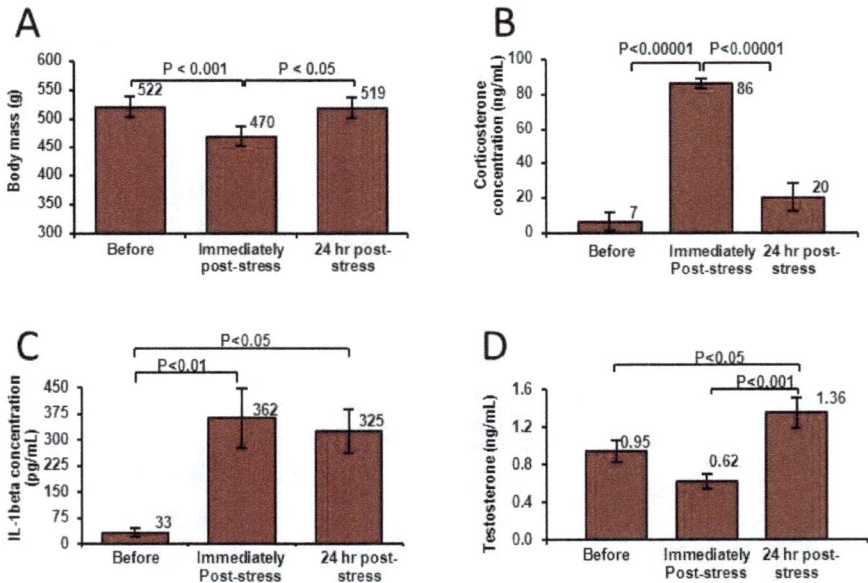

Figure 3. Effects of acute short-term restraint stress (1 hour) and recovery from stress on mean a) body mass, b) serum corticosterone, c) serum interleukin-1β and d) serum testosterone concentrations. Bars on graphs illustrate mean values, while error bars indicate standard deviations.

Body mass decreases significantly, but only transiently, in response to acute stress as applied by our group. This is mainly the result of increased defecation and urination. In terms of corticosterone, an acute increase of between 8-12-fold is seen. This response plateaus after one hour, and rats are able to recover from one exposure to restraint within one day. Testosterone concentrations are not acutely affected by acute stress, but it may increase during the recovery period. This effect is similar to that seen in athletes after a stressful bout of exercise, and may suggest an ability to cope and resist the stressful effects of the particular stressor.

In the chronic model, since the rat is not able to fully recover between stress exposure sessions when done daily for an extended time, testosterone levels do decrease with this model, resulting in a more catabolic state, and even up-regulation of the proteolytic pathways. In other words, although only mild in severity, this model is severe enough to result in undesirable side-effects in the longer term, making it an excellent simulation for chronic stress such as occupation-related stress in humans. From the cytokine data, restraint stress clearly has a pro-inflammatory effect as well, which makes this a particularly suitable model for investigations into the efficacy of e.g. anti-inflammatory interventions. Note that the IL-1β levels are still significantly elevated even after the recovery period – this is most likely due to the relatively long half-life of the cytokine. Again, in the long term, a shift toward a pro-inflammatory status is achieved.

Some groups have used involuntary swimming (forced swimming in a 1m³ swimming pool warmed to 24°C) as stressor. Although acute forced swimming is a recognised test to assess depressive-like behaviour (although this is being disputed), rats are natural swimmers, so it is doubtful whether this method – when applied chronically - is really a significant stressor. In fact, in the discipline of exercise science, researchers train rats to swim in order to study hypertrophy and metabolic adaptation to exercise training. These anabolic responses are the direct opposite of the catabolic response that is the stress response, further placing doubt on the use of this technique to realistically simulate chronic stress. Furthermore, in our experience, females are more willing swimmers than males. Males were found to simply climb onto the most submissive animal, which would then literally be drowned without investigator intervention. Alternatively, they might hold their breath and sit at the bottom of the pool for as long as they can before jumping/swimming up for a breath of air, rather than exercising the whole time. Although females tend to actually swim a lot better without the constant prodding required with males, their voluntary exercise capacity/willingness to exercise also varies dramatically. Therefore, as with voluntary running models (using purpose-designed running wheels), the "natural athletes" have to be selected from a larger cohort prior to the study. This then has the disadvantage of possible genetic pre-selection, which may yield data that is not widely applicable across the whole population. It is clear therefore, that this model has many limitations and should not be a first choice for simulation of psychological stress.

A number of other stressors may be employed, and some of these are not very labour-intensive, so that they are commonly used in combination with the stressors discussed above, to prevent adaptation, as mentioned earlier. These include soiled bedding, tail flick, and inversion or cage tilt. Bedding is soiled with water by simply pouring 300ml of water onto cage bedding and leaving rats to endure this discomfort for an hour before changing the bedding again. For the tail flick protocol, a rat is manually restrained and its tail placed in a water bath kept at 49 °C until the rat voluntarily flicks it out. For the cage tilt, the restraint cage is turned upside down for the duration of a restraint session which usually lasts from 30 minutes to an hour when used in combination with cage tilt. These are all examples of mild severity stressors. Extreme heat or cold are also referred to as stress models, but these stressors are more metabolic than psychological in nature.

3.2. Keeping experimental animal stress free

Although left for last in this section, the following point is perhaps the most important. When conducting any experiment investigating the response to stress, it is of major importance to keep all animals "otherwise" stress free. In other words, one has to ensure that rats are only exposed to the standardised stressors used as interventions in the study. Several precautions may be needed to prevent other stressors from confounding data. For example, vibration has recently been identified as a stressor in terms of the immune system. Animals exposed to constant low grade vibration may deplete their lymphocytes in as little as two to three weeks. Considering that lymphocytes make up the bulk of rat white blood cells (about 75%), it is clear that the end result is an immune-compromised animal with very abnormal cytokine profile. Therefore, while it may seem like a good idea to have a generator handy, the constant vibration it causes, may in fact be detrimental to your study.

Furthermore, new male rats should never be introduced to existing housing groups (e.g. if one rat dies, it should not be replaced with another adult rat), and adult male rats should not redistributed between cages after they have established their hierarchy. They have a social hierarchy and such changes will result in social stress, the result of which is difficult to determine before it is too late. Lastly, rodents in particular have to be handled to accustom them to their handlers. During this time, they also become used to the sounds and smells associated with their housing environment. Introduction of a new sound or smell may result in an uncontrolled, unstandardized stress response. In our laboratory, the simple guideline during acclimation of rats after arrival from the breeding unit, is to expose them to all sounds, smells (e.g. disinfectants used both during every day maintenance and during sample collection procedures), actions (e.g. weighing, sham injections, oral gavage with tap water only) and people required for the intervention study, with the exception of the intervention itself. During sacrifice, a meticulous procedure has to be followed: Firstly, all surfaces should be disinfected with a disinfectant the animal has been habituated to, in order to disguise any body odour from the previously sacrificed animal. Then, the rat is taken from its cage and euthanasia applied as soon as possible. Rats still in line for sacrifice have to be protected from any sound or smell that could alert them to what is happening; otherwise they will have a severe acute stress response. Sprague-Dawley rats for example has been shown to have increased heart rate and mean arterial blood pressure when present in the same room where other rats were being exposed to a variety of interventions, which included routine actions such as cage changes, but also experimental interventions such as decapitation (Sharp et al., 2002).

Interestingly in this study, witness rats that were individually housed, showed a greater stress response than rats group housed, further illustrating the additive effect of different stressors. The magnitude of this acute stress response can indeed be enormous. In a study by our group, corticosterone responses were determined in rats that could smell and hear experimental procedures for sacrifice. When sorted according to the order of sacrifice, it is clear that the rats waiting their turn were experiencing acute stress that accumulated with time (Figure 4).

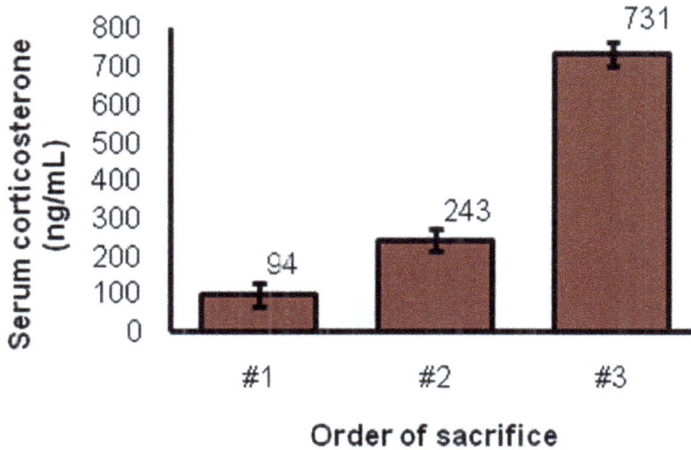

Figure 4. Cumulative corticosterone levels in an acute stress response that was elicited by witnessing the experimental killing of littermates in male Wistar rats killed approximately 15-20 minutes apart.

4. Quantifying stress responses

In terms of psychological stress, an obvious and very popular assessment technique in humans are the use of validated, standardised questionnaires designed to assess levels of perceived stress, anxiety, depression, hardiness, job satisfaction, etc. Quite clearly this method is not of use in animal models. Instead, tests to analyse and quantify stressed behaviour have been developed. The most common techniques in this context are the open field and elevated plus maze tests, as well as the forced swimming test mentioned earlier. To increase the accuracy of interpretations made from behavioural tests, it is advised to combine at least two behavioural tests, rather than to rely on the results from only one technique.

For the open field test, the researcher relies on the fact that rats naturally fear large open spaces, since this would expose them to predators. For this test, an "open field" of 1m^2 with gridlines, with high walls around all sides, are used (Figure 5). The rat to be assessed is simply placed in the centre of the open field, and its exploratory behaviour assessed by quantification of movement frequency and distance. A variation of this test is to have a second open field test on a separate day, which involves placing a novel object in the centre of the open field – the number of approaches made to this object is recorded. The interpretation of the results is not without complexity though. While a greater degree of locomotor activity and more time spent in the inner zone is usually seen as indicative of a relaxed emotional state, this same result is obtained in young rats after the traumatic experience of maternal separation. The latter condition is seen as an anxious, hyperreactivity or hyperarousal state. The "novel object" open field test can distinguish between these two explanations for the same behavioural test result: while an emotionally relaxed rat would approach the novel object often to investigate, the hyperaroused rat would be much less keen to explore the novelty.

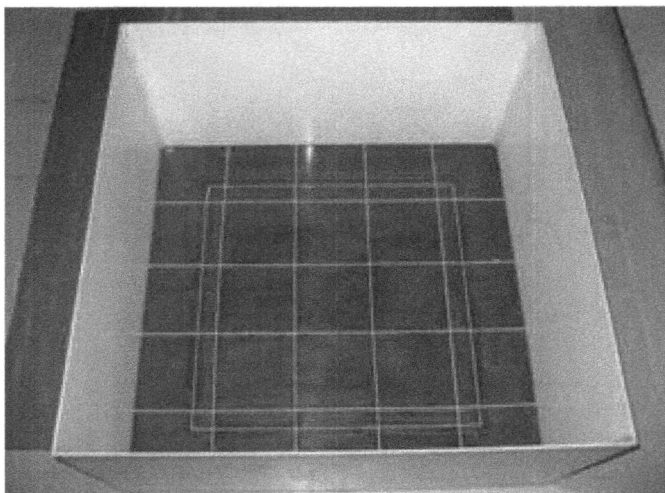

Figure 5. The open field test platform

The elevated plus maze test uses this same basic principle. The maze consist of a platform in the shape of a plus sign (+), with two opposite arms open (i.e. looking a bit like a diving platform) and the other arms closed along the sides. This platform is placed at a height of 0.5 m off the floor (Figure 6). Similar to the open field test, the rat is placed in the centre of the plus, and its courage to enter the open arms, *versus* the relatively safer closed arms (at least as perceived by a rodent), is assessed in terms of not only the number of times an open or closed arm is entered, but also the time spent in the respective arms, either moving about or sitting in one position, as well as the rat's aggressive (rearing) or self-soothing (grooming) behaviour while in the arms. In this way, a lot of data on behavioural changes may be generated, to use on its own, or to correlate with physiological data such as hormone levels. However, as with the open field test, the data is not easy to interpret. Therefore, again, no one measure should be considered as a stand-alone result.

It is of importance to note that the intervention protocol, or stress model used, may also dictate or limit the assessment techniques that are possible. Firstly, the behavioural tests are performed over the space of a few minutes. Therefore, if the investigation was related to the upstream stress responses to acute stress on the level of the brain, the physiological aspects of these responses need to be assessed immediately after exposure to the stressor. Doing a behavioural test first will result in central effects being missed, because the tissue sample will be collected too late. A suggestion to get around this is to perform the behavioural tests one day prior to the collection of tissue and blood samples for physiological and/or biochemical analyses. The use of appropriate control animals will prevent the behavioural tests from confounding results in such cases.

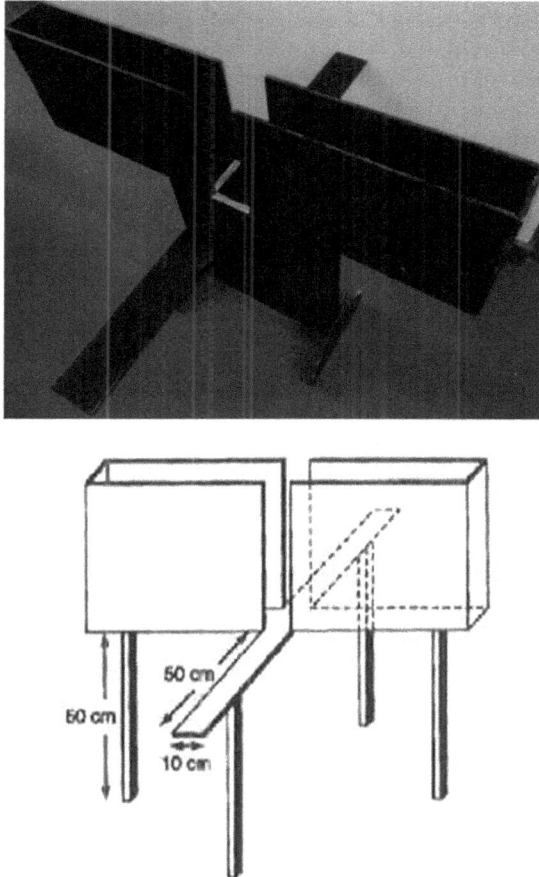

Figure 6. The elevated plus maze, with a technical drawing below to indicate dimensions.

Secondly, the type of stress intervention chosen may influence behaviour quite dramatically. For example, when considering the elevated plus maze, an anxious or stressed rat does not move about freely and would prefer the closed arms of the elevated plus maze, while an emotionally relaxed animal will exhibit more exploratory behaviour, and be more willing to enter and explore the open arms. However, when testing stressed or anxious behaviour in a rat that has just been restrained for an hour, the opposite effect is seen: an example of behavioural data illustrating this phenomenon in an elevated plus maze test is provided in Table 1. Data show that stressed rats chose to enter open arms more frequently than controls, which in this case may be interpreted as a counter reaction to having been confined to a small space during restraint. The latter explanation is very feasible, since the restraint stressed rats entered the closed arms less frequently than the controls. Although this decision would normally indicate a relaxed state, one has to keep in mind that the normally comforting closed arms would now resemble the restraint cage unit the rat had just "escaped" from, so that the rat, even though stressed, decided that the open arms are the safer option. The third parameter illustrated in Table 1, grooming, which is a self-soothing behaviour as stated earlier, clearly shows that despite the atypical result just described, the restrained rats were indeed stressed, since they spent more than four times as long trying to calm themselves than the control animals.

	Number of entries into open arms	Number of entries into closed arms	Time spent grooming (in seconds)
Control	4.3 ± 0.5	8.3 ± 0.7	11.3 ± 2.3
Stressed	5.9 ± 0.6*	6.1± 0.5*	49.8 ± 8.5**

Table 1. Selected parameters indicating behavioural responses to repeated restraint stress in male Wistar rats. Asterisks indicate values significantly different from controls (ANOVA with Bonferroni *post hoc* tests: *$P<0.05$; **$P<0.001$).

In terms of physiological assessment, stress can be assessed in terms of neuronal and endocrine pathways, as well as signalling proteins such as cytokines. Factors which may impact significantly on the quality of data is the method and timing of sacrifice and of sample collection. Recent studies on rodents commonly use intraperitoneal injection of a sodium pentabarbitone overdose. This is relatively painless and the animal loses consciousness fairly quickly. This method is also useful in the context of stress, with the exception of studies with the aim of investigating central changes. The reason for this is that the rodent will perceive the "loss of control" when losing consciousness, resulting in a central stress effect. While this effect may not reach downstream tissues in time to affect the outcome of analyses significantly, definite changes will be seen in the brain itself. Therefore, when conducting *in vivo* studies in the field of neurophysiology, it may be advisable to rather use cervical dislocation or decapitation techniques. The timing of sample a sample is of course vital. Sample collection for hormones should take into account diurnal variation in glucocorticoid levels, as discussed earlier. (For rodents, corticosterone is the glucocorticoid produced in highest quantities, whereas in humans it is cortisol.) For example, samples for determination of corticosterone levels should all be taken at the same time of day AND at the same period of recovery after the last stress exposure, so that the experiment may require quite a bit of logistical synchronisation. Also, the biological half-life of parameters of interest should be considered. For example, while corticosterone is a down-stream output of the stress pathways and has a relatively long half-life, ACTH is secreted fairly early in the stress response and has a half-life of less than 15 minutes, so that samples obtained at the end of a two-hour restraint protocol will probably not have detectable levels of ACTH, but sufficient corticosterone to be able to quantify the stress response. The design of stress protocols will therefore have different endpoints, depending on the aim of the investigation, for example a short restrain period may be more ideal for detection of upstream events in the stress pathways, while a longer one may be required for down-stream parameters to become available in circulation. Therefore, in order to time the sacrifice of an animal and collection of samples optimally, it is necessary to understand the basic biochemistry and/or pharmacology of parameters of interest.

In some instances it may be even more useful to determine down-stream effects related to earlier events, rather than trying to "catch" upstream parameters in circulation at an optimal time. This is also true when the parameter of interest can have its origin from more than one source. For example, when considering the inflammatory component of the response to stress – which has been linked to many chronic diseases recently – it is difficult to pinpoint the origin of cytokines when only assessed in blood, since most of them are released from a wide variety of cells. Also, since some cytokines, such as IL-6, have an autocrine-type action, its level in circulation is often not indicative of events at cellular level. In these instances, immunostaining of tissue levels of these parameters are very useful. Indirect measurements of e.g. inflammatory responses can also inform on the response to stress. For example, instead of measuring TNF-α levels in blood, activity of the proteolytic pathways in tissue may be employed as indirect indicator of TNF-α activity, which known to play an important role in muscle wasting, or cachexia. In this way, the timing of sampling become less critical, and the effect at the level of the target tissue, may be directly elucidated.

5. Characterisation and standardisation of stress models

The severity of the stressor will determine the extent of acute activation of the HPA-axis and/or SAM pathway, as well as the adaptability of the animal to the stressor, i.e. the chronic response to any particular stressor. This necessitates the standardisation and characterisation of any particular model by researchers prior to its application for research purposes. Our group have characterised our model of restraint stress in terms of a variety of parameters. One of these is the corticosterone response, which is presented for protocols of different durations in Figure 7.

This figure illustrates the significant difference in the response to a specific stressor acutely, and after chronic intermittent exposure, after which one may expect habituation to the stressor. One can see from these data that the stressor employed was indeed mild; although there was a substantial increase in corticosterone concentration in serum immediately after the restraint (at the "acute" time point), the rat was able to completely recover its corticosterone levels to control levels one day after the single restraint session. The data further indicates the effectiveness of this model to induce chronic stress: the value labelled "4 days" indicates that 3 restraint stress sessions over 3 days resulted in a corticosterone response that the rats could not completely recover from overnight, resulting in a significantly elevated corticosterone level even after a period of recovery, albeit not as highly elevated as in the acute version of the model.

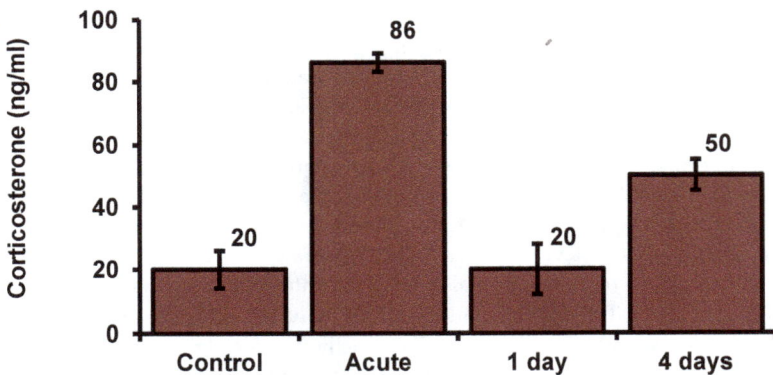

Figure 7. Corticosterone responses to one hour of restraint stress daily, for protocols of different durations. Values are means for at least n=10 rats per experimental group.

However, as discussed earlier, these results in its entirety will probably only be valid for the model as executed in our hands. Although the same trend should be seen – e.g. the increased corticosterone levels in stressed rats – the magnitude of this response as well as the animal's ability to habituate to it, is largely dependent on the execution of the model by various research groups, who each adapts the protocol to be best suited for their own particular research interests. Therefore, it is vital to include sufficient control groups for all interventions, in order to facilitate cross-group comparisons of results.

6. Conclusion

Conducting research using experimental animal models is a complex endeavour, with many considerations, adaptations to make and precautions to take. However, when applied by researchers with the ability to adapt a protocol to make the most of it, results achieved are very satisfactory in terms of quality, repeatability and direct applicability to actual physiological situations. Therefore, in conclusion, cell-based scientists and systems biologists should combine efforts to successfully counter the effects of stress.

Author details

Carine Smith

Stellenbosch University, South Africa

Acknowledgement

I would like to acknowledge all the postgraduate students and collaborators of the Interdisciplinary Stress Biology Group at the Department Physiological Sciences at Stellenbosch University, South Africa, who contributed to the experience gained and lessons learnt through working in rodent models of stress.

7. References

Allen C and Kendall JW (2005) Maturation of the circadian rhythm of plasma corticosterone in the rat. *Endocrinology* 80 (5): 926-930.

Christiansen S, Bouzinova EV, Palme R, Wiborg O (2012) Circadian activity of the hypothalamic-pituitary-adrenal axis is differentially affected in the rat chronic mild stress model of depression. *Stress* (epub Feb 23) PMID 22217141.

Ellenbroek BA, Geven EJ, Cools AR (2005) Rat Strain Differences in Stress Sensitivity, In: *Handbook of Stress and the Brain*, volume 15, chapter 14, Steckler T, Kalin NH, Reul JMHM, Elsevier B.V.

Garcia A, Marti O, Valles A, Dal-Zotto S, Armario A (2000) Recovery of the Hypothalamic-pituitary-adrenal Response to Stress. Effect of Stress Intensity, Stress Duration and Previous Stress Exposure. *Neuroendocrinology* 72(2): 114-125.

Gomez F, Lahmane A, de Kloet ER, Armario A (1996) Hypothalamic-pituitary-adrenal Response to Chronic Stress in Five Inbred Rat Strains: Differential Responses are Mainly Located at the Adrenocortical Level. *Neuroendocrinology* 63(4):327-337.

Hashimoto M, Kuwahara M, Tsubone H, Sugano S (1999) Diurnal Variation of Autonomic Nervous Activity in the Rat. *Journal of Electrocardiology* 32(2):167-171.

Miki S and Sudo A (1996) Adaptation of circadian corticosterone and catecholamine rhythms to light-dark cycle reversal in the rat. *Industrial Health* 34: 134-138.

Selye H. (1956). *The Stress of Life*, McGrawHill, New York. (Revised edition: 1976)

Sharp J, Zammit T, Azar T, L. Dawson D (2002) Does Witnessing Experimental Procedures Produce Stress in Male Rats? *Contemp Top Lab Anim Sci* 41: 8 -12.

Chapter 10

Glucocorticoids in Mate Choice

Fhionna R. Moore

Additional information is available at the end of the chapter

1. Introduction

Choosing the right mate is fundamental to reproductive success. Selecting the right genes with which to combine one's own increases the chances of offspring survival and reproduction. Choosing wisely, then, can increase the number of copies of genetic material being passed on to future generations. This means that it serves an individual well to signal their own strengths and qualities in order to attract mates, and it serves the opposite sex well to express preferences for honest signals of mate quality. As opposed to natural selection (the process by which traits which confer a survival advantage are selected for [1]), sexual selection is selection for those traits that confer benefits in terms of attracting, and mating with, members of the opposite sex [2]. Such sexually selected traits often serve to reduce the chances of survival and their adaptive function is solely to increase an individual's mating success. Classic examples are the peacock's extravagant tail plumage that dramatically increases chances of predation [3], and the display of the bowerbird, which bears a heavy energetic cost to construct [4]. These traits have evolved as the benefits of attracting members of the opposite sex outweigh the associated costs to survival. In order for these social signalling systems to work, however, the signal must provide an honest indication of quality [5, 6]. If it is possible to cheat, the system could not function: elaborate displays would no longer signal a genetic benefit for offspring.

Honest signals of mate-choice relevant qualities fall into two broad categories, both of which are impossible to fake. These are qualities that infer "indirect" benefits, which include heritable traits such as a strong immune system [7, 8], and those that infer "direct" benefits, such as the ability and willingness to provide resources and parental care. Over the last decade evidence has accumulated to suggest that the physiological stress response may be linked to both sets of characteristics. For one, the glucocorticoid hormones modulate the immune system, meaning that stress may influence health and condition which, in turn, influence the ability of an individual to mate successfully or to provision and care for offspring [9, 10]. Alternatively, between-individual variation in dimensions of the stress response such as the peak levels of glucocorticoids secreted in response to a stressor and the time taken for levels to return to baseline are heritable, meaning that individuals are likely to differ in their ability to cope effectively and efficiently with stress [11, 12]. There is a growing body of evidence that demonstrates that females assess the glucocorticoid status of potential opposite sex partners, and express preferences for cues to low stress.

Given the role of hormones in directing the allocation of energy to different physiological and behavioural functions, it is not surprising that they have received attention in the context of mate choice and sexual signalling. Testosterone has received by far the most attention in this domain due to evidence for its role in the development of those male traits used to attract females. Among many other traits testosterone is, for example, consistently found to relate to the vitality of sexually selected plumage colouration in birds (see for example [13, 14]), the size and strength of antlers in red deer stags (*Cervus elaphus*; see for example [15, 16]) and the intensity and complexity of bird song (see for example [17, 18]). In essence, high testosterone results in a strong signal that, in turn, translates into mating success. In the Immunocompetence Handicap Hypothesis of sexual selection [7], testosterone-dependent traits are proposed to provide an honest signal of the strength of a male's immune system due to the hormone's immunosuppressive actions. In other words, only those males who have inherited a robust immune system can afford the costs of the elevated testosterone required for development of extravagant sexual signals. A large antlered red deer stag, then, is signalling his superior immune system. This, in turn, should attract female mates who seek to acquire such "good genes" for their offspring. In the years since its inception, this model has generated a huge body of research, with a Google Scholar search for "Immunocompetence Handicap" returning ~2, 500 publications.

Despite providing an elegant explanation for the maintenance of variation in the expression of sexual signals as honest indicators of quality, and good evidence that such traits are linked to parasite resistance, however, one of the Immunocompetence Handicap model's fundamental assumptions fails to receive adequate support. Reviews show inconsistency in evidence for immunosuppression by testosterone [19]. As a consequence, biologists have attempted to address this weakness by identifying additional or alternative endocrinological factors that may contribute to the system. And this is where the glucocorticoids have attracted attention. These stress hormones are correlated with testosterone across species (albeit the direction of the relationship is variable; see for example [11, 20 – 23]) and modulate immune function [24] and body condition [9, 10]. In [11], for example, the authors demonstrated that an immunosuppressive effect of testosterone in the house sparrow (*Passer domesticus*) disappeared when the effects of the primary avian glucocorticoid corticosterone were controlled for statistically. They concluded that the effects of testosterone on the immune system may be mediated or moderated by co-occurring levels of glucocorticoids. More recently, it has been suggested that low levels of glucocorticoids may be preferable due to detrimental effects of high levels on body condition and health [10]. The following discussion addresses the evidence to date to suggest functions of glucocorticoids in mate choice and sexual selection.

2. How do glucocorticoids influence mate choice?

Human research offers excellent opportunities to test roles of stress in mate choice. There is evidence that cortisol (the primary human glucocorticoid) and testosterone are positively correlated [25], although this finding is not consistent (see for example [26, 27]) and may depend upon, for example, the intensity of recent exercise [28]. Sexually dimorphic facial characteristics derive from sex differences in the ratio of the male and female sex hormones that emerge at puberty (see for example [29]). A surge of testosterone in males during adolescence promotes cranio-facial bone growth resulting in heavier jaws and eyebrow ridges. These changes are inhibited in females by the action of oestrogen. In adulthood there are positive relationships between both circulating testosterone [30] and testosterone response to a challenge [31] and masculinity of the male face, as well as between oestrogen and femininity in female faces [32]. This means that there are cues to testosterone in the male face that we can parametrically manipulate using sophisticated digital face morphing techniques. Circulating levels of cortisol and testosterone can be measured using non-invasive methods that reduce activation of the stress response to provide an accurate estimate of baseline levels of the hormones. Furthermore, it is possible to obtain ratings by women of perceptions of facial stimuli that differ in cues to the hormones. These are luxuries not so easily afforded by work with other species and mean that we are able to identify any mediating or moderating role of cortisol on relationships between testosterone and attractiveness in a uniquely controlled way.

The relationship between sexual dimorphism and attractiveness is fairly consistent for female faces, with both men and women agreeing that the more feminine a face, the more attractive it is (see for example [33, 34]). For male faces, however, the story is more complicated, with variation in women's preferences suggestive of a trade-off in the relative importance of a committed, reliable partner versus a partner who signals "good genes". Given the relationship between testosterone and masculinity of the male face, masculine faced males may signal a robust immune system. While this is likely to be attractive to women seeking to secure a strong immune system for offspring, it must be balanced up against the negative personality characteristics that are attributed to the owners of masculine male faces, including dishonesty, low likelihood to commit to a relationship and aggression (see for example [35, 36]). This perhaps explains why women tend to prefer feminine-faced men who are attributed with honesty, commitment and good parenting in general, but to switch to preferences for more masculine faces at times when the chances of conception are high including the fertile phase of the menstrual cycle (see for example [37]), when commitment is less important to mate choice decisions, such as when faces are judged for a short term rather than a long term relationship (see for example [38]) and in societies in which there is greater competition for resources [39] or in which the costs of ill health are high [40].

In a sample of 69 Scottish male students, my colleagues and I measured testosterone and cortisol from saliva samples collected by passive drool at two time-points (one in the morning and one in the afternoon), to control for circadian fluctuations in both hormones, using enzyme-linked immunosorbant assays. Mean testosterone leves ranged from 0.07 – 0.63 ng/mL, and mean cortisol from 3.7 – 24.04 nmol/L. We also took facial photographs of participants under standardized conditions (e.g. with diffuse flash lighting, at the same distance from the camera and with glasses removed and neutral expression). We assessed the effects of testosterone and cortisol on facial attractiveness in two ways. First, we asked a sample of female participants to rate the faces for attractiveness, masculinity and health on 1 – 7 scales (1 = not at all attractive/masculine/healthy, 7 = extremely attractive/masculine/healthy). The faces of males with low cortisol were rated as significantly more attractive than those with high cortisol (r^2 = -0.36, p = 0.027). There were no relationships between cortisol, health and masculinity and, unlike previous studies ([37] for example), testosterone was not related to women's perceptions of the faces (all p > 0.3). Next, we used the face morphing software *Psychomorph* to create "composite" facial images which contained cues to combinations of high and low levels of testosterone and cortisol [41]. For this, we identified groups of 5 – 6 males with the following combinations of hormones, based on median splits: high testosterone and high cortisol, high testosterone and low cortisol, low testosterone and high cortisol, low testosterone and low cortisol. We then "averaged" together the faces of the participants in each of these groups to give composite stimuli containing cues to the 4 combinations of hormones (see Figure 1).

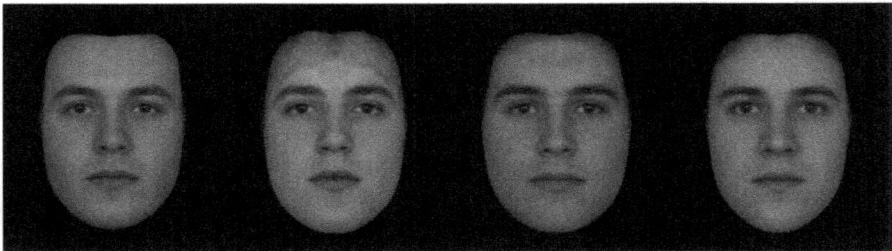

Figure 1. Composite male faces constructed to differ in combinations of testosterone and cortisol. From left to right: high testosterone with high cortisol, high testosterone with low cortisol, low testosterone with high cortisol, low testosterone with low cortisol. Taken from Moore et al. 2011. Proceedings of the Royal Society of London Series B, doi:10.1098/rspb.2010.1678.

The stimuli were then rated by a novel sample of female participants during the fertile and non-fertile phases of their menstrual cycles. Using mixed model Anova, we found that women consistently preferred the low cortisol composites ($F_{(1, 42)}$ = 5.11, p = 0.029). Post hoc analyses revealed that this effect was significant in the fertile ($F_{(1, 42)}$= 6.44, p = 0.015), but not the non-fertile (p > 0.1) cycle phase (see Figure 2). We concluded that women can detect cues to cortisol in the male face, and that low cortisol is desirable in a male partner. We also suggested that low cortisol may be associated with beneficial heritable characteristics as women expressed the strongest preferences for facial cues to low cortisol at times when they were most likely to conceive [26].

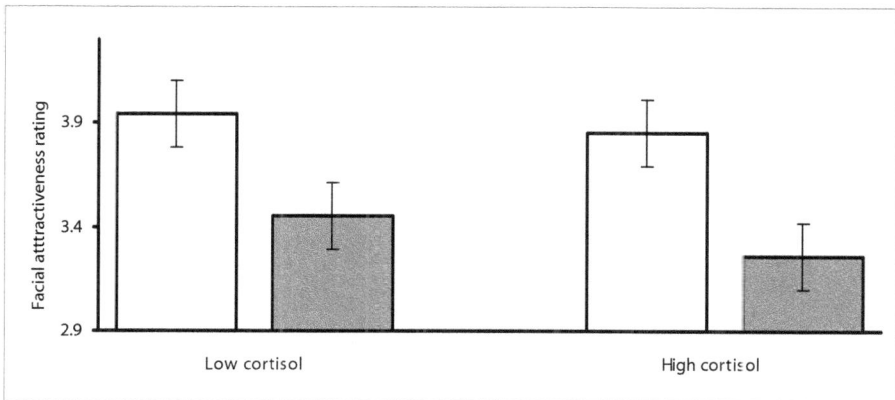

Figure 2. Mean attractiveness ratings of composite male faces constructed to differ in cues to cortisol by women during the non-fertile (empty bars) and fertile (filled bars) phases of their menstrual cycles with error bars showing +- 1 SE. In a mixed model anova there was a significant effect of cortisol on attractiveness ($F_{(1, 42)}$ = 5.11, p = 0.029). Post hoc tests revealed that this effect was significant only during the fertile phase of the cycle ($F_{(1, 42)}$= 6.44, p = 0.015) [26].

We replicated this pattern of results in a different sample of faces with a novel sample of female raters, again recruited from UK student populations. Once again, women preferred the faces of males with low cortisol, and didn't express preferences for testosterone. In this second study, we also tested the effects of the hormones on perceived dominance and health, finding that low cortisol faces were also rated as more dominant and healthy than high cortisol faces [26, 27]. The findings of both studies are consistent with work in other species that shows that females prefer males with low levels of glucocorticoids. In [12], for example, the authors found that female zebra finch (*Tynopygea guttatta*) preferred males with low corticosterone, and expressed no preference for cues to testosterone. Spectrophotometric measures of plumage suggested that dimensions of plumage colour and brightness provided cues to the stress status of the male. Similarly, in [42] Leary and colleagues found that female great plains toads (*Bufo cognatus*) preferred the calls of males with low glucocorticoids. There is growing evidence, then, that glucocorticoids play a role in mate choice. Why this may be, however, is unclear.

Glucocorticoids and testosterone

One possibility is that the hormonal underpinnings in expression of sexual traits that have previously been attributed to testosterone are, in fact, due to the effects of the glucocorticoids (see for example [11]). If this were the case, however, we would expect to find effects of testosterone that disappear once glucocorticoids are controlled for statistically. Although this pattern of results was reported for a study of effects of the hormones on the immune function of the house sparrow, this has not been replicated in other species. It seems unlikely, then, that the role of stress is so straightforward. Rather than simple mediation of effects of testosterone by those of cortisol, in both of our studies described above we found an interaction between testosterone and cortisol, such that the detrimental effects of cortisol were stronger in those males with low testosterone compared to those with high testosterone (See Figure 3). We proposed that high testosterone males (i.e. those signalling the strength of their immune system) are better able to cope with the detrimental effects of stress [26, 27]. In order to test this explanation, however, it is necessary to experimentally manipulate stress in males who differ in their level of testosterone and test for any divergent effects on immune system and/or sexual signals.

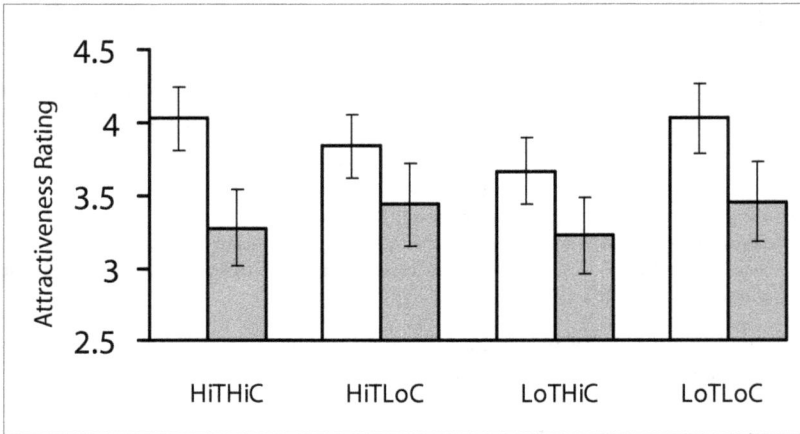

Figure 3. Mean attractiveness ratings of composite faces that differ in combinations of testosterone and cortisol (+1 s.e.) by women during the non-fertile (empty) and fertile (filled) phases of their menstrual cycles. The figure shows an interaction between the hormones, such that cortisol reduces attractiveness in males with low testosterone, but enhances it in males with high testosterone. Taken from Moore et al. 2011. Proceedings of the Royal Society of London Series B, doi:10.1098/rspb.2010.1678.

While we have replicated the interaction between testosterone and cortisol in two UK samples, in a recent attempt to determine whether our results extend across human populations, we found evidence to suggest that the effects of combinations of sex and stress hormones on facial appearance are population-dependent. In a third study, we tested relationships between testosterone, cortisol and facial attractiveness in a sample of 74 male students. This time we tested relationships across the faces of individual males, rather than in digitally manipulated composite faces and measured testosterone and cortisol from intravenous blood samples rather than from saliva as this allowed us to take simultaneous measurements of immune function. Contrary to previous studies, we found a positive relationship between testosterone and men's facial attractiveness, but no relationship between cortisol and attractiveness. While we found an interaction between testosterone and cortisol in effects on facial attractiveness, it's nature differed to that reported in our previous studies such that this time the positive relationship between testosterone and attractiveness was strongest in those males with low cortisol [43]. See Figure 4.

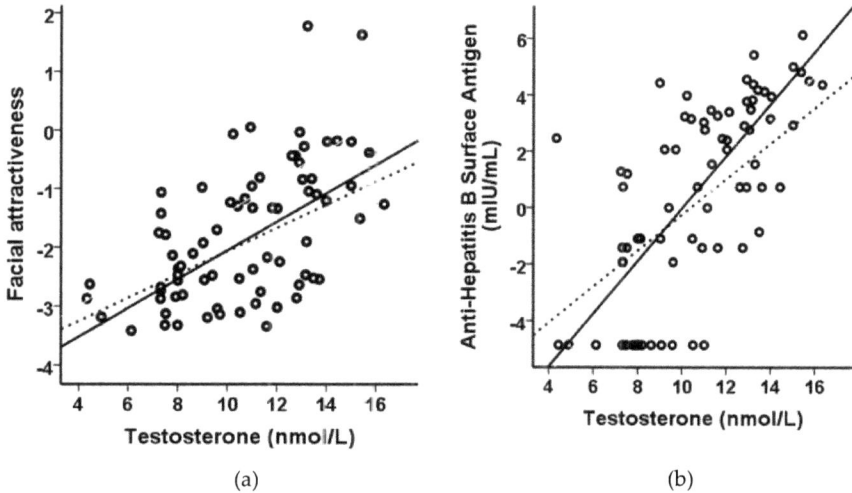

(a)   (b)

Figure 4. Relationships between testosterone and (a) facial attractiveness in a sample of Latvian male students rated by female participants drawn from the same population, showing an interaction with cortisol such that the relationship was strongest in those males with low cortisol (solid line) and weakest in those with high cortisol (broken line) and (b) antibody response to a hepatitis B vaccine, showing an interaction with cortisol such that the relationship was strongest in those males with low cortisol (solid line) and weakest in those with high cortisol (broken line). From [43].

Why should we find differences in the nature of the interaction between testosterone and cortisol on facial attractiveness between our samples? It seems unlikely that we can attribute this to differences in our methods. In all 3 studies we tested for relationships between the hormones and face perceptions across individual faces and failed to find interactions between testosterone and cortisol in either of the first two studies. Does the construction of composites result in spurious results? Only further testing will adequately test this, but an alternative possibility is that societal-level factors cause systematic variation in the effects of sex- and stress- hormones (and combinations of the two) on attractiveness. While the samples in our first two studies were taken from populations of UK students, the sample for our third study – the one in which we found a different interaction between the hormones – was drawn from a sample of male students and female raters from the University of Daugavpils in Latvia. Could societal-level differences in the strategies employed by women to assess the attractiveness of male faces underpin the differences we report in the effects of sex- and stress-hormones on facial attractiveness? There is evidence to suggest that this could be the case. In [40], for example, Debruine and colleagues reported that societal level health measures were related to women's preferences for cues to testosterone in the male face. That is, women in societies in which the costs of ill health are high express stronger preferences for cues to high testosterone. Perhaps, then, cultural differences in the provision of healthcare, or in other social and economic factors, cause the female raters in our samples to express divergent preferences for cues to testosterone and/or cortisol, which in turn will influence the nature of the interaction between the two. This is insightful as identification of the socioecological factors that underpin variation in preferences for cues to the hormones can contribute to our understanding of the traits and characteristics that they signal. My collaborators and I are currently conducting further cross-cultural research to achieve this.

That population-level differences in socioecology could influence the nature of the role of stress in mate choice is further supported by cross-species differences in interactions between testosterone and glucocorticoids on sexual traits. Such interactions have been reported in several avian species. In the red grouse, for example, a positive relationship between testosterone and comb area was stronger in males with low levels of co-occurring glucocorticoids than in those with physiological markers of high stress [44]. Conversely, in the red bishop (*Euplectes orix*), the relationship between testosterone and plumage colour was inverse under high stress, but positive or non-significant under low stress [45]. Despite evidence, then, that testosterone-dependent signalling is contingent upon concurrent stress, the nature of interactions between sex and stress hormones is inconsistent.

In order to begin to interpret the meaning of this inconsistency, it is necessary to understand a little more about how the two hormones interact at a physiological level. One way is through competition for binding sites on the two types of glucocorticoid receptor. The first of these has a high affinity for the stress hormones, so glucocorticoids tend to bind to these first, meaning that the receptors are typically saturated at peak points in the circadian cycle and therefore serve primarily to regulate circadian rhythms. The second type, although more abundant, have a lower binding affinity, so tend to bind once all the first type are engaged. These, then, are the receptors that are bound during response to a stressor and regulate the stress response [46]. This means that baseline and peak response glucocorticoids can be conceptualized as different hormonal systems as their binding to different types of receptors results in divergent effects on physiology and behaviour [46]. As the proteins which bind glucocorticoids (corticosteroid binding globulins) can also bind testosterone, there may be competition between the hormones for binding sites – particularly in avian species who lack independent sex steroid binding globulins [47, 48]. It is possible, for example, that elevated glucocorticoids reduce the numbers of receptors available for testosterone, reducing bound levels and increasing free levels which may influence effects of testosterone on behaviour and signalling. Perhaps, then, relationships between testosterone and glucocorticoids, and their combined effects on sexual signals, depend upon the species and the dimension of the stress response that is measured (e.g. peak versus baseline).

Immunocompetence

The "stress-linked" model of hormonally-mediated sexual selection as originally proposed over a decade ago [11, 49], in acknowledgement of increasing awareness that extant endocrinological models did not sufficiently explain variation in the cross-species data, proposed that effects of glucocorticoids on sexual traits were likely to occur through their effects on the immune system. Despite evidence for an immunomodulatory role of stress, meaning that this seems to be a viable possibility, it poses a difficult problem to address, and an even more difficult system to model, as it is not simply the case that stress suppresses the immune system. Depending upon the nature, duration and predictability of a stressor, for example, stress can enhance, suppress or redistribute immune activity [24]. How, then, can we model and test roles of stress in sexual selection that are mediated by effects on the immune system? To date, a handful of studies of avian species have tested inter-relationships between stress, immune function and sexual signalling demonstrating complex relationships between immune function, stress and sexual signals. A study of red grouse, for example, reported a positive relationship between glucocorticoids and parasite load and an inverse relationship between parasite load, and testosterone-dependent ornament (i.e. supraorbital comb) area [44]. Similarly, a study of blue tits (*Cyanistes caeruleus*) demonstrated parasite load to be positively related to a physiological marker of stress (heat shock proteins) and inversely to sexually selected colouration [50]. Conversely, a study of song sparrows (*Melospiza melodia*) reported no relationship between stress and immune function [51], meaning that detrimental effects of stress on song repertoire were not mediated by immunocompetence. In our work with human faces, my colleagues and I found that the pattern of the interaction between testosterone and cortisol on attractiveness was mirrored by the same pattern in effects on antibody response to a vaccine [43]. See Figure 4b. While there is some evidence, then, to suggest that the combined effects of testosterone and cortisol on sexual signalling are concurrent with those on immune function, it seems likely that such results are dependent upon the arm of the immune system that is assessed as well as the measurement of stress.

Stress and body condition

Husak and Moore [10] suggested that glucocorticoids could influence the intensity of sexual signals via their detrimental effects on body condition. If stress reduces body condition (e.g. body mass and/or fat stores), an individual who is experiencing stress is less likely to be able to afford to allocate energy and metabolic resources to sexual signalling. Effects of stress on body condition, however, are inconsistent, with studies from some species showing that stress reduces body condition (song sparrow (*Melospiza melodia*) [51]; upland geese (*Chloephaga picta*) [52]; zebra finches [53]), others showing stress to increase body condition (Beldings ground squirrels (*Spermophilus beldingi*) [54]) and still others showing no effect (e.g. mallard ducks (*Anas platyrhynchos*) [55]). Furthermore, few studies have shown effects of stress on sexual signals that were consistent with those on condition. An exception is the red grouse, in which parasite load was shown to reduce body condition, increase physiological markers of stress and reduce the expression of plumage colouration [56]. The evidence, then, suggests that any effects of stress on sexual signals do not occur via its action on body condition. In fact, in some cases, stress may cause a reallocation of resources away from body condition and into sexual signalling. Positive relationships between stress and the expression of carotenoid – based colouration at the cost of condition have been reported in the zebra finch [53] and the common lizard [57]. This suggests that, in some cases, stress causes a redistribution of energy and resources away from long term goals and instead to short term priorities (e.g. mating). This would seem to be a sensible strategy when, for example, survival was threatened, which may be signalled by elevated stress hormones.

Stress &behaviour

In addition to sexual signals such as ornaments, colouration or song, stress also impacts upon behaviours relevant to reproduction. There may, then, be behavioural cues to glucocorticoid status which females make use of in their mate choice decisions, or stress-dependent sexual signals may provide insight into an individual's likely behaviour. Activation of the hypothalamic-pituitary-adrenal axis in response to stress suppresses the hypothalamic-pituitary-gonadal axis which is responsible for mediating sexual behaviour [58], resulting in reduced expression of sexual behaviours. One mechanism, for example, by which stress suppresses reproductive behaviour is via inhibition of the gonadotropin protein hormones which regulate reproductive function by glucocorticoids [59, 60]. It is well known that chronically elevated stress suppresses reproduction by, for example, reducing sex drive, courtship behaviour and fertility(see for example [61 - 63]). There is also evidence that acutely elevated glucocorticoids have a similar outcome with, for example, glucocorticoids elevated by fasting reducing courtship behaviour such as singing in the male zebra finch [64] and the locomotor activity that contributes to foraging and reproduction in male Allegheny dusky salamanders (*Desmognathus ochrophaeus*;[65]). Elevated glucocorticoids are also associated with reduced provisioning of offspring (see for example [66]).It is possible, then, that females attend to behavioural indications of high stress, or that stress-dependent sexual signals provide an indication of reproductive function and/or ability to provision offspring. Avoiding individuals who are currently experiencing stress will reduce the chances of attempting to mate with a member of the opposite sex with reduced reproductive function and/or ability to provision offspring, thereby allowing the female to maximise her reproductive success.

There are also relationships between stress and dominance, although these are typically complex and dependent upon, among many others, both the status of an individual in a hierarchy and the stability of the social structure. Attention to cues to stress, then, may enable an individual to select an opposite sex partner who occupies a high status position in a dominance hierarchy, with associated high status and access to premium resources, ensuring high status, well-provisioned offspring. It is not simply the case, however, that high stress is a cue to low rank in a hierarchy. Creel [67], for example, demonstrates that, although agonistic social interactions can provoke a large glucocorticoid response, in established social groups, where individuals know the hierarchy, such responses are not necessarily the case and in some cooperative breeding species (i.e. a social system in which individuals contribute to the care of others' offspring) such as the meerkat (*Suricata suricatta*), for example, dominant individuals may have higher glucocorticoids that subordinates. It seems likely that divergent levels of stress hormones in accordance with strata of the social structure are dependent upon both the nature of the hierarchy which is, in turn, dependent upon species socioecology but also upon stability of the hierarchy. In unstable structures, if dominant individuals are involved in the most agonistic encounters, then it is the dominant individuals who experience the highest levels of stress. In mallards and pintails (*Anas acuta*; [55]), bison (*Bison bison*; [68]) and ring necked pheasants (*Phasianus colchicus*; [56]), for example, dominant males have higher levels of glucocorticoids than subordinate males. It seems likely, then, that if cues to stress are used to infer information about a potential partner's dominance status or, vice versa, if dominance status influences stress levels, the direction of such relationships will be species dependent.

Future research

Despite evidence to suggest that glucocorticoids play a role in sexual selection and mate choice, the nature and function of that role remains unclear. The effects of stress, while typically serving to reduce male attractiveness and the expression of sexual signals, are not consistent with some studies showing positive effects. Furthermore, despite proposals that the effects of stress occur through its action on immune function and/or body condition, there is little evidence to support this. Therefore, while we know that females prefer males with cues to low levels of stress hormones, we do not yet know what cues they attend to or what is signalled by "low stress". Despite a growing body of research, then, we are still confronted by a number of unknowns. Is it the case, for example, that males signal their current stress status? Or do they rather signal their ability to respond optimally to a stressor (i.e. an adaptive response which promotes survival but reduces the detrimental costs to health)? Are all sexual traits and signals similarly influenced by stress? That is, does stress affect those traits which show great plasticity during adulthood (e.g. plumage colouration in birds, or skin health in humans) differently to those which emerge at set developmental stages (e.g. bird song or human facial sexual dimorphism). Is the link with immune function so complex that we have to look at redistribution of resources across the arms of the immune system in response to chronic versus acute, and predictable versus unpredictable stressors? To begin to answer these questions, and to model roles of stress in mate choice, it is now necessary to test the effects of baseline stress, and of dimensions of the stress response (e.g. total amount of glucocorticoids produced in response to a standardised stressor and time to return to baseline) on different types of sexual signals (e.g. those that are typically dependent upon current condition versus those that develop at set life history stages) and to interpret findings in the context of species and population ecology [69]. Cross-cultural and cross-species comparisons can likewise contribute to our understanding of the traits signalled by low glucocorticoids.

3. Conclusion

To summarise, then, there is a growing body of evidence to show that the glucocorticoid hormones are implicated in mate choice and sexual selection. Women prefer the faces of males with low levels of cortisol, for example, and female zebra finch prefer males with low levels of corticosterone. We do not know, however, why females express these preferences as it is not yet clear what characteristics are signalled by cues to low glucocorticoids. Suggestions in the literature are that stress reduces body condition or suppresses the immune system which, in turn, reduce the extent to which individuals seek to attract members of the opposite sex. The extant evidence, however, does not consistently support these theories. It has also been proposed that stress mediates the effect of testosterone on sexual signals. Again, there is little support for this with results instead suggesting an interaction between testosterone and glucocorticoids – the nature of which is dependent upon the species, population and, in all likelihood, current socioecological conditions. What is clear is that there is increasing evidence for stress in sexual selection. It is now necessary to seek to better understand and model its precise roles and functions by conducting research which clearly operationalises the dimension of the stress response and the type of trait under investigation.

Author details

Fhionna R. Moore
School of Psychology, College of Art and Social Science, University of Dundee, UK

Acknowledgement

I am grateful to Kate Buchanan for insightful comments on a related draft and to Indrikis Krams, Markus Rantala and Vinet Coetzee for interesting discussions on the roles of stress in sexual selection.

4. References

[1] Darwin C (1859) On the Origin of Species by Means of Natural Selection, or the Preservation of Favoured Races in the Struggle for Life. John Murray, London; modern reprint Charles Darwin, Julian Huxley.

[2] Darwin C (1871) The Descent of Man and Selection in Relation to Sex. John Murray, London

[3] Petrie M, Halliday T, Sanders C (1991) Peahens prefer peacocks with elaborate trains. Anim. Behav. 41: 323-331.

[4] Borgia G (1985) Bowers as markers of male quality. Tests of a hypothesis. Anim. Behav. 33: 266-271.

[5] Grafen A (1990) Biological signals as handicaps. J. Theor. Biol 144:517-546.

[6] Zahavi A (1975) Mate selection - a selection for a handicap. J. Theor. Biol. 53: 205-214.

[7] Folstad I, Karter A J (1992) Parasites, bright males and the immunocompetence handicap. Am. Nat. 139: 603-622.

[8] Hamilton W D, Zuk M (1982) Heritable true fitness and bright birds: a role for parasites? Science 218: 384-387.

[9] Buchanan K L (2000) Stress and the evolution of condition dependent signals. Trends Ecol. Evol. 15: 156-160.

[10] Husak J F, Moore I T (2008) Stress hormones and mate choice. Trends Ecol. Evol. 23: 532-534.

[11] Evans M R, Goldsmith A R, Norris, S R A (2000) The effects of testosterone on antibody production and plumage colouration in male house sparrows (*Passer domesticus*). Behav. Ecol. Sociobiol. 47: 156-163.

[12] Roberts M L, Buchanan K L, Bennett A T D, Evans M R (2007) Mate choice in zebra finches: does corticosterone play a role? Anim. Behav. 74: 921-929.

[13] Hill G E, McGraw K J (2006). Bird Coloration. Vol. 2: Function and Evolution. Cambridge, Massachusetts: Harvard University Press

[14] Lindsay W R, Webster M S, Schwabl H (2011) Sexually selected male plumage colouration is testosterone dependent in a tropical passerine, the red-backed fairy wren (*Malanus melanocephalus*). PLoS One 6: e26067.

[15] Malo A F, Roldan E R S, Garde J J, Soler A J, Vicente J, Gortazar C, Gomendio A (2009) What does testosterone do for red deer males? Proc. Roy. Soc. B 276: 971-980.

[16] Price J, Allen S (2004) Exploring the mechanism regulating regeneration of deer antlers. Phil. Trans. R. Soc. B 359: 809–822.

[17] Ritschard M, Laucht S, Dale J, Brumm H (2011) Enhanced testosterone levels affect singing motivation but not song structure in Bengalese finches. Physiol. Behav. 102: 31-35.

[18] Saldanha C, Clayton N, Schlinger B (1999) Androgen metabolism in the juvenile oscine forebrain: a cross-species analysis at neural sites implicated in memory function J. Neurobiol. 33: 619–631.

[19] Roberts M L, Buchanan K L, Evans M R (2004) Testing the immunocompetence handicap hypothesis: a review of the evidence. Anim. Behav. 68: 227-239.

[20]. Deviche P J, Hurley L L, Fokidis H B, Lerbour B, Silverin B, Silverin B, Sabo J, Sharp (2010). Acute stress rapidly decreases plasma testosterone in a free-ranging male songbird: Potential site of action and mechanism. Gen. Compar. Endocrin. 169: 82-90.

[21] Gratto-Trevor C L, Oring L W, Fivizzani A J (1991) Effects of blood sampling stress on hormone levels in the semipalmated sandpiper. J. Field Ornithol. 62: 19–27.

[22] Owen-Ashley N T, Hasselquist D, Wingfield J C (2004) Androgens and the immunocompetence handicap hypothesis: unravelling direct and indirect pathways in song sparrows. Am. Nat. 164: 490-505.

[23] Moore I T, Lerner J P, Lerner, D T, Maso R T (2000) Relationships between Annual Cycles of Testosterone, Corticosterone, and Body Condition in Male Red-Spotted Garter Snakes, *Thamnophis sirtalis concinnus*. Physiolog. Biochem. Zool. 73:307–312.

[24] Martin L B (2009) Stress and immunity in wild vertebrates: timing is everything. Gen. Compar. Endocrinol. 163: 70-76.

[25] Mehta P H , Josephs R A (2010) Testosterone and cortisol jointly regulate dominance: Evidence for a dual-hormone hypothesis. Horm. Behav.58: 898–906.

[26] Moore F R, Cornwell R E, Law Smith M J, Al Dujaili E A S, Sharp M, Perrett D I (2011) Tests of the stress-linked immunocompetence handicap hypothesis in human male faces. Proc. Roy. Soc. B278: 774-780.

[27] Moore F R, Al Dujaili E A S, Cornwell R E, Law Smith M J, Lawson J F, Sharp M, Perrett D I (2011) Cues to sex and stress hormones in the human male face: functions of glucocorticoids in the immunocompetence handicap hypothesis. Horm. Behav. 60: 269-274.

[28] Brownlee K K, Moore A W, Hackney A C (2005) Relationship between circulating cortisol and testosterone: influence of physical exercise. J. Sports Sci. Medicine 4: 76-83.

[29] Enlow D H (1990) Facial growth, 3rd edn. Philadelphia, PA: Harcourt Brace Jovanovich

[30] Penton-Voak I S& Chen J Y (2004) High salivary testosterone is linked to masculine male facial appearance in humans.Evol. Hum. Behav. 25: 229-241.

[31] Pound N, Penton Voak I S, Surridge A K (2009) Testosterone responses to competition in men are related to facial masculinity. Proc. Roy. Soc. B. 276: 153-159.

[32] Law Smith M J, Perrett D I, Jones B C, Cornwell R E, Moore F R, Feinberg D R, Boothroyd L G, Stirrat M R, Whiten S, Pitman R M, Hillier S G (2006) Facial appearance is a cue to oestrogen levels in women. Proc. Roy. Soc. B 273: 135-140.

[33] Perrett D I, Lee K J, Penton-Voak I, Rowland D R, Yoshikawa S, Burt D M, Henzi S P, Castles D L, Akamatsu S (1998) Effects of sexual dimorphism on facial attractiveness. Nature 394: 884-887.

[34] Moore F R, Taylor V, Law Smith M J, Perrett D I (2011) Sexual dimorphism in the female face is a cue to health and social status but not age. Pers. Ind. Diff. 50: 1068-1073.

[35] Boothroyd L G, Jones B C, Burt D M, Perrett D I (2007) Partner characteristics associated with masculinity, health and maturity in male faces. Pers. Ind. Diffs. 43: 1161-1173.

[36] Swaddle J, Reierson G (2002) Testosterone increases perceived dominance but not attractiveness. Proc. Roy. Soc. B 269: 2285–2289.

[37] Penton Voak I S, Perrett D I, Castles D L, Kobayashi T, Burt D M, Murray L K, Minamisawa R (1999). Menstrual cycle alters face preferences. Nature 399: 741-742.

[38] Waynforth D, Delwadia S, Camm. (2005). The influence of women's mating strategies on preference for masculine facial architecture. Evol. Human Behav. 26: 409–416.

[39] Brooks R, Scott I M, Maklakov A A, Kasumovic M M, Clark A P, Penton-Voak I S. 2011. National income inequality predicts women's preferences for masculinised faces better than health does. Proc. R. Soc. B 278: 810–812.

[40] DeBruine L M, Jones B C, Crawford J R, Welling L L M, Little A C (2010) The health of a nation predicts their mate preferences: cross-cultural variation in women's preferences for masculinized male faces. Proc. R. Soc. B 277: 2405–2410.

[41] Tiddeman B, Burt, M, Perrett, D I (2001) Prototyping and Transforming Facial Textures for Perception Research. IEEE Computer Graphics and Applications 21: 42-50.

[42] Leary C J, Jessop T S, Garcia A M, Knapp R (2004). Steroid hormone profiles and relative body condition of calling and satellite toads: implications for proximate regulation of behavior in anurans. Behav. Ecol. 15: 313-320.

[43] Rantala M J, Moore F R, Skrinda I, Krama T, Kivleniece I, Kecko S, Krams I (2012) Evidence for the stress-linked immunocompetence handicap hypothesis in humans. Nature Comms. DOI: 10.1038/ncomms1696.

[44] Bortolotti G R, Mougeot F, Martinez-Padilla J, Webster L M I, Piertney S B (2009) Physiological stress mediates the honesty of social signals. PloS One 4: e4983.

[45] Edler A V, Friedl T W P (2010) Individual quality and carotenoid-based plumage ornaments in male red bishops (Euplectes orix): plumage is not all that counts. Biol. J. Linn. Soc. 99: 384-397.

[46] Romero L M (2004) Physiological stress in ecology: lessons from biomedical research. Trends in Ecol Evol. 19: 249-255.

[47] Klukowski L A, Cawthorn J M, Ketterson E D, Nolan Jr. V (1997) Effects of experimentally elevated testosterone on plasma corticosterone and corticosteroid-binding globulin in dark-eyed juncos (*Junco hyemalis*). Gen. Comp. Endocrinol. 108: 141–151.

[48] Swett MB, Breuner CW (2008) Interaction of testosterone, corticosterone and corticosterone binding globulin in the white-throated sparrow (*Zonotrichia albicollis*). Comp Biochem Physiol A Mol Integr Physiol. 151: 226-31.

[49] Møller A P (1995) Hormones, handicaps and bright birds. Trends Ecol. Evol. 10: 121.

[50] del Cerro S, Merino S, Martinez-de la Puerte J, Lobato E, Ruiz-de-Castañeda Rivero-de Aguilar J Martinez J, Morales J, Tomás G, Moreno J (2010). Carotenoid-based plumage colouration is associated with blood parasite richness and stress protein levels in blue tits (*Cyanistes caeruleus*). Oecologia 162: 825-835.

[51] Pfaff J A, Zanette L, MacDougall-Shackleton S A, MacDougall-Shackleton E A (2007) Song repertoire size varies with HVC volume and is indicative of male quality in song sparrows (*Melospiza melodia*). Proc. R. Soc. B. 274: 2035-2040.

[52] Gladbach A, Gladbach D J, Quillfeldt P (2010) Variations in leukocyte profiles and plasma biochemistry are related to different aspects of parental investment in male and female upland geese *Chloephaga picta leucoptera*. Comp. Biochem. Physiol. A. 156: 269-277.

[53] McGraw K J, Lee K, Lewin A (2011) The effect of capture-and-handling stress on carotenoid-based beak coloration in zebra finches. J. Comp. Physiol. A. 197: 683-691.

[54] Nunes S, Pelz K M, Muecke E-M, Holekamp K E, Zucker I (2006). Plasma glucocorticoids concentrations and body mass in ground squirrels: seasonal variation and circannual organisation. Gen. Compar. Endocrin. 146: 136-143.

[55] Poisbleau M, Fritz H, Guillon N, Chastel O (2005) Linear social dominance hierarchies and corticosterone responses in male mallards and pintails. Horm. Behav. 47: 485-492.

[56] Mateos C (2005) The subordination stress paradigm and the relation between testosterone and corticosterone in male ring-necked pheasants. Anim. Behav. 69: 249-255.

[57] Cote J, Meylan S, Clobert J, Voituron Y (2010) Carotenoid-based colouration, oxidative stress and corticosterone in common lizards. J. Experiment. Biol. 213: 2116-2124.

[58] Breen K M, Stackpole C A, Clarke I J, Pytlak A V, Tilbrook, A J, Wagenmaker E R, Young E A, Karsch F J (2004) Does the type II glucocorticoid receptor mediate cortisol-induced suppression in pituitary responsiveness to gonadotropin-releasing hormone? Endocrinology 145: 2739–2746.

[59] Attardi B, Klatt B, Hoffman G E, Smith M S (1997) Facilitation or inhibition of the estradiol-induced gonadotropin surge in the immature rat by progesterone: regulation of GnRH and LH messenger RNAs andactivation of GnRH neurons. J. Neuroendocrinol. 9: 589–599.

[60] Attardi B, Pfaff D W, Fink G (1995) Actions of progesterone on the pituitary in relation to facilitation of the estradiol induced gonadotropin surge in the immature rat. Soc. Neurosci. Abstr. 582: 13.

[61] Greenburg N, Wingfield J C (1987) Stress and reproduction: reciprocal relationships. D.O. Norris, R.E. Jones (Eds.), Reproductive Endocrinology of Fishes, Amphibians and Reptiles, Wiley, New York, pp. 389–426

[62] Menendez-Patterson A, Florez-Lozano J A, Fernandez S, Marin B (1980) Stress and sexual behavior in male rats. Physiol. Behav. 24: 403–406.

[63] Moberg GP (1991) How behavioral stress disrupts the endocrine control of reproduction in domestic animals J. Dairy Sci. 74: 304–311.

[64] Lynn S E, Stamplis T B, Barrington W T, Weida N, Hudak C A (2010) Food, stress, and reproduction: Short-term fasting alters endocrine physiology and reproductive behavior in the zebra finch. Horm. Behav. 58: 214–222.

[65] Ricciardella L F, Bliely J M, Feth, C C, Woodley, S K (2010). Acute stressors increase plasma corticosterone and decrease locomotoractivity in a terrestrialsalamander (*Desmognathus ochrophaeus*). Physiol. Behav. 101: 81-86.

[66] Tilgar V, Moks K, Saag P (2011) Predator-induced stress changes parental feeding behavior in pied flycatchers.Behav. Ecol. 22:23-28.

[67] Creel S (2001) Social dominance and stress hormones. Trends in Ecol Evol. 18: 491-198.

[68] Mooring M S, Patton M L, Lance V A, Hall B M, Schaad E W, Fetter G A, Fortin S S, McPeak K M   Glucocorticoids of bison bulls in relation to social status. Horm. Behav. 49: 369-375.

[69] Evans M R (2010) Why does testosterone influence morphology, behaviour and plasticity? Open Ornithol. J. 3: 21-26.

Glucocorticoids in Metabolism and Energy Cycling

Role of Glucocorticoids in Regulation of Iodine Metabolism in Thyroid Gland: Effects of Hyper-And Hypocorticism

Liliya Nadolnik

Additional information is available at the enc of the chapter

1. Introduction

A close relationship between the key bodily regulatory systems, hypophysis-adrenal and hypophysis-thyroid systems, is fairly well-known.

However, the mechanisms of their interaction at different levels have not been conclusively established. This is of considerable interest due to glucocorticoids and thyroid hormones playing a key role in regulation of the most important systems of vital activity and adaptation. The role of glucocorticoids in regulation of thyroid cell function is interesting due to marked growth of thyroid pathology in different world's regions, along with considerably improved iodine prevertion [1], as well as an increased level of environmental stressogenicity. One should also note an increased tension in life of the individual and the society on the whole (psychological, social and other types of stress). The development of the society has actually created a new human environment with a raised level of stressogenic factors. The chronic stress –induced development of hypercorticism can play a significant pathogenetic role in the changed thyroid function which does not only depend on bodily iodine allowances.

Thyroid-stimulating hormone (TSH) [2, 3, 4], iodine [4, 5], thyroglobulin (ThG) [6], estrogens [7], cytokines [8] and other biologically active molecules play an important role in regulation of thyroid cell functions. It is interesting that deficiency of iodine, the key substrate for synthesis of thyroid hormones, decreases the activity of the HPA-axis. It was found [9] that rats with chronic iodine deficiency showed the absence of a normal circadian rhythm of corticosterone secretion and a weakened secretory rise of a corticosterone level under stress that remains to be diminished in amplitude during a month following restoration of the iodine status.

Thyroid cell function can be regulated by glucocorticoids via changes in the concentrations of the pivotal bioregulators: thyroid-stimulating hormone, TSH, iodine and thyroglobulin. The mechanisms and effects of these interactions call for further studies. Thyrocytes express glucocorticoid receptors, alpha (GR-alpha) and beta (GR-beta), which seem to play an important role in differentiation of thyroid cells since cells of thyroid adenoma demonstrated a decrease of mRA GR-alpha and an increase in GR-beta [10].

1.1. Relationships between regulatory effects of hypothalamic and hypophyseal hormones of hypothalamo-hypophyseal-adrenal and hypothalamo-hypophyseal-thyroid axes

Relationships between the hypothalamo-hypophyseal-adrenal (HHA) and hypothalamo-hypophyseal-thyroid (HHT) systems were established at different regulatory levels. Administration of a thyrotropin-releasing hormone (TRH) was accompanied by a decreased adrenocorticotropic hormone (ACTH) level in blood serum of stressed rats [11]. Corticotropin-releasing hormone (CRH) increased plasma TSH and T4 [12]. Banos C. et al. [13] demonstrated that administration of 2 mg ACTH to healthy volunteers decreased the TSH response to TRH. These results characterize certain antagonism between TSH and ACTH.

1.2. Effects of glucocorticoids on TRH and TSH levels

TSH synthesis is determined by balance of positive regulation and negative regulation by TRH and triiodothyronine (T3), respectively; in addition, somatostatin and dopamine also exert inhibitory control (Diagram 1). Glucocorticoids decreased serum TSH in animals and humans. Administration of a high dose of dexamethasone not only suppressed TSH but also decreased the TSH response to TRH administration [14]; the suppressive effect of dexamethasone on TSH decreased in elderly people [15].

Administration of a single dose of hydrocortisone (500 mg) increased both TSH production and stimulation by TRH [16]; only long-term hypocorticism (Cushing's disease) may be a cause for decreased TSH level. The earlier recovery (up to control values) of the diurnal rhythm of TSH than that of cortisol suggests that the TSH rhythm is not under the direct control of circulating cortisol [17]. In adrenalectomized rats the TSH level decreased in serum but not in the pituitary gland [18]. Glucocorticoids decrease blood serum TSH concentrations in humans and animals. Dexamethasone administration to hypothyroid rats decreased serum TSH; dexamethasone augmented a T3-induced decrease of TSH. However, changes in pituitary TSH α- and β-subunit mRNA concentrations were not found [19].

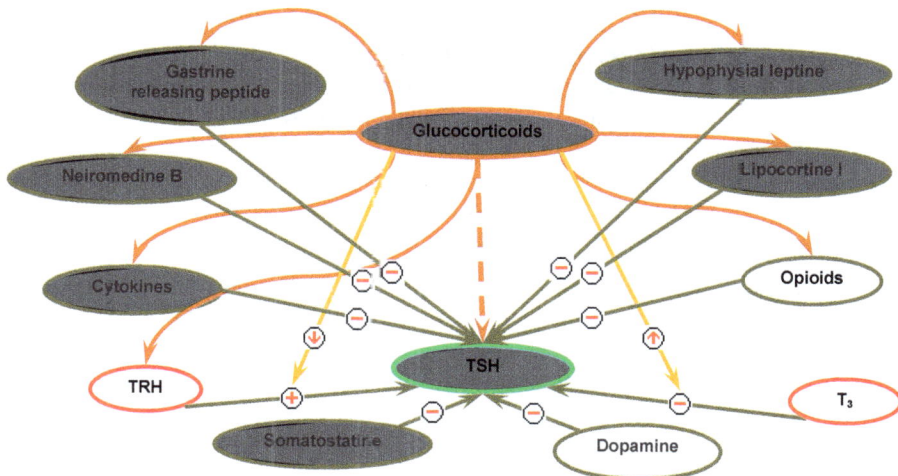

Scheme 1. Effect of glucocorticoids on TSH. +, stimulatory effect; -, inhibitory effect; ↓– weakening of stimulatory effect; ↑– enhancement of inhibitory effect

Kakucska I. et al. obtained clearer results on the effects of glucocorticoids on the hypothalamo-pituitary-thyroid axis [20]. In the paraventricular hypothalamic nuclei of adrenalectomized rats, an increase in corticotropin releasing hormone (CRH) mRNA occurred in parallel to the increase (68.3%) in pro-TRH mRNA. On the contrary, administration of corticosterone or dexamethasone caused a marked decrease in CRH mRNA and pro-TRH mRNA by 43.2 and 73.3%, respectively. Insignificant changes in pro-TRH mRNA were found in the lateral hypothalamus.

Mechanisms of the stress-induced decrease in TRH/TSH secretion possibly involve glucocorticoids, cytokines, and opioids. Recently, a new regulatory mechanism, involving pituitary neuromedin B, gastrin-releasing peptide, and pituitary leptin, acting as local inhibitors of TSH release, has been proposed [21]. In vitro studies have shown that the lipocortin-1 (LC1) protein is a mediator of the glucocorticoid-induced suppression of TSH secretion by the anterior pituitary [53]. Treatment of anterior pituitary cells with 0.1 µM dexamethasone significantly increased the amount of LC1, associated with the outer surface of the pituitary cells and decreased the intracellular content of LC1. Addition of an N-terminal LC1 fragment (residues 1-188) decreased TSH release mediated by vasoactive intestinal peptide and forskolin, but failed to influence those initiated by 10 µM BAYK 8644, the calcium channel stimulator. The inhibitory action of dexamethasone was substantially reversed by a specific monoclonal anti-LC1 antibody [22]. The inhibitory effect of dexamethasone was used for monitoring of subclinical hypothyroidism in obese patients. Administration of TRH after dexamethasone increased the TSH level only in hypothyroid patients but not in euthyroid obese patients [23].

1.3. Effect of glucocorticoids on iodine uptake by the thyroid gland

Iodine uptake is the most important function of thyroid cells; it is controlled by TSH, which stimulates ^{131}I uptake in vivo and in vitro and also expression of sodium-iodide symporter (NIS) in the culture of human thyrocytes [24]. Sodium-iodide symporter (NIS) is located on the apical membrane of thyrocytes; its activity is coupled to Na+,K+-ATPase. TSH influences transcription of NIS gene through Pax-8 and factors activated by intercellular interaction during folliculogenesis [25]. High iodine doses directly inhibit iodide uptake by influencing regulation of NIS protein and mRNA expression [26, 27].

Immobilization stress and also ACTH administration to rats with pituitary damages increased ^{131}I uptake by the thyroid gland in vitro [28]. Cultivation of FRTL-5 thyrocytes under hypoxic conditions was accompanied by increase iodide uptake [29]; heat stress (15 min at 45°C) eliminated this effect. Using culture of ewe thyroid gland follicles it was found that combination of TSH and 10 nM cortisol was optimal for stimulation of iodide uptake without additive and synergistic effects; this effect was also reproduced by combination of TSH with dexamethasone [30]. In addition, the stimulating effect of TSH was potentiated by physiological concentrations of insulin and insulin-like growth factors (IGF I and IGF II). Subsequent studies demonstrated a direct biphasic effect of hydrocortisone on metabolism of thyroid gland cells. Physiological concentrations of hydrocortisone ($1-1000$ nM) in a dose-dependent manner stimulated TSH- and 8-bromo-cAMP-induced iodide uptake, realized via increased production of cAMP and activation of cAMP-dependent metabolic pathways in the primary cultures of porcine thyrocytes [31]. The stimulating effect of hydrocortisone in combination with TSH was inhibited by the glucocorticoid antagonist RU486; the specific hydrocortisone effect appears to be mediated by a thyrocyte glucocorticoid receptor.

It is suggested that the stimulating effect of glucocorticoids on ^{131}I uptake may be used for treatment for breast cancer [32] and prostate cancer [33]. Incubation of NP-1 cells with dexamethasone (10^{-8}–10^{-6} M) caused a 1.5-fold increase in iodide uptake, and a 1.7-fold increase in expression of Na^+/I^-- simporter (NIS) mRNA and protein concentration; NP-1 cell death increased from 55 to 95%, thus suggesting increased cytotoxicity of [131]I. These studies (employing clonogenic assay and nonradioactive proliferation assay) also revealed that treatment of NP-1 cells decreased proliferation of prostate cancer cells. Thus, stress (at least acute stress) may be considered as a factor activating iodide content in the thyroid gland; however, univocal solution of this problem requires further investigations because of multilevel effects of glucocorticoids on thyroid homeostasis

1.4. Effects of glucocorticoids on iodine oxidation and organification in thyrocytes

Single reports on the effect of stress or glucocorticoids on iodide oxidation by thyroperoxidase (TPO), thyroglobulin iodination and subsequent thyroid hormone secretion are available in the literature. Corticosterone administration for 10 days in three different doses (25, 50, 100 mg per 100 g of body weight) inhibited thyroid gland TPO of juvenile female turtles [34], but the mechanism of the inhibitory effect was not studied. Studies in this direction are especially important due to the key role of TPO in thyroid hormone biosynthesis.

The electron microscopy study of thyrocytes revealed accumulation of colloidal droplets in follicle cytoplasm; this suggests that prednisone may decrease basal secretion of thyroid hormones by inhibiting lysosomal hydrolysis of colloid in the follicular cells [35].

1.5. Role of glucocorticoids in the regulation of thyroid hormone receptors

It is known that most of T3 effects are realized via nuclear receptors of thyroid hormones. T3 and glucocorticoid hormones synergistically interact in biosynthesis of growth hormone in the rat pituitary and in the T3-induced metamorphoses in amphibians. Glucocorticoid hormones potentiated metabolic effect of T3 [36]. Dexamethasone increased rat liver specific receptor binding of thyroid hormones. Dexamethasone administration to adrenalectomized rats increased the concentration of protein and mRNA of beta 1 receptor [36]. Molecular studies employing transfection of COS-7 cells revealed that dexamethasone increased transcription activity of thyroid hormone receptor beta 1 promoter [36].

1.6. Effect of stress on peripheral metabolism of thyroid hormones (deiodinase activity in target tissues)

Brain, liver, kidney, heart, muscles, and immune system are the most important targets for thyroid hormones. It is possible that glucocorticoids control tissue levels of T3. Acute stress (footshock) increased the brain T3 content in male and female rats by 12−19% [37]. Two days of total water and food deprivation as stress increased the thymus lymphocyte T3 content in weanling and adult female rats [38], which was normalized after 48 h [39]. It is known that thyroxine (T4) is the main hormone produced by the thyroid gland, however, since it does not exhibit biological activity and therefore thyroxin may be considered as a prohormone or a plasma storage form of thyroid hormones, which plays an important physiological role. A family of selenocysteine oxidoreductases known as iodothyronine deiodinases (D) plays the major role in T4 activation. Three types of these enzymes (mainly determining realization of the hormonal effect of thyroid hormones) have been identified. Their localization and activity are tissue-specific (Scheme 2, 3).

Glucocorticoids exhibit differentiated tissue- and age-specific effects on various tissue deiodinases [40, 41]; they also regulate deiodinases during embryogenesis. Dexamethasone administration to pregnant ewes increased activity of DI in the fetal liver and decreased DIII activity in fetal kidneys [42]. In 20-day-old fetuses, glucocorticoids had no effects on circulating thyroid hormone levels despite their clear decrease in the activity of hepatic and renal deiodinases and an increased activity in the brain, thereby indicating that in this age

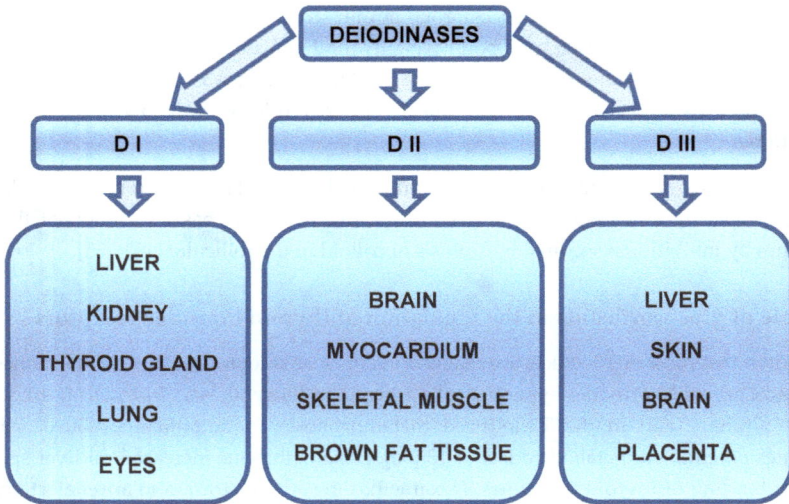

Scheme 2. Tissue distribution of deiodinases

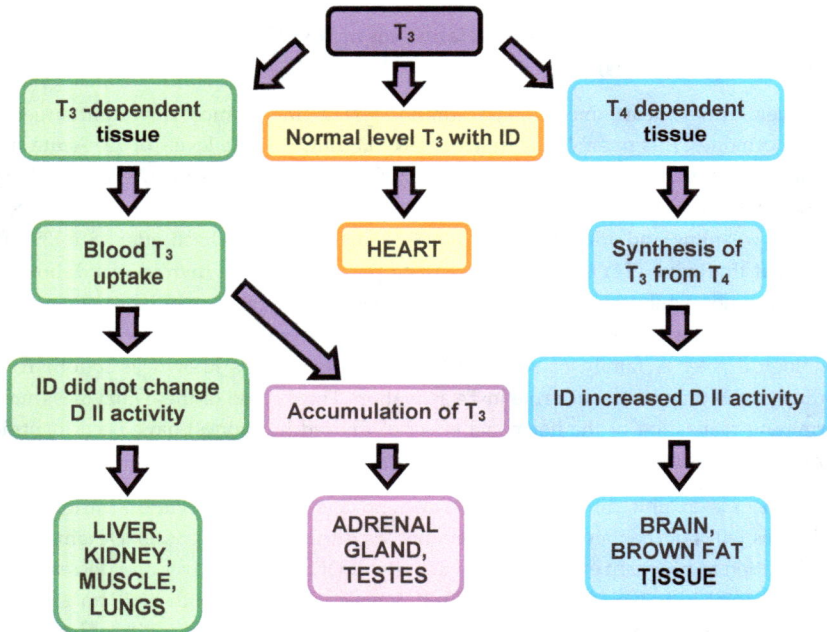

Scheme 3. Forms of thyroid hormone utilization by various

Types of deiodinases	Target tissues	Effect	Reference
DI	fetal liver, ewes	↑	[42]
DIII	fetal kidneys, ewes	↓	[42]
DIII	5-day-pups liver, rat	↑	[43]
DIII	5-day-pups kidneys, rat	↑	[43]
DIII	5-day-pups brain, rat	–	[43]
DIII	brown adipose tissue, rat	↓	[58]
DII	brain, rat	↑	[44]
DI	liver, rat	↓	[51]
DI	kidneys, rat	↓	[52]
DI	hepatocytes in vitro	↑	[54]

Table 1. Effect of GC and stress on activities of various types of deiodinases in rat tissues (↑– stimulatory effect; ↓ inhibitory effect; – no effect)

thyroid circulating thyroid hormone levels are more dependent on thyroidal secretion than on peripheral deiodination. In 5-day-pups, dexamethasone increased blood T3 and T4 and DII activity in the liver, kidney but not in the brain; however, in 12-day-old pups, the dexamethasone effects were maintained only on liver and kidney DIII activity [43].

Effects of stress on deiodinase activity in various tissues still require better elucidation. The most significant effect of glucocorticoids was found on brain DII activity. Even mild, short-term stress (intraperitoneal injection of saline, intragastric intubation, and two different forms of handling (being grasped as for intraperitoneal injection and being moved from one cage to another, and a 2-h period spent in a slowly rotating drum) caused a significant increase in brain DII activity [44]. this was accompanied by a 300%-increase in T3 concentration. These effects were not found in the liver and no changes of DI activity were found in the brain and liver. Dexamethasone caused up-regulation of DII activity [45]. Administration of steroidogenesis inhibitors (aminoglutethimide and metyrapone) to rats decreased adrenal DII activity both in physiological rest and under stress [46]; this suggests normal corticosterone levels required for a deiodinase response to the stress treatment. It appears that the glucocorticoid regulation of DII is the most differentiated. Recent in vitro data obtained using mouse and rat pituitary cells demonstrated that addition of glucocorticoids increased the activity of this enzyme and its mRNA [47], whereas the opposite effect was obtained in mouse mammary gland epithelial cells [48]. In the AtT-20 mouse pituitary tumor cells, glucocorticoids and CRH stimulated expression of mRNA and activity of DII [49]. Effects of glucocorticoids, found in experiments on cultivated hypophyseal cells, confirm their important stimulatory role in the metabolism of thyroid hormones in the CNS.

A decrease in blood thyroid hormones and TRH mRNA seen in fasting and food deprivation was accompanied by the increase DII activity and DII mRNA. Studies of mechanisms of DII activation during fasting revealed that the decrease in leptin levels plays a permissive role during glucocorticoid-induced regulation of the DII enzyme [50].

There are contradictory data on the effects of glucocorticoids on DI activity in various tissues. Cold stress of rats either for 24 h or 28 days (as well as that combined with immobilization) significantly reduced DI activity in the liver [51]. Immobilization of rats for 6 - 8 h was accompanied by the decrease in DI activity in the liver and kidneys; this was attributed to the decrease in the enzyme activity rather than to decreased substrate availability because serum T4 concentration remained unchanged [52]. In adult rats, glucocorticoids decreased DI activity in the liver [53]. In vitro studies on the cultured rat hepatocytes revealed the opposite effects: glucocorticoids increased DI activity and expression of DI mRNA [54]. In kidney NRK 52E cells, dexamethasone increased DI activity and expression of DI mRNA, while in cultured pituitary tumor cells, glucocorticoids did not influence DI mRNA [55]. In the fish *Nile tilapia*, dexamethasone decreased activity of DI and DII in the liver; long-term administration of this hormone increased availability of circulating T3 [56].

The decrease in plasma T3 and the increase in rT3 concentrations observed in stress may be associated with glucocorticoid stimulation of DIII [57]. Regulatory mechanisms of effects of thyroid hormones in various tissue cells have not been conclusively established. Glucocorticoids decreased DIII expression in rat brown adipose tissue [58]. The study of deiodinase activities in human cell lines revealed that estradiol increased DIII activity in ECC-1 cells, dexamethasone inhibited DIII in WRL-68 cells only in the presence of fetal calf serum in the medium [59]. Dexamethasone in a dose-dependent manner decreased the stimulatory effect of T3 on ICAM-1 protein in human ECV 304 cells [74].

All these results indicate that glucocorticoids modulate effects of thyroid hormones by influencing deiodinase activity in various target tissues. They cause significant increase of DII activity in the brain (and thus increase brain T3 level); stress exhibited inhibitory effect on DI activity in the liver and kidneys. Nevertheless, mechanisms underlying glucocorticoid regulation of T4 deiodination in various tissues require further investigation.

1.7. Thyroid gland function under impaired adrenal functions

Taking into consideration the multilevel effects of glucocorticoids on the thyroid status and peripheral metabolism of thyroid hormones, a study of functional activity of the thyroid gland under conditions of adrenal impairments appears to quite reasonable.

Adrenalectomy in rats increased thyroid gland stimulation by TSH and its secretory activity [60]. In patients with adrenal insufficiency cessation of replacement glucocorticoid therapy resulted in an increase of T3 and a decrease of (reversive triiodothyronine) rT3 concentrations, whereas the level of T4 and TSH remained basically unchanged [61].

There are clinical case reports on impairments of thyroid function in patients with hypercorticism before and after adrenalectomy and with adrenal insufficiency. The state of the pituitary-adrenal axis mainly determines the thyroid status in humans. Under hypercorticism in patients with Cushing's syndrome there were decreased serum concentrations of thyroid hormones and TSH; in addition, in 56.2--66.6% there was a prevalence of thyroid nodular disease; this was significantly higher than in the control group [63]. Long-term hypercorticism in patients with Cushing's syndrome was accompanied by inhibition of basal and TRH-stimulated TSH secretion [62]. These patients had an attenuated pituitary response to TRH administration and there was a negative correlation between plasma levels of TSH and cortisol (but not T3); after convalescence the reaction to TRH normalized [64]. There was a single case report on the development of Graves's disease characterized by pronounced hyperthyroidism after a successful surgical operation in a patient with Cushing's syndrome [65]. Authors suggest that suppression of hypercorticism activated latent autoimmune processes in the thyroid gland. Graves's disease with hyperthyroidism manifestations was diagnosed 9 months after unitaleral adrenalectomy in a woman with Cushing's syndrome [66]. In some patients subjected to surgical adrenalectomy for hypercorticism transitory dysfunction of the thyroid gland with symptoms of hypo- or hyperthyroidism developed [67]. Silent thyroiditis developed in a female patient after unilateral adrenalectomy for treatment of Cushing's syndrome followed by a gradual tapering of replacement dose of prednisolone to 5 mg/day; thus thyroiditis was characterized by low TSH, increased thyroid hormone levels, extremely low iodine uptake and increased titers of antimicrosomal and antithyroglobulin antibodies [68]. Recent observations have demonstrated that secondary hypothyroidism and hypercalciemia are consequences of the glucocorticoid deficiency developed after adrenalectomy for Cushing's syndrome [69].

In 103 patients with ACTH deficiency Murakami T. et al. [70] found signs of hypothyroidism (a decrease in free T3 and T4 concentrations, high TSH) and characteristic symptoms of clinical manifestations of thyroid insufficiency (cold intolerance, muscle rigidity, loss of interest in life). After hydrocortisone therapy all signs of impairments of the pituitary-thyroid axis disappeared in more than 70% cases; this suggests that glucocorticoid insufficiency is one of reasons underlying thyroid dysfunction. A high TSH level was found in patients with Addison's disease; administration of glucocorticoids caused dose-dependent inhibition of TRH-induced stimulation of TSH secretion; it is possible that glucocorticoids regulate pituitary sensitivity to TRH [71].

Moderate hypothyroidism is a consequence of exogenous or endogenous hypercorticism. In prepubertal children with nonclassical congenital adrenal hyperplasia (NCCAH) TSH and cortisol were secreted in a pulsatile and circadian fashion with a clear nocturnal TSH surge; daytime TSH levels were lower in the NCCAH group than in control children. The cross-correlation analysis of the 24-h raw data demonstrated that TSH and cortisol were negatively correlated, with a 2.5-h lag time [72].

Adrenalectomy not only reduced plasma corticosterone levels to almost zero, but also decreased plasma T3 and T4 levels, but diurnal rhythms of the HPT axis did not depend on rhythms of the HPA axis [73]. In pregnant female rats adrenalectomized on gestation day 8 there was a decrease in TRH mRNA, increase in serum TSH, and a decrease of T3 only in females [74]; it appears that maternal glucocorticoids determine the development of the hypothalamic-pituitary-thyroid axis in progeny.

Conclusion. The analysis of the literature data shows that the role of glucocotricoids in regulation of iodine metabolism in thyroid cells as well as their effects on the HHT system have not been conclusively established. Very few data are available on early changes in thyrocyte iodine metabolism induced by psychoemotional stress which characterize triggering of adaptation in metabolic systems. The idea is very important of the mechanisms of iodine oxidation and organification and the function of the key enzyme in thyroid hormone biosynthesis, TPO, with the activity governing synthesis of thyroid hormones. This seems to be especially topical in relation to increased levels of stressogenic factors in human environment and functions of all the systems under the stress of hypocoticism.

The goal of the above research is to assess the effects of glucocorticoids on the activities of the main steps of thyroid iodine metabolism and to study the features of iodine metabolism under exposure to short-term and chronic psychoemotional stresses.

2. Materials and methods

Experimental animal models. All the experiments were carried out on Wistar female rats (160-180g body weight) which were fed on a standard laboratory diet. Control and experimental groups contained 10-12 animals.

Acute unavoidable psychoemotional stress. This model was aimed at simulation of negative emotions in rats (fear, alarm, anger and aggression). To this end, we used the modified techniques of Desiderato O. [75] and Tolmachev D.A. [76]. The rats were exposed to a combined stress (each animal was placed in an individual box) in a special chamber whose metallic floor was penetrated with 5-mA electric current. The mild painless irritation of the low extremities was accompanied by interrupted noise (electric bell) and light (100-Wt electric bulb) during 20 min or 5-60 min singly. Stress was always given at the same time from 9.00 to 10.00 o'clock in the morning. No manipulations were carried out before placing the animals to penal cells and taking them out. The number of animals in the groups was 8 to 10.

Short-term repeated psychoemotional stress was simulated using the modified techniques of Desiderato O. [75] and Tolmachev D.A. [76] but the exposure was repeated: 20 min daily during 28 days. Animals with normal thyroid status were subjected to multiple exposures to psychoemotional stress.

Simulation of hypocorticism in rats. To simulate glucocorticoid deficiency, the animals were subjected to bilateral adrenalectomy (AE) (n=10). The surgery was performed by a conventional method [30] under ester anaesthesia. After the surgery, the animals were fed on the standard laboratory diet and received a 0.9 sodium chloride solution as a drinking fluid. The animals were selected for experimental groups after a 3-day recovery period following the surgery.

Administration of high doses of potassium iodide to animals with normal and reduced glucocorticoid status.

Single administration. A KI solution was administered by a gastric tube at doses of 0.7; 7.0 and 70.0 mg/kg B.W. (which corresponds to 10, 100 and 1000 daily KI doses [77] or 0.54; 5.35; 53.51 mg iodide/kg B.W.) in the volume of 0.4-0.6 ml. The control rats received distilled water (0.5 ml). The animals were decapitated after 24 h following the administration.

Multiple administration. Potassium iodide was administered by a gastric tube at doses of 0.07, 0.21, 0.70 and 7.0 and 35 mg/kg body weight (which corresponds to 1, 3, 10, 100 and 500 daily doses of potassium iodide or 0.05, 0.16, 0.64, 5.35 and 27.76 mg iodine / kg body weight) in a volume of 0.4-0.6 ml at 9 o'clock daily over 14 days. The control rats received distilled water in a volume of 0.5 ml. After 24 h following the last (14th) administration of KI, the animals were decapitated.

Studies on thyroid iodine metabolism. Determination of total (It), protein-bound (Ib) and free iodine (If) in rat thyroid tissue. The method for determination of total iodine and its protein-bound and free fractions in thyroid tissue was developed directly for this research applying a commonly used catalytic cerium-arsenite method for measurement of iodine in the urine [78]. To determine the total iodine content, 0.125 ml of thyroid homogenate (1:2000) was placed to a test-tube and 0.3 ml of concentrated $HClO_3$ and $HClO_4$ (5:1) was added. The samples were incubated at 110°C for 60 min. They were cooled to a room temperature and 1 ml of a 0.5% sodium arsenite solution was added. The samples were shaken, and after 20 min, 0.5 ml of 1.2% cerium ammonium sulfate was added. Optical density was measured after 20 min at a wavelength of 400 nm. Iodine concentration was calculated by a calibration curve. To construct the calibration curve, we used KIO_4 at concentrations of 0, 20, 50, 100, 150 and 200 µg/l.

To measure the contents of protein-bound and free iodine in the thyroid homogenate, the proteins were sedimented with 5.2% perchloric acid and 0.125 ml of the supernatant was used to determine free iodine concentration, the sediment was used to measure protein-bound iodine concentration. After the separation of the iodine fractions, the procedure of measurement corresponded to that described above (I total).

Determination of urinary total iodine concentration in rats. To determine urinary iodine concentration, 0.125 ml of urine from the morning portion (collected between 7 and 9 a.m.) was used. At high iodine concentrations, the samples were diluted 5-, 10-fold and over. Then the urine was burned in a mixture of concentrated $HClO_3$ and $HClO_4$ and the sample was assayed for iodine content as was described above.

Determination of TPO activity. To determine TPO activity, we used the method based on reactions of iodine enzymatic oxidation [79]. 2.8 ml of 0.05 M of sodium phosphate buffer,

0.05 ml of 0.6 M KI and 0.1 ml of thyroid homogenate (1:80) or its microsomal fraction were placed in a 1-cm thermostatically controlled cell. The reaction mixture was stirred and incubated for 15 min at temperature of 28°C. The reaction was started by addition of 0.05 ml of 12 µM H_2O_2. The reaction rate was recorded for 1 min at a wavelength of 353 nm using a Cary-100 spectrophotometer. The TPO activity was calculated using the molar extinction coefficient of ε =22900 M^{-1} x cm^{-1} for the product formed [77]. Enzyme activity was expressed as µmol/min x g protein.

Determination of thyroid hormone concentration in blood serum. The concentrations of total T_4 and total and free blood serum T_3 were measured radioimmunologically using RIA-T4 –CT and RIA-T3-CT kits (Institute of Bioorganic Chemistry, National Academy of Sciences of Belarus, Republic of Belarus).

Determination of total corticosterone concentration in rat blood serum. Blood serum total corticosterone concentration was measured by high performance liquid chromatography (HPLC). The assay was carried out using 0.2 ml of blood serum which was placed to a test-tube with a ground stopper, 1.0 ml of chloroform and 10 µM dexamethasone solution were added (as an internal standard) followed by addition of 40 µl of fresh 1.0 M solution of sodium hydroxide. Corticosteroids were extracted for 1 min. The test-tubes were centrifuged for 3 min at 600 g and then the lower (chloroform) fraction was carefully collected. The chloroform fraction was evaporated to dryness in a nitrogen flow. The samples were dissolved in 20 µl of the mobile phase and applied on a column. The steroids were separated on KAX-1-64-3 columns (2x64 mm) filled with a Silasorb -600 (LC) normal-phase sorbent with the particle diameter of 5 µm (Lachema, Czech Republic). The mixture of hexan-chloroform-methanol in the volume ratio of 7:1:1 was used as the mobile phase [80]. A Milikhrom liquid microcolumn chromatograph (Russia) was used for detection in a UV-detector at a wavelength of 246 nm. The rate of the eluent supply was 200 µl/min. Steroids were identified from the retention time. Corticosterone concentration was calculated from the calibration curve and expressed as nM. A corticosterone (Sigma) solution was used to construct the calibration curve and a dexamethasone (Sigma) solution was used as an internal standard.

Statistical analysis. The data were processed statistically using Mann-Whitney's U-test. The results are presented as means (M) ± standard deviation of the mean. * P<0,05; ** P<0,01; *** P<0,001. The critical value for the significance level was taken to be 5%.

3. Results

3.1. Studies on iodine metabolism under hypercorticism (stress and post-stress periods)

Under psychoemotional stress, the corticosterone content was most elevated (405.8-447.7%) for 15-60 min. It was decreased following 2 hours after stress cessation (2.9-fold) and increased after 6 hours (2.1-fold) at the post-stress period (Fig. 1). Analysing the wave-like dynamics of changes in corticosterone concentration at the post-stress period, we should note that the rats were stressed in the morning (9.00 to 10.00 a.m.) and the rise in corticosterone concentration at the post-stress period was not related to its circadian rhythm (since the circadian rhythm of corticosterone is characterized by maxima per 20.00 hour). The corticosterone concentration was observed to increase in the afternoon (16.00 p.m.) after 6 hours following the post-stress period, and this elevation of serum corticosterone is a characteristic manifestation of a regulatory feedback mechanism. As a response to a marked reduction of corticosterone concentration after 2 hours following stress, the ACTH concentration elevated, which induced a new wave in increasing blood and adrenal corticosterone concentration that is a manifestation of the adaptation syndrome.

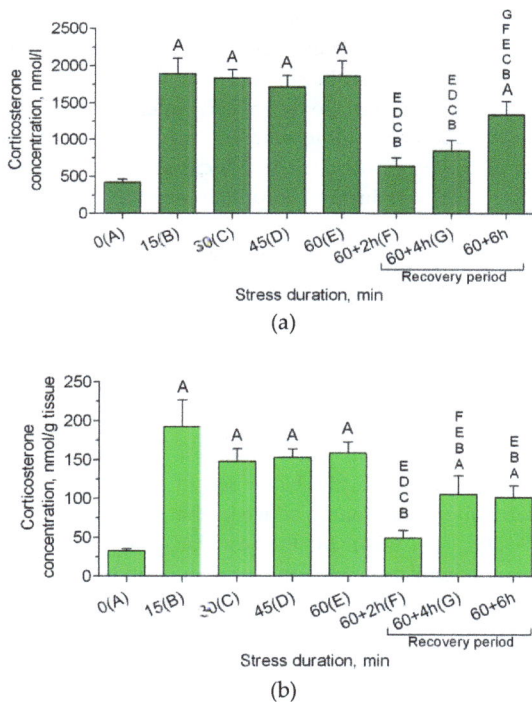

Figure 1. Blood serum (A) and adrenal (B) corticosterone concentrations in rats at acute stress and post-stress periods, after exposure to psychoemotional stress (n=8).

A, B, C, D, E, F, G are groups of animals, respectively. The letters under each column indicate statistically significant changes in the parameter (p<0.05) compared to the corresponding group (e.g., in Fig.1A, the parameter for Groups 15B, 30C, 45D, 60E is statistically significant compared to Group A). The same designations are in Figures 2-4.

The dynamics of changes in the parameters characterizing thyroid iodine metabolism was of a wave-like pattern, which indicates a pronounced response of the rat thyroid to stress. This was most pronounced for changes

in the index If, which is quite explicable. During 15-30 min of stress the thyroid total iodine concentrations remained unchanged (176.9-234.9 μg/g tissue). However, after 60 min, its content was 39.3% decreased in comparison with 15-and 30-min stress (Fig. 2A). During the acute stress phase (15-30 min), intensification of iodide organification was noticed: the concentration of its protein-bound fraction was 37.6% elevated, and the ratio of protein-bound I to total I was 1.2-fold increased (Fig. 2B). The 70.5% elevation of free iodide concentration in the thyroid gland (Fig. 2C) was probably due to activation of proteolytic processes in thyroglobulin and thyroid hormone formation. We cannot also exclude activation of iodine uptake with consideration for the absence of iodine supply to the body during stress, which can be due to increased activities of tissue deiodinases. Along with this, in spite of the evidence for Na^+/I^- simporter expression in some cells (salivary and mammary glands) the literature lacks information about other iodine depots in addition to the TG. After 60-min stress, the thyroid showed diminished concentrations of free and protein-bound iodine, which seemed to be a consequence of highly active secretory processes and inhibition of iodine organification, TPO activity (Fig. 3) remained at a level of control values during 30-min exposure to stress, decreasing by 34.8% after 45 min, which was accompanied by a 16.8% reduction of protein-bound I concentration. The stress-induced drop in TPO activity can be due to changed kinetic parameters of the enzyme. TPO was found to be sensitive to elevation of ROS concentrations and aldehyde products of lipid peroxidation in thyroid cells [81]. Moreover, an important role in this case can be played by a decreased TSH level that regulates key processes in the TG. Taking into consideration the antagonistic relations between ACTH and TSH, one can suggest the metabolic changes in the TG to be caused by a stress-induced increase of the ACTH level which can induce a decrease of TSH production.

The correlation analysis of the results did not show a correlation between thyroid TPO activities and glucocorticoid levels in the blood serum and adrenal glands. After 60-min stress, a negative correlation was found between the total thyroid iodide and adrenal corticosterone (r= –0.952, p=0.003). In the control group, the content of adrenal corticosterone positively correlated with the protein-bound I to total I ratio (r=0.955, p=0.01), which indicates involvement of glucocorticoids in regulation of iodine homeostasis in the TG.

The decrease in corticosterone concentration after 2 h following the stress exposure was followed by activation of TPO (3.6-fold) as opposed to 60-min stress and control (3.4-fold). The TPO activation at the post-stress period suggests the presence of regulatory mechanisms for its activity which are related to a corticosterone level since it is at that period that its blood and adrenal concentrations were diminished most appreciably. The subsequent elevation of corticosterone concentrations in 4 and 6 h within the recovery period was followed by a dramatic decrease of thyroid TPO activity.

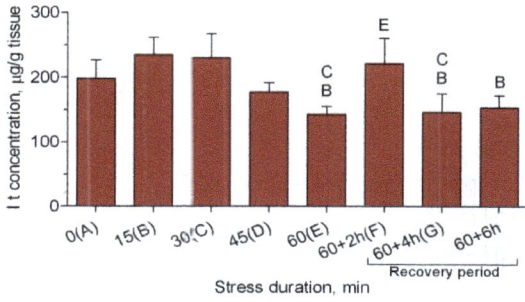

(a)

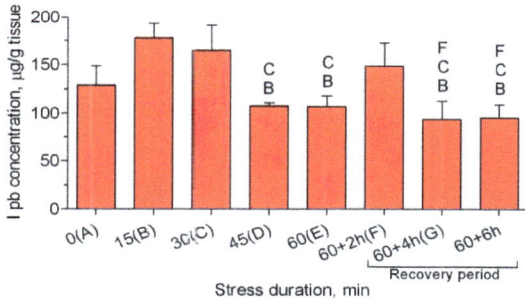

(b)

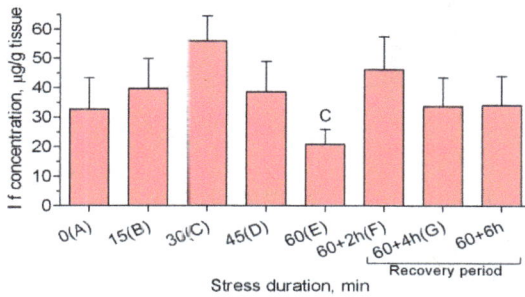

(c)

Figure 2. Rat thyroid total (A), protein-bound (B), and free (C) concentration of iodine during acute stress and post-stress periods.
A, B, C, D, E, F, G represent respective designations for groups of animals.
B, C, E. F represent statistically significant change in the parameter (p< 0.05) compared to the corresponding group

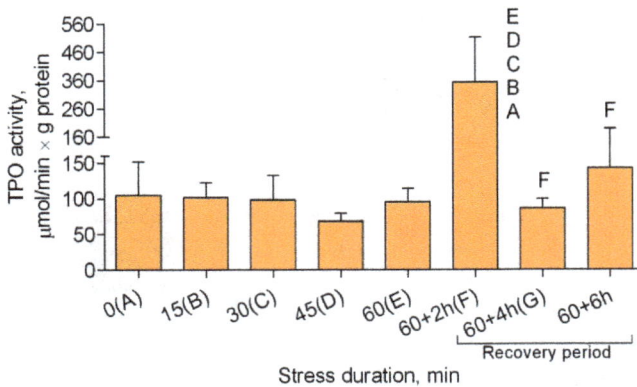

Figure 3. Rat thyroid TPO activity at acute stress and post-stress periods.
A, B, C, D, E, F, G represent corresponding designations for animal groups.
A, B, C, D, E represent statistically significant changes in parameter (p<0.05) compared to the corresponding group.

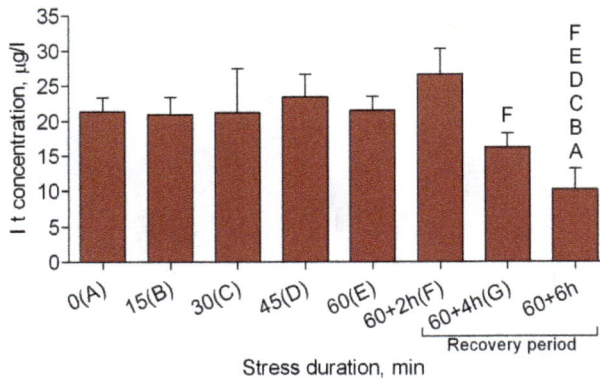

Figure 4. Rat blood iodine concentration at acute stress and post-stress periods.
A, B, C, D, E, F, G represent corresponding designations for animal groups.
A, B, C, D, E, F represent statistically significant changes in the parameter (p<0.05) compared to the corresponding group.

The iodine status restoration after the 2- h post-stress period is characterized by elevated concentrations of total I, protein-bound I and free I (55.5, 38.3 and 40.8%, respectively). A marked restoration to the control values of all the thyroid parameters studied was noticed after 4-6 h following the cessation of stress exposure. Under physiological conditions, the blood serum iodine content was not high (approx. 20 µg/l). However, acute stress diminished its level (52.3%) at the post-stress recovery period (after 6 h following stress), which can be a consequence of restoration of the iodine status in the thyroid (Fig. 4).

	Control	Stress, 15 min	Stress, 30 min	Stress, 45 min
Groups	A	B	C	D
T₄ total, nM	59.4±4.1	60.6±3.6	60.5±2.4	59.09±4.4
T₃ free, nM	2.9±0.22	2.9±0.21	2.3±0.12	2.3±0.20^A,B

	Stress, 60 min	Stress, 60 min + 2-hour post-stress periods	Stress, 60 min + 4-hour post-stress periods	Stress, 60 min + 6-hour post-stress periods
Groups	E	F	G	H
T₄ total, nM	58.7±3.5	59.1±2.2	64.8±6.0	51.6±4.5
T₃ free, nM	2.1±0.21 ^A,E	2.7±0.29	2.1±0.13^A,B,F	2.0±0.26^A,B,E

A,B,F $P<0.05$ compared to control.

Table 2. Rat blood T₄ and T₃ concentrations at acute stress and post-stress periods

The stress exposure did not produce significant changes in the concentration of blood serum total T₄. However, the free T₃ content lowered at the 30th minute of stress and remained to be 18.6 to 28.5% lowered throughout the experiment. It was not until 2 hours later that it increased up to the control values (Table 1).

Our findings show involvement of the TG in adaptation of the body to acute stress. We should note the thyroid ability to a rapid recovery of the iodine status at the post-stress period. Throughout a short period of time (15-30 min), the acute stress induced activation and uptake of iodide and thyroid hormone secretion.

However, oxidation of iodide was inhibited and the contents of total I, protein-bound I and free I were decreased after 45 and, significantly, after 60 min.

The 60-min exposure to psychoemotional stress revealed a negative correlation between the concentration of total I in the thyroid and the corticosterone concentration in the adrenals (r= –0.952, p=0.003). This shows that overproduction of glucocorticoids under stress induces a decrease of thyroid iodine content, resulting in a negative iodine balance at the post-stress period. The 2-hour recovery period is characterized by a pronounced activation of thyroid iodine metabolism (TPO activity rose over 3-fold), and the partial restoration of the thyroid iodine status (after 4-6 hours) was accompanied by a decreased blood serum iodine content.

The following correlations were established at the post-stress recovery period:

- after 4 hours, the blood serum iodide concentration negatively correlated with the corticosterone concentration (r= –0.831, p=0.040);
- after 6 hours, there was a highly significant correlation (r=0.937, p=0.006) between the blood corticosterone level and the ratio of protein-bound I to total I;

The data for the recovery period demonstrate that the blood corticosterone level can be viewed as a factor inducing a decrease of blood iodine concentration in rats.

Thus, the short-term stress (5-30 min) induced activation of biosynthesis and secretion of thyroid hormones. The most important regularity of the post-stress period is restoration of the thyroid iodine status due to activation of iodine uptake and organification as well as the presence of a close negative correlation between the thyroid concentration of I total and the adrenal corticosterone concentration (r= –0.956, p=0.003). After 6 h of the recovery period, the concentration of blood corticosterone was positively correlated to the ratio of protein-bound I/total I in the TG (r=0.937, p=0.006). A close correlation found between the levels of corticosterone and iodine in the thyroid gland may primarily show possible regulatory effects of glucocorticoids on iodine uptake. But no effects of glucocorticoids on TPO were found, which definitely indicates the absence of direct interactions. However, elevation of thyroid iodine concentration, induced by glucocorticoids, can activate TPO.

The above findings show that the exposure to stress induced a marked imbalance in the thyroid iodine status which was rapidly recovered at the post-stress period due to the decreased blood serum iodine concentration and that the restoration of the thyroid iodine status is most closely related to the glucocorticoid status.

3.2. Studies on the effect of acute exposure to stress on the kinetics of iodine metabolism in rats after administration of physiological potassium iodide doses

We studied the effects of 30-min psychoemotional stress on the iodine metabolism after administration of three daily doses of potassium iodide (KI was administered directly before the exposure to stress). The administration of three daily doses of KI increased 4.3-fold the blood iodine level within 6 hours. This concentration was decreased to the control values after 24 h (Fig. 5). In the group of rats subjected to stress, the iodine content also increased (296.7%) after 30 min following the administration of 3 daily doses of KI. In contrast to the control rats, the stressed rats showed a pronounced maximum of blood iodine concentration after 6 h (839.4% elevation, 170.7µg/l). After 24 h, the level of blood iodine in the stressed rats did not differ from that in the controls. The stress-induced changes in the kinetics of blood iodine concentration are a consequence of a disturbed regulation of iodine homeostasis. The dramatic, over 800%, elevation of blood iodine concentration can be due to an imbalance in the activity of its uptake: lowering of uptake in the TG and activation of uptake in the gastrointestinal tract at the post-stress period. It should be noted that it is at that period that the rat blood showed an increase in the corticosterone concentration (Table 2). A comparative examination of the curves characterizing changes in thyroid iodine concentrations in two animal groups (Fig. 5 B) shows that after 24 h, the thyroid iodine concentration elevated 1.7-fold in the control rats and remained essentially unchanged in the stressed rats (1.2-fold increase).

The 30-min psychoemotional stress leveled off the increase in the thyroid iodine status after administration of 3 daily KI doses. The changed concentrations of thyroid protein-bound I and free I (Fig. 5, B and C) reflect changes in TPO activity in the thyroid gland (Fig. 5D). The administration of 3 daily KI doses was accompanied by activation of its organification in the group of control rats within 1 h (the level of protein-bound I was increased by 54.1%) and elevation of its concentration by 74.3% after 24 h.

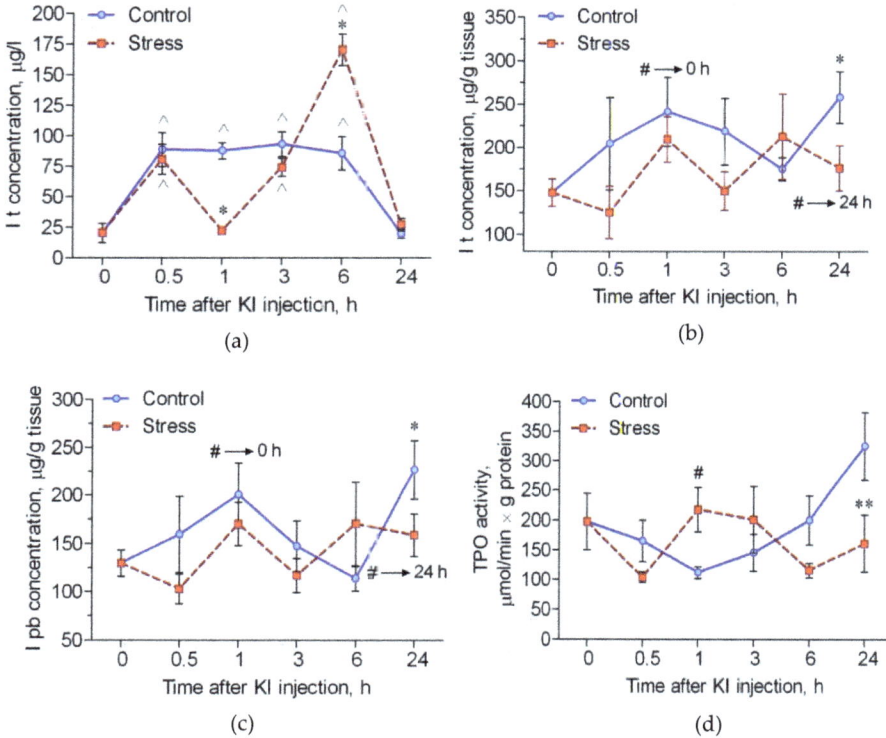

Figure 5. Effect of 30-min exposure to psychoemotional stress on iodine content in rat blood serum (A), total iodine (B), protein-bound iodine (C), activity of TPO (D) in rat thyroids after administration of 3 daily doses of KI within 24 h of the post-stress period (^ P<0.05 compared to the initial level (0 h); * P<0.05 when comparing the indices in control and stressed rats; $ P<0.05; #→0 – 0.1<p<0.05 compared to group of 0 h; #→24 – 0.1<p<0.05 when comparing the indices in stressed rats to controls (24 h).

The dynamics of changes in TPO activity in the stressed animals treated with 3 daily doses of KI had an essentially opposite character in comparison with the controls (Figure 5D). The post-stress increase in TPO activity after 1 h was accompanied by 41.5% decrease of its activity by 6 h as opposed to the initial level. As compared to the control animals, the activity of TPO in the thyroid of the stressed rats diminished over 2-fold , whereas the concentration of protein-bound I decreased 1.4-fold after 24 h following the administration of 3 daily KI doses.

The data obtained indicate that the 30-min exposure to stress after the administration of 3 daily KI doses changed the kinetics of iodine metabolism in rats within 24 h of the post-stress period. These data reflect complex relationships between the regulatory effects of the pituitary-thyroid and pituitary-adrenal systems as well as the whole complex of metabolic stress changes in the organism in respect to the key steps in thyroid iodine metabolism. Stress enhances the iodine inhibitory effect.

	Before KI administration	After KI administration				
		30 min	1 h	3 h	6 h	24 h
Blood corticosterone, nM	302.8±28.5	1279.1± 101.6*	1580.4± 118.9*	2135.8± 260.7*	1778± 194.9*	472.7± 47.4
	Before stress	After administration of KI and exposure to stress				
		30 min	1 h	3 h	6 h	24 h
Blood corticosterone, nM	302.8±28.5	2571.6± 282.7*	867.8± 104.5*	664.3± 100.5*	1661.8± 272.5*	697.7± 75.9*

Table 3. Effect of 30-min stress exposure on corticosterone concentration in rat blood after administration of 3 daily doses of KI within 24 h of post-stress period

The most pronounced stress-induced changes in iodine metabolism after administration of physiological KI doses (3 daily doses) are characterized by:

• abnormal kinetics of changes in blood iodine concentration within 24 h after administration of KI, which was manifested by accumulation of blood iodine (839.4% elevation) after 6 h at the post-stress period;

• changes in the kinetics of iodine uptake and oxidation in the TG, which results in a decreased content of total I and protein-bound I in thyroids of stressed rats after administration of 3 daily doses of KI as opposed to the control group which showed an increase of these parameters.

3.3. Effect of unavoidable repeated short-term psychoemotional stress on the functional activity of the rat thyroid

A research was carried out into a short-term stress effect (daily, over a long period of time) on the activities of the key steps in iodine metabolism in the rat thyroid. The data obtained indicate that daily 20-min exposure to stress (4 weeks) induced pronounced changes in thyroid iodine metabolism.

Figure 6 shows that the total thyroid iodine content in stressed animals was elevated 1.97-fold as opposed to controls and amounted to 491.8±15.5 µg/g tissue. The contents of its protein-bound and free fractions corresponded to 329.9±8.3 µg/g tissue and 161.8±18.4 µg/g tissue, which was 1.6-and 3.1-fold higher compared to the controls. The increased thyroid iodine concentration was accompanied by a changed ratio of its various fractions (Table 3). The 2-fold elevated free I/protein-bound I ratio and the lowered protein-bound I/total I ratio

(1.18-fold) are indicative of a lowered efficiency of thyroid iodine organification under stress.

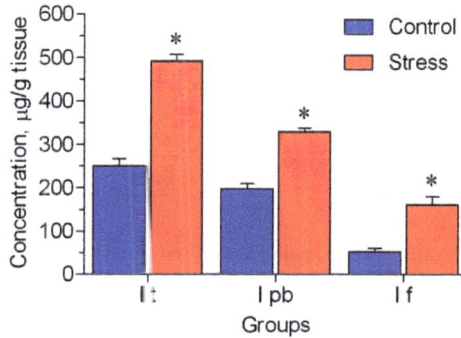

*statistically significant changes vs control group (p<0.05)

Figure 6. Effect of 4-week psychoemotional stress (20 min, daily) on contents of total I, protein-bound I and free I in the rat thyroid

Indices	Control	Stress
Free I/protein-bound I	0.26±0.034	0.50±0.066*
Protein-bound I/total I	0.79±0.021	0.67±0.028*
Urinary I, µg/l	17.9±2.29	22.2±1.94

* P<0.05 compared to control.

Table 4. Effect of short-term daily psychoemotional stress on the ratio of different rat thyroid iodine fractions and urinary iodine excretion

Indices	Control	Stress
T4 total, nM	49.2±2.82	51.7±3.34
T3 total, nM	1.2±0.06	1.3±0.07
TPO, µmol/min x g tissue	23.4±2.70	20.9±2.91
Thyroid weight, mg	15.7±0.63	13.3±0.47*
Thyroid cytosolic protein, mg/g tissue	158.5±3.6	137.9±5.3*

* P<0.05 compared to control.

Table 5. Effect of short-term daily psychoemotional stress on the concentration of blood thyroid hormones, TPO activity, thyroid weight and thyroid protein concentration

No changes were found in the activity of TPO, the key enzyme of thyroid hormone biosynthesis (Table 5). The thyroid weight in stressed rats was lowered by 18%, whereas the protein concentration in the thyroid cytosolic fraction – by 13%. The blood thyroid hormone content at the post-stress period was maintained at the level of control values (Table 5), the level of corticosterone was increased by 32.8% (Table 6) and the weight of the adrenal glands rose by 13%.

Indices	Control	Stress
Blood serum corticosterone, nM	383.2±65.9	509.2±90.0#
Adrenal corticosterone, nmol/g tissue	152.8±17.9	176.2±30.8
Adrenal weight, mg	46.6±1.9	52.7±2.5*

* P<0.05; # P<0.1 compared to control.

Table 6. Effects of short-term daily psychoemotional stress on adrenal weight, blood corticosterone concentration and corticosterone concentration in rat adrenals.

As our data show, stress caused multidirectional changes in the activities of the key steps of thyroid iodine metabolism. The elevated content of the total and free iodine is a consequence of stimulation of its absorption at the post-stress period [28]. The decreased efficiency of iodine organification may be due to TPO inhibition and lowering of thyroglobulin concentration. The stress-induced lowering of thyroid TPO activity was shown earlier. As Table 7 demonstrates, the repeated exposure to short-term stress during 7 days and over was accompanied by a decrease of thyroid TPO activity both directly after exposure to stress (46.9-56.6%) and after 24 h following its cessation (59.2-60.7%).

Index	Control	Stress, 7 days		Stress, 14 days	
		A	Б	A	Б
TPO, μmol/min g protein	153.5±15.2	81.4±21.43*	60.2±4.9*	66.6±9.4*	62.6±18.22*

Group A animals were decapitated directly after the last exposure to stress; Group B animals were decapitated 24 h after the last exposure to stress. * P<0.05 compared to control.

Table 7. Effect of short-term (20 min) psychoemotional stress (daily, 7, 14 days) on thyroid TPO activity

Effects of stress on iodine oxidation and organification in thyroid cells have not been virtually investigated. We found only one study on female tortoises. Thyroid TPO activity in young female tortoises was lowered after ten-fold administration of corticosterone (25, 50, 100 μg/100 g body weight) [34]. Nothing has been known of the effect of stress on thyroglobulin biosynthesis. However, the diminished level of thyroid protein-bound I can be stipulated by its impaired biosynthesis. Moreover, a consequence of stress was a 13%-decreased total protein concentration in the thyroid cytosolic fraction. This certainly applies to thyroglobulin, taking into consideration that it amounts to 75-80% and up of the total thyroid protein.

The main regulator of TPO and thyroglobulin synthesis is TSH whose secretion is inhibited by glucocorticoids [20], which can induce depression of thyroid hormone synthesis. Stress is suggested to cause a decrease of TSH production via pituitary neuromedin B, gastrin-releasing peptide and pituitary leptin acting as local inhibitors of TSH release under stress [21]. It was found that lipocortin -1 is a mediator of glucocorticoid-induced suppression of TSH secretion by the anterior lobe of the pituitary gland [21].

The inhibitory effect of stress seems to be followed by activation of thyroid metabolism at the post-stress period and the restoration of thyrocyte function is related to activation of thyroid hormone secretion, which is confirmed by resorption of colloid and depletion of thyroid follicules. These conditions disturb the thyroglobulin synthesis/secretion balance. As a result, the thyrocytes and follicular lumen accumulate a considerable amount of non-organified iodine, which is confirmed by our findings. Stress decreases thyroid weight, which can be both a consequence of its hypersecretion and destructive processes; the mechanism of this change is certainly interesting.

The experimental findings show that a consequence of the repeated exposures to psychoemotional stress are pronounced structural and metabolic changes in the TG that are characterized by an elevated iodine content, a decreased extent of its organification, development of oxidative stress and lymphocyte infiltration along with the impaired thyroid follicular structure. The mechanisms of the regularities found call for detailed research and are of great interest to disclose the pathogenesis of autoimmune thyroiditis, thyroid carcinoma as well as the contribution of the thyroid component to development of endemic and nodular goiters.

There are presently no unambiguous data on the role of stress in induction of thyroid pathology in humans. Individual cases have been described of autoimmune thyroiditis developed after surgical treatment of hypercorticism (Cushing's syndrome) [65]. A pronounced stress effect can be an onset of Graves' disease [82]. There were reports about relationships between stress and Hashimoto's thyroiditis [83]. According to Polish researchers [84] secondary adrenal deficiency can be a cause of autoimmune thyroid diseases in humans: stress affects the immune system, and immunologic modulations are considered to be a factor inducing autoimmune thyroiditis in genetically prone individuals [85]. Stress hormones, affecting antigen-presenting immune cells, can influence the differentiation of bipolar T-helpers from Th1 to Th2 phenotype, which causes suppression of cellular immunity and enhancement of humoral immunity. Stress is likely to contribute to the development of Graves' disease by shifting the Th1/Th2 ratio from Th1 to Th2. Recovery after stress or immunosuppressive effect of pregnancy can induce a "reverse shift" in Th2 → Th1, causing autoimmune (sporadic) thyroiditis [85].

Stress-induced impairment of thyroid function characterized by development of oxidative and iodine stress is likely to be viewed as a main mechanism of thyroid ageing in humans and, consequently, to be a cause of diseases of age related to thyroid deficiency [86, 87]. Further studies are needed to disclose the mechanisms of stress-induced impairment of thyroid functions.

3.4. Studies on rat thyroid iodine metabolism under hypocorticism (after adrenalectomy)

The above findings confirm that stress considerably changes thyroid iodine metabolism, affecting its uptake and organification. Since all the experimental studies were carried out using models characterizing hyperfunction of the adrenal glands (stress), a comparative investigation of iodine metabolism in rats with adrenal deficiency should be done in order to establish the biochemical mechanisms.

The glucocorticoid status in rats was assessed by the level of corticosterone which was lowered 4.4 to 6.4-fold in adrenalectomized (AE) rats compared to controls. Adrenal deficiency was a cause of 44.2 % - decreased thyroid TPO activity (Fig. 7B). The administration of 1000 daily doses of KI (a dose=70 mg/kg) decreased thyroid TPO activity in the TG of the control rats and elevated it in the glucocorticoid-deficient animals with to the control values. The administration of 1000 daily doses of KI was accompanied by increases in thyroid total I (42.2%), protein-bound I (19.1%) and free I (90.6%) in AE rats (Fig. 8). This indicates that under hypocorticism the regulatory mechanisms for thyrocyte functions can be disturbed by high iodine doses.

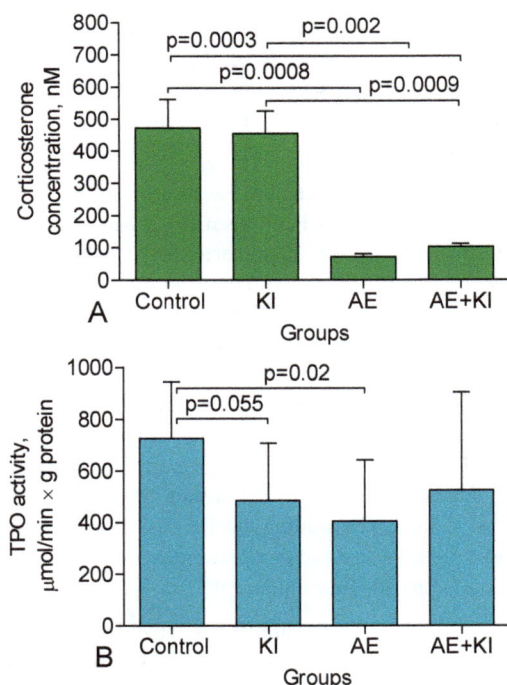

Figure 7. Effect of single administration of 1000 daily doses of KI on concentration of blood serum corticosterone (nM) (A) and TPO activity (μmol/min x g protein) in thyroids of intact and AE rats (B)

(a)

(b)

(c)

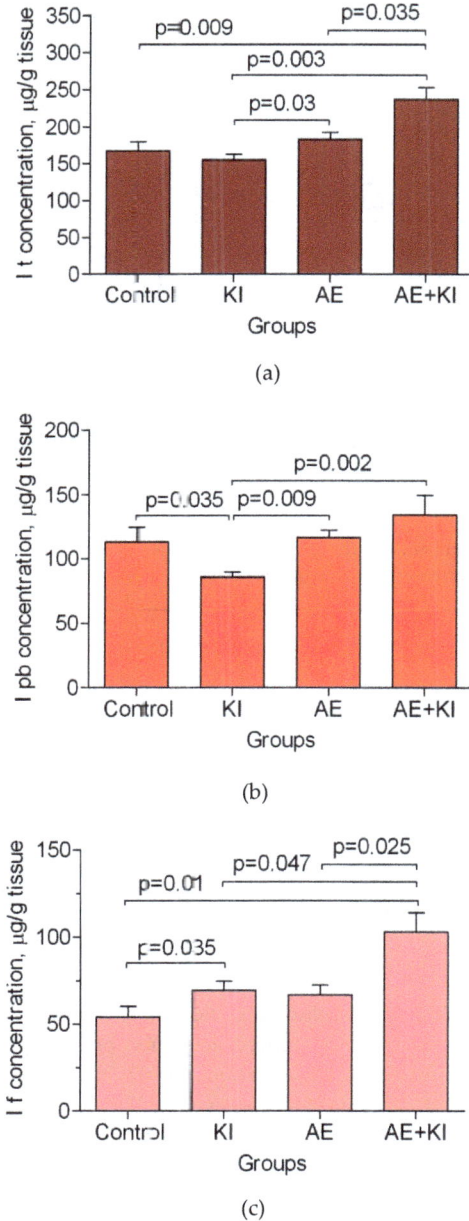

Figure 8. Effect of single administration of 1100 daily KI doses on contents of total I, protein-bound I and free I in thyroids of rats with normal and decreased glucocorticoid statuses

The blood thyroid hormone levels in AE rats were above the control values (27% for T4 and 35% for T3), but administration of KI lowered the concentrations of T4 by 41.1% and T3 by 34% compared to the AE animals. T4 was 29% decreased even in comparison with the controls (Fig. 9).

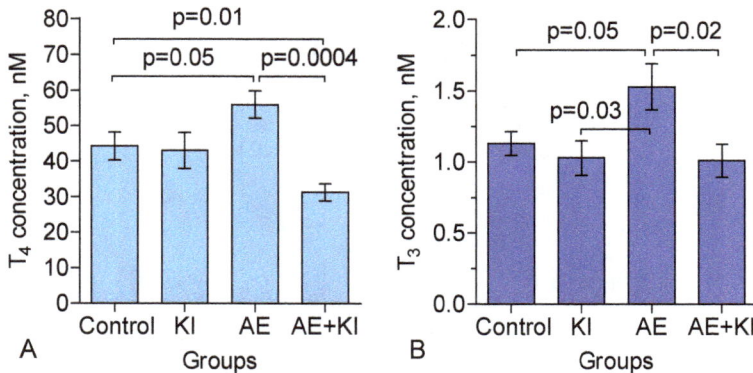

Figure 9. Effect of single administration of high KI dose on concentrations of total blood serum T4 and T3 in rats with normal and decreased glucocorticoid statuses

Index	Control	1000 daily doses of KI	AE	AE+1000 daily doses of KI
	A	B	C	D
TBARS, nmol/g tissue	131.2±8.9	212.5±22.9A	150.4±15.0	115.5±9.6B,C
Catalasa, μmol/min×g protein	36.8±1.3	40.0±1.6	32.2±0.8A,B	33.7±1.7B
SOD, activity u./min×g protein	43.2±4.2	56.8±1.4A	51.1±2.0A,B	48.9±2.9B
GR, μmol/min×g protein	24.0±1.2	22.7±1.0	26.7±1.0B	25.5±1.5

Table 8. Effect of single administration of 1000 daily doses of KI on TBARS levels and antioxidant enzyme activities in thyroids of rats with normal and decreased glucocorticoid statuses

In contrast to the rats with the normal glucocorticoid status, in which the administration of KI inhibited the thyroid function and induced activation of oxidative processes (62.0% elevation of TBARS concentration, 54.3% activation of SOD), the adrenalectomized rats did not show activation of lipid peroxidation (the level of TBARS was decreased by 23.2%, Table 8).

The AE animals demonstrated elevated concentrations of T3 and T4 in the blood serum (Fig. 9). These changes seemed to be caused by alterations in thyroid iodine metabolism since the contents of its different fractions did not change under decreased glucocorticoid status (Fig. 8). It was found earlier that AE caused enhancement of liver thyroxin-binding globulin synthesis and its binding capacity in the blood [88] as well as inhibition of the peripheral metabolism of thyroid hormones. Enhancement of deposition of blood thyroid hormones and, consequently, inhibition of their metabolism may cause elevation of thyroid hormone concentrations.

Most interesting changes were found after administration of high iodine doses to rats. In contrast to control animals with the characteristic acute Wolff – Chaikoff's effect, we did not observe inhibition of iodide organification in this group. Moreover, a pronounced lowering of T_4 and T_3 concentrations in the blood serum of AE rats after the administration of high iodine doses suggests that the cause of the absence of the Wolff-Chaikoff's effect under hypocorticism can be impaired maturing of the prohormone, thyroglobulin, and abnormal secretion of thyroid hormones to the blood, which provides for elevated concentration of protein-bound I in this group. Elevated TSH concentrations and enhanced NIS expression and, consequently, increased uptake of iodide absorption by the TG are also possible.

Our findings show that the effects of the single administration of the high KI dose on the activity of hormonogenesis in thyroids from normal and AE animals are multidirectional. Thyroids from the intact rats show inhibition of iodide organification accompanied by induction of oxidative stress, whereas the hypocorticoid rats demonstrate a reverse effect: activation of iodide uptake and organification as well as a decrease in the intensity of lipid peroxidation. These results are of a considerable interest in relation to some clinical studies which prove that impairments in the glucocorticoid status can be linked to development of autoimmune thyroid diseases. Lowering of the functional activity in the hypophyseal link (ACTH) and/or the adrenal (cortisol) link was noted in patients with autoimmune tyroiditis [89, 90]. It was shown that autoimmune tyroiditis and diabetes mellitus are developed on the average 7 years after autoimmune damage of the adrenal glands [91]. In patients suffering from hypercorticism of different genesis, AE contributes to development of autoaggression in their thyroids [68, 66, 92]. It is suggested that puerperal thyroiditis, as a consequence of a temporary decrease of the glucocorticoid status in females at the puerperal period [93], is due to ACTH-releasing hormone inhibition of the synthesis and secretion of maternal hypothalamic ACTH-releasing hormone and that this inhibition is of a placental origin. It should be mentioned that impaired functional activities of the pituitary-adrenal axis are also noted in other autoimmune diseases [94]. The mechanisms of the regularities found certainly require further studies since the literature lacks information on this problem.

3.5. Excess administration of iodine induces development of hyperthyroiditis in rats with glucocorticoid deficiency

Glucocorticoid deficiency is a cause for impairments of the adequate regulation of the thyroid status and thyroid iodine metabolism. It was interesting to study the properties of the iodine metabolism after its repeated administration to rats with adrenal deficiency.

After 2 weeks following AE, the blood serum thyroid hormone concentrations in operated animals were partially restored and amounted to 23.7-42.3% of the control values (Fig. 10)

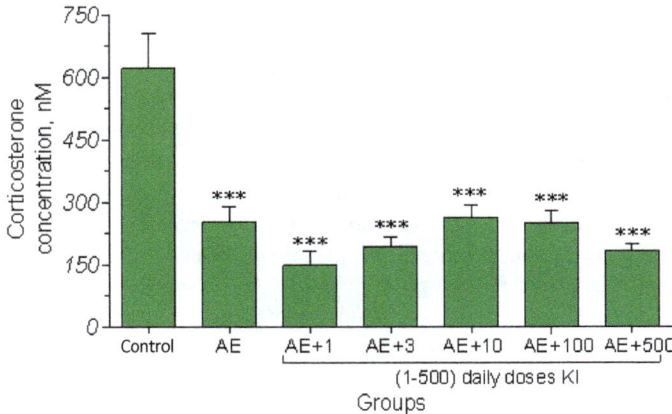

*** statistically significant changes vs control group (p<0.001)

Figure 10. Effect of 14-day administration of 1-500 daily doses of KI on blood serum corticosterone concentration in AE rats.

Studies on the thyroid iodine metabolism showed that repeated administration of high KI doses resulted in 46.9-115.7% increased concentrations of total I and caused 120.4 to 223.9% elevations of free I in all the experimental groups (Fig. 11). Glucocorticoid hormones are likely to inhibit iodide uptake by erythrocytes since the levels of nonorganified iodine were 1.2-fold increased after AE in rats which did not receive supplementary KI. One more confirmation is a more considerable growth of free I concentrations in thyroids of rats with hypocorticism (120.4-223.9%, Fig. 11) compared to controls (94.8-128.0%) after administration of KI at the same doses. Iodine organification in AE rats was enhanced by 32-86% in rats treated with 3 to 500 daily doses of KI (Fig. 11). TPO activity in AE rats was 29.4% elevated and 2.4, 3.9 and 3.7-fold increased (Table 9) after administration of 3, 100 and 500 KI daily doses.

	Control	Daily doses of KI administered to AE animals				
		No administration	1	3	100	500
TPO, μmol/min× g protein	173.9±22.5	193.8±10.3	275.4±77.4	387.9±78.4*	616.5±178.1*	579.7±120.6*

Table 9. Effect of 2-week administration of 1 to 500 daily doses of potassium iodide on TPO activity (μm/min×g tissue) in thyroids of AE rats

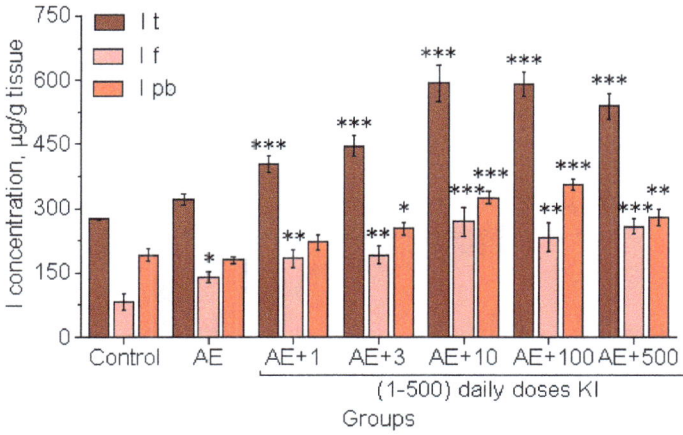

*statistically significant changes vs control group (p<0.05), **p<0.01; ***p<0.001

Figure 11. Effect of 14-day administration of 1-500 daily doses of KI on the concentrations of total I, protein-bound I and free I in thyroids of AE rats

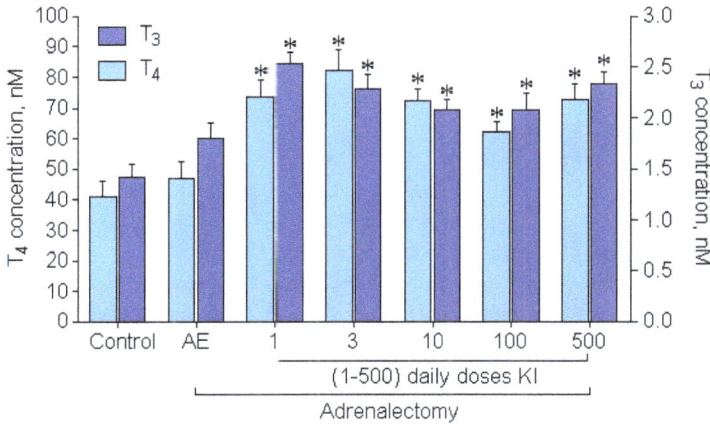

* statistically significant changes vs control group (p<0.05)

Figure 12. Effect of 14-day administration of 1 to 500 daily doses of potassium iodide on the concentrations of total T_4 and T_3 in the blood serum of rats with normal and lowered glucocorticoid statuses

The repeated and single administrations of excess potassium iodide to rats with hypocorticism were characterized by activation of iodide metabolism in the TG, which was followed by development of pronounced hyperthyroidism in AE animals. The blood serum total T_4 concentration (Fig. 12) was increased by 52-100% in rats with adrenal deficiency treated with KI for 14 days compared to control animals. The T_3 concentration (Fig. 12) reached 145.5-177.5% of the control level.

In this situation, a pronounced disturbance in the regulatory mechanisms of the pituitary-thyroid axis may be observed, which is accompanied by development of hypothyroidism and indicates a permissive (coordinating) role of glucocorticoids in regulation of thyroid homeostasis.

Our findings indicate that regulation of iodide uptake is very closely related to the state of the pituitary-adrenal system. Excess iodine intake under hypocorticism causes development of hyperthyroiditis.

4. Conclusion

1. Short-term stress (5-30 min) induced activation of biosynthesis and secretion of thyroid hormones. The most important established regularity of the post-stress period is restoration of the iodine thyroid status due to activation of uptake and organification of iodine as well as a negative correlation between the total thyroid concentration and adrenal corticosterone concentration (r= –0.952, p=0.003), which indicates participation of glucocorticoids in regulation of iodine thyroid homeostasis.

2. The most pronounced stress-induced changes in iodine metabolism after the treatment by physiological KI doses (3 daily doses) are characterized by:
    -   disturbed kinetics of blood iodine content within 24 h following the KI treatment, which was characterized by accumulation of blood iodine (826%) after 6 hours following the post-stress period;
    -   changed dynamics of thyroid uptake and oxidation of iodine, which caused a decrease in the concentrations of total I and protein-bound I in thyroids of stressed rats after the treatment with 3 daily doses of KI in contrast to the control group which showed elevation of these indices.

3. It was shown that repeated exposure to short-term psychoemotional stress (for 4 weeks) induced pronounced structural and metabolic changes in the thyroid gland that were characterized by elevated iodine content, as well as a decrease of the extent of its organification and development of oxidative stress.

4. The lowered glucocorticoid status in rats is characterized by increased blood thyroid hormone concentrations and decreased TPO activity (44.2%). In contrast to the animals with normal glucocorticoid status, the AE rats did not show any inhibitory effect of high iodine doses (Wolff-Chaikoff's effect) after the single administration of 1000 daily doses of KI, and activation of thyroid iodide uptake and organification was observed.

5. The 2-week administration of KI (1-500 daily doses) to rats with glucocorticoid deficiency increased the levels of free iodine (120-224%) and protein-bound iodine (32-86%) as well as thyroid TPO activity. In contrast to controls, this was followed by development of pronounced hyperthyroiditis (T_4 amounts to 152-200% and T_3 – 145 to

177% of the control values), which is a consequence of impairments in the key mechanisms of thyrocyte regulation and shows a permissive (coordinating) role of glucocorticoids in respect to the given effects.

The state of chronic stress may be a cause of impaired iodine metabolism in thyroid cells, which can induce development of hypothyroiditis and autoimmune thyroid pathology. Deficiency of the pituitary-adrenal system enhances the probability of development of hyperthyroiditis.

Author details

Liliya Nadolnik

Department of Bioregulators, Institute of Bioorganic Chemistry National Academy of Sciences of Belarus, Belarus

Acknowledgement

We are grateful to her colleagues and post –graduate students at the Institute of Pharmacology and Biochemistry of the National Academy of Sciences of Belarus, Dr. Sergey Chumachenko (Ph.D. in Biology), Dr. Sergey Lupachik (Ph.D. in Biology), Ms. Daria Goreva and Ludmila Kiryukhina for the assistance in the implementation of this project.

5. References

[1] Derwahl M, Seto P, Rapoport B (1989) Complete nucleotide sequence of the cDNA for thyroidperoxidase in FRTL-5 rat thyroid cells. Nucleic Acids Res. 17: 8380-8384.

[2] Kaminsky S, Levy O, Salvador C, Dai G, Carrasco N (1994) Na+/I- symporter activity is present in membrane vesicles from TSH-deprived non I- transporting cultured thyroid cells. Proc. Natl. Acad. Sci. USA. 91: 3789-3793.

[3] Nikiforov Y (2006) Radiation-induced thyroid cancer: what we have learned from Chernobyl. Endocr. Pathol. 17: 307-317.

[4] Uyttersprot N, Pelgrims N, Carrasco N, Gervy C, Maenhaut C, Dumont J, Miot F (1997) Moderate doses of iodide in vivo inhibit cell proliferation and the expression of thyroperoxidase and Na+/I- symporter mRNAs in dog thyroid. Mol. Cell Endocrinol. 131: 195-203.

[5] Espinoza C, Schmitt L, Loos U (2001) Thyroid transcription factor 1 and Pax8 synergistically activate the promot er of the human thyroglobulin gene. J. Mol. Endocrinol. 27: 59–67.

[6] Lagorce J, Thomes J, Catanzano G, Buxeraud J, Raby M, Raby C (1991) Formation of molecular iodine during oxidation of iodide by the peroxidase/H2O2 system. Implications for antithyroid therapy. Biochem. Pharmacol. 42: S89-S92.

[7] Hahn F, McClellan R, Boecker B, Muggenburg B (1988) Future development of biological understanding of radiation protection: implications of nonstochastic effects. Health. Phys. 55: 303-313.

[8] Schumm-Draeger P (2001) Sodium/iodide symporter (NIS) and cytokines. Exp. Clin. Endocrinol. Diabetes. 109: P. 32-34.

[9] Bjorkman U, Ekholm R, Denef J (1981) Cytochemical localization of hydrogen peroxide in isolated thyroid follicles J. Ultrastruct. Res. 74: 105-115.

[10] Zang X, Li Y, Wang Z, Li P (2006) Glucocorticoids receptor subunit gene expression in thyroid gland and adenomas. Acta Oncol. 45: 1073-1078.

[11] Liu Z (1992) Effect of TRH on anti-restraint stress in rats. Zhongguo Yi Xue Ke Xue Yuan Xue Bao. 14: 118-121.

[12] Kuhn E, Geris K, Van der Geyten S, Mol K, Darras V (1998) Inhibition and activation of the thyroidal axis by the adrenal axis in vertebrates. Comp. Biochem. Physiol. A Mol. Integr. Physiol. 120: 169-174.

[13] Bános C, Takó J, Salamon F, Györgyi S, Czikkely R (1979) Effect of ACTH-stimulated glucocorticoid hypersecretion on the serum concentrations of thyroxine-binding globulin, thyroxine, triiodothyronine, reverse triiodothyronine and on the TSH-response to TRH. Acta Med. Acad. Sci. Hung. 36: 381-394.

[14] Re R, Kourides I, Ridgway E, Weintraub B, Maloof F (1976) The effect of glucocorticoid administration on human pituitary secretion of thyrotropin and prolactin. J. Clin. Endocrinol. Metab. 43: 338-346.

[15] Iovino M., Steardo L, Monteleone P (1991) Impaired sensitivity of the hypothalamo-pituitary-thyroid axis to the suppressant effect of dexamethasone in elderly subjects Psychopharmacology (Berl.). 1105: 481-484.

[16] Rubello D, Sonino N, Casara D, Girelli M, Busnardo B, Boscaro, M (1992) Acute and chronic effects of high glucocorticoid levels on hypothalamic-pituitary-thyroid axis in man. J. Endocrinol. Invest. 15: 437-441.

[17] Azukizawa M, Mori S, Ohta H, Matsumura S, Yoshimoto H, Uozumi T, Miyai K, Kumahara Y (1979) Effect of a single dose of glucocorticoid on the diurnal variations of TSH, thyroxine, 3,5,3'-triiodothyronine, 3,3',5'-triiodothyronine and cortisol in normal men. Endocrinol. Jpn. 26: P. 719-723.

[18] Fang V, Shian L (1981) Adrenal influence on pituitary secretion of thyrotropin and prolactin in rats. Endocrinology. 108: 1545-1551.

[19] Ahlquist J, Franklyn J, Ramsden D, Sheppard M (1989) The influence of dexamethasone on serum thyrotrophin and thyrotrophin synthesis in the rat. Mol. Cell Endocrinol. 64: 55-61.

[20] Kakucska I, Qi Y, Lechan R (1995) Changes in adrenal status affect hypothalamic thyrotropin-releasing hormone gene expression in parallel with corticotropin-releasing hormone. Endocrinology. 136: 2795-2802.

[21] Van der Geyten, S., Byamungu, N., Reyns, G.E., Kühn, E.R., and Darras, V.M (2005) Iodothyronine deiodinases and the control of plasma and tissue thyroid hormone levels in hyperthyroid tilapia (Oreochromis niloticus). J. Endocrinol. 184: 467-479.

[22] Taylor A, Flower R, Buckingham J (1995) Dexamethasone inhibits the release of TSH from the rat anterior pituitary gland in vitro by mechanisms dependent on de novo protein synthesis and lipocortin 1. J. Endocrinol. 147: 533-544.

[23] Coiro V, Volpi R, Capretti L, Speroni G, Pilla, S, Cataldo S, Bianconcini M, Bazzani E, Chiodera P (2001) Effect of dexamethasone on TSH-secretion induced by TRH in human obesity. Investig. Med. 49: P. 330-334.

[24] Saito T, Endo T, Kawaguchi A, Ikeda M, Nakazato M, Kogai T, Onaya T (1997) Increased expression of the Na/I symporter in cultured human thyroid cells exposed to thyrotropin and in Graves' thyroid tissue. J. Clin. Endocrinol. Metab. 82: 3331-3336.

[25] Bernier-Valentin F, Trouttet-Masson S, Rabilloud R, Selmi-Ruby S, Rousset B (2006) Three-dimensional organization of thyroid cells into follicle structures is a pivotal factor in the control of sodium/iodide symporter expression. Endocrinology. 147: 2035-2042.

[26] Ferreira A, Lima L, Araújo R, Müller G, Rocha R, Rosenthal D, Carvalho D. (2005) Rapid regulation of thyroid sodium–iodide symporter activity by thyrotrophin and iodine. J. Endocrinol. 184: P. 69-76.

[27] Tonacchera M, Pinchera A, Dimida A, Ferrarini E, Agretti P, Vitti P, Santini F, Crump K, Gibbs J (2004) Relative potencies and additivity of perchlorate, thiocyanate, nitrate, and iodide on the inhibition of radioactive iodide uptake by the human sodium iodide symporter. Thyroid. 14: 1012-1019.

[28] Knopp J, Kvetnansky R, Murgas M, Knopp J. (1978) The changes of in vitro [131]-iodine uptake in the thyroid gland of rats exposed to septal lesions and immobilization stress. Physiol. Bohemoslov. 27: 329-332.

[29] Kiang J, Wang X, Ding X, Gist I, Smallridge R (1996) Heat shock inhibits the hypoxia-induced effects on iodide uptake and signal transduction and enhances cell survival in rat thyroid FRTL-5 cells. Thyroid. 6: 475-483.

[30] Becks G, Buckingham D, Wang J, Phillips I, Hill D (1992) Regulation of thyroid hormone synthesis in cultured ovine thyroid follicles. Endocrinology. 130: 2789-2794.

[31] Takiyama Y, Tanaka H, Makino I (1994) The effects of hydrocortisone and RU486 (mifepristone) on iodide uptake in porcine thyroid cells in primary culture. Endocrinology. 135: 1972-1979.

[32] Unterholzner S, Willhauck M, Cengic N, Schütz M, Göke B, Morris J, Spitzweg C (2006) Dexamethasone stimulation of retinoic Acid-induced sodium iodide symporter expression and cytotoxicity of 131-I in breast cancer cells. J. Clin. Endocrinol. Metab. 91: 69-78.

[33] Scholz I, Cenqic N, Göke B, Morris J, Spitzweg C. (2004) Dexamethasone enhances the cytotoxic effect of radioiodine therapy in prostate cancer cells expressing the sodium iodide symporter. J. Clin. Endocrinol. Metab. 89: 1108-1116.

[34] Ray P, Sarkar S, Sengupta A, Chaudhuri-Sengupta S, Maiti B (2006) Roles of thyroid, adrenal and pancreatic hormones on thyroid activity of the soft-shelled turtles Lissemys punctata punctata Bonnoterre. Folia Biol. (Krakow). 54: 93-102.

[35] Woltz H, Thompson F, Kemppainen R, Munnell J, Lorenz M (1983) Effect of prednisone on thyroid gland morphology and plasma thyroxine and triiodothyronine concentrations in the dog. Am. J. Vet. Res. 44: 2000-2003.

[36] Montesinos M, Pellizas C, Velez M, Susperreguv S, Masini-Repiso A, Coleoni A (2006) Thyroid hormone receptor beta 1 gene expression is increased by Dexamethasone at transcriptional level in rat liver. Life Sci. 78: 2584-2594.

[37] Friedman Y, Bacchus R, Raymond R, Joffe R, Nobrega J (1999) Acute stress increases thyroid hormone levels in rat brain. Biol. Psychiatry. 45: 234-237.

[38] Csaba G, Kovacs P, Tothfalusi L, Pallinger E. (2005) Prolonged effect of stress (water and food deprivation) at weaning or in adult age on the triiodothyronine and histamine content of immune cells. Horm. Metab. Res. 37: 711–715.

[39] Pallinger E, Csaba G (2005) Influence of acute stress on the triiodothyronine (T3) and serotonin content of rat's immune cells. Acta Physiol. Hung. 92: 47-52.

[40] Darras V, Kotanen S, Geris K, Berghman L, Kühn E (1996) Plasma thyroid hormone levels and iodothyronine deiodinase activity following an acute glucocorticoid challenge in embryonic compared with posthatch chickens Gen. Comp. Endocrinol. 104: 203-212.

[41] Van der Geyten S, Segers I, Gereben B, Bartha T, Rudas P, Larsen P, Kühn E, Darras V (2001) Transcriptional regulation of iodothyronine deiodinases during embryonic development. Molecular and Cellular Endocrinology. 183: 1-9.

[42] Forhead A, Jellyman J, Gardner D, Giussani D, Kaptein E, Visser T, Fowden A (2007) Differential effects of maternal dexamethasone treatment on circulating thyroid hormone concentrations and tissue deiodinase activity in the pregnant ewe and fetus. Endocrinology. 148: 800-805.

[43] Van der Geyten S, Darras V (2005) Developmentally defined regulation of thyroid hormone metabolism by glucocorticoids in the rat. J. Endocrinol. 185: 327-336.

[44] Baumgartner A, Hiedra L, Pinna G, Eravci M, Prengel H, Meinhold H (1998) Rat brain type II 5'-iodothyronine deiodinase activity is extremely sensitive to stress. J. Neurochem. 71: 817-826.

[45] Verhoelst C,Van der Geyten S, Roelens, S, Darras V, (2005) Regulation of thyroid hormone availability by iodothyronine deiodinases at the blood-brain barrier in birds. Ann. N.Y. Acad. Sci. 1040: 501-503.

[46] Anguiano B, Valverde C (2001) Cold-induced increment in rat adrenal gland type II deiodinase is corticosterone dependent. Endocrine. 15: 8-91.

[47] Kim S, Harney J, Larsen P (1993) Hormonal regulation of thyroglobulin export from the endoplasmic reticulum of cultured thyrocytes. J. Biol. Chem. 268: 4873-4879.

[48] Song S, Oka T (2003) Regulation of type II deiodinase expression by EGF and glucocorticoid in HC11 mouse mammary epithelium. American Journal of Physiology Endocrinology and Metabolism. 284: E1119-E1124.

[49] Araki O, Morimura T, Ogiwara T, Mizuma H, Mori M, Murakami M (2003) Expression of type 2 iodothyronine deiodinase in corticotropin-secreting mouse pituitary tumor cells is stimulated by glucocorticoid and corticotropin-releasing hormone. Endocrinology. 144: 4459-4465.

[50] Coppola A, Meli R, Diano S (2005) Inverse shift in circulating corticosterone and leptin levels elevates hypothalamic deiodinase type 2 in fasted rats. Endocrinology. 146: 2827-2833.

[51] Brtko J, Macejova D, Knopp J, Kvetnansky R (2004) Stress is associated with inhibition of type I iodothyronine 5'-deiodinase activity in rat liver. Ann. N.Y. Acad. Sci. 1018: P. 219-223.

[52] Bianco A, Nunes M, Hell N, Maciel R (1987) The role of glucocorticoids in the stress-induced reduction of extrathyroidal 3,5,3'-triiodothyronine generation in rats. Endocrinology. 120: 1033-1038.

[53] Balsam A, Ingbar S (1978) The influence of fasting, diabetes, and several pharmacological agents on the pathways of thyroxine metabolism in rat liver. Joural of Clinical Investigation. 62: 415-424.

[54] Menjo M, Murata Y, Fujii T, Nimura Y, Seo H (1993) Effects of thyroid and glucocorticoid hormones on the level of messenger ribonucleic acid for iodothyronine type I 5_-deiodinase in rat primary hepatocytes grown as spheroids Endocrinology. 133: 2984-2990.

[55] Maia A, Harney J, Larsen P, Maia A (1995) Pituitary cells respond to thyroid hormone by discrete, gene-specific pathways. Endocrinology. 136: 1488-1494.

[56] Walpita C, Grommen S, Darras V, Van der Geyten S (2007) The influence of stress on thyroid hormone production and peripheral deiodination in the Nile tilapia (Oreochromis niloticus). Gen. Comp. Endocrinol. 150: 18-25.

[57] Van der Geyten S, Darras V (2005) Developmentally defined regulation of thyroid hormone metabolism by glucocorticoids in the rat. J. Endocrinol. 185: 327-336.

[58] Hernandez A, St Germain D (2002) Dexamethasone inhibits growth factor-induced type 3 deiodinase activity and mRNA expression in a cultured cell line derived from rat neonatal brown fat vascular-stromal cells. Endocrinology. 143: 2652-2658.

[59] Kester M, Kuiper G, Versteeg R. Visser T (2006) Regulation of type III iodothyronine deiodinase expression in human cell lines. Endocrinology. 147: 5845-5854.

[60] Malendowicz L, Filipiak B (1975) The effects of adrenalectomy and hydrocortisone replacement on the thyroid of the adult male rat I. Morphometrical data and histochemistry of some oxidative enzymes. Endokrinologie. 64: 223-231.

[61] Grubeck-Loebenstein B, Vierhapper H, Vierhapper H, Waldhäusl, W., Nowotny P (1983) Thyroid function in adrenocortical insufficiency during withdrawal and re-administration of glucocorticoid substihetion. Acta. Endocrinol. (Copenh). 103: 254-258.

[62] Rubello D, Sonino N, Casara D, Girelli M, Busnardo B, Boscaro M, Acute and chronic effects of high glucocorticoid levels on hypothalamic-pituitary-thyroid axis in man. J. Endocrinol. Invest. 15: 437-441.

[63] Invitti C, Manfrini R, Romanini B, Cavagnini F (1995) High prevalence of nodular thyroid disease in patients with Cushing's disease. Clin. Endocrinol. (Oxf.). 43: 359-363.

[64] Benker G, Raida M, Olbricht T, Wagner R, Reinhardt W, Reinwein D (1990) TSH secretion in Cushing's syndrome: relation to glucocorticoid excess, diabetes, goitre, and the - sick euthyroid syndrome. Clin. Endocrinol. (Oxf.). 33: 777-786.

[65] Morita H, Isaji M, Mune T, Daido H, Isomura Y, Sarui H, Tanahashi T, Takeda N, Ishizuka T, Yasuda K (2002) Transient Graves disease developing after surgery for Cushing disease. Am. J. Med. Sci. 323: 162-165.

[66] Arikan E, Guldiken S, Altun B.U, Kara M, Tugrul A (2004) Exacerbations of Graves' disease after unilateral adrenalectomy for Cushing's syndrome. J. Endocrinol. Invest. 27: 574-576.

[67] Takasu N, Ohara N, Yamada T, Komiya I (1993) Development of autoummune thyroid dysfunction after bilateral adrenalectomy in a patient with Corney's complex and after removal of ACTH-producing pituitary adenoma in a patient with Cushing's desease. J. Endocrinol. Invest. 16: 697-702.

[68] Yamakita N, Sakata S, Hayashi H, Maekawa H, Miura K (1993) Case report: silent thyroiditis after adrenalectomy in a patient with Cushing's syndrome. Am. J. Med. Sci. 305: 304-306.

[69] Katahira M, Yamada T, and Kawai M (2004) A case of cushing syndrome with both secondary hypothyroidism and hypercalcemia due to postoperative adrenal insufficiency. Endocr. J. 51: P. 105-113.

[70] Murakami T, Wada S, Katayama Y, Nemoto Y, Kugai N, Nagata N (1993) Thyroid dysfunction in isolated adrenocorticotropic hormone (ACTH) deficiency: case report and literature review. Endocr. J. 40: 473-478.

[71] Hangaard J, Andersen M, Grodum E, Koldkjaer O, Hagen C (1996) Pulsatile thyrotropin secretion in patients with Addison's disease during variable glucocorticoid therapy. J. Clin. Endocrinol. Metab. 81: 2502-2507.

[72] Ghizzoni L, Mastorakos G, Street M.E, Vottero A, Mazzardo G, Vanelli M, Chrousos G, Bernasconi S (1997) Spontaneous thyrotropin and cortisol secretion interactions in patients with nonclassical 21-hydroxylase deficiency and control children. J. Clin. Endocrinol. Metab. 82: 3677-3683.

[73] Ooka-Souda S, Draves D, Timiras P (1979) Diurnal rhythm of pituitary-thyroid axis in male rats and the effect of adrenalectomy. Endocr. Res. Commun. 6: 43-56.

[74] Slone-Wilcoxon J, Redei E (2004) Maternal-fetal glucocorticoid milieu programs hypothalamic-pituitary-thyroid function of adult offspring. Endocrinology. 145: 4068-4072.

[75] Desiderato O,. MacKinnon J, Hissom H (1974) Devolopment of gastric ulcers in rats following stress termination. J. Compar. Physiol. Psychol. 87: 208-214.

[76] Tolmachev D (1991) A technique for modelling chronic psychoemotional stresses in experimental toxicological conditions. Gig. Tr. Prof. Zabol. 8: 26-28.

[77] Boltze C, Brabant G, Dralle H, Gerlach R, Roessner A, Hoang-Vu C (2002) Radiation–induced thyroid carcinogenesis as a function of time and dietary iodine supply: an in vivo model of tumorigenesis in the rat. Endocrinology. 143: 2584-2592.

[78] Dunn J, Crutchfield H, Gutekunst R, Dunn A (1993) Two simple methods for measuring iodine in urine. Thyroid. Summer. 3:119-123.

[79] Alexander N (1962) Spectrophotometric assay for iodide oxidation by thyroid peroxidase. Analytical Biochem. 4: 341-345.

[80] Yamada Y, Aizawa A (1984) Simple and convenient method for quantitation of corticosterone by high–performance liquid chromatography – ultraviolet detection. J. Pharmac. Methods. 11: P. 291-297.

[81] Sugawara M, Sugawara Y, Wen K, Giulivi C (2002) Generation of oxygen free radicals in thyroid cells and inhibition of thyroid peroxidase. Exp Biol Med (Maywood). 22: 141-146.

[82] Mizokami T, Wu Li A, El-Kaissi S, Wall J. (2004) Stress and thyroid autoimmunity. Thyroid. 14: 1047–1055.

[83] Klecha A, Barreiro Arcos M, Frick L, Genaro A, Cremaschi G. (2008) Immune-endocrine interactions in autoimmune thyroid diseases. // Neuroimmunomodulation. 15: 68–75.

[84] Kasperlik-Laluska A, Czarnocka B, Czech W (2003) Autoimmunity as the most frequent cause of idiopathic secondary adrenal insufficiency: report of 111 cases. Autoimmunity. 36: 155-159.

[85] Tsatsoulis, A. (2006) The role of stress in the clinical expression of thyroid autoimmunity. Ann. N.Y. Acad. Sci. 1088: 382-395.

[86] Imaizumi M, Akahoshi M, Ichimaru S, Nakashima E, Hida A, Soda M, Usa T, Ashizawa K, Yokoyama N, Maeda R, Nagataki S, Eguchi K (2004) Risk for ischemic heart disease and all-cause mortality in subclinical hypothyroidism. J. Clin. Endocrinol. Metab. 89: 3365-3370.

[87] Crunkhorn S, Patti M (2008) Links between thyroid hormone action, oxidative metabolism, and diabetes risk? Thyroid. 18: 227-237.

[88] Emerson C, Seiler C, Alex S, Fang S, Mori Y, DeVito W (1993) Gene expression and serum thyroxine-binding globulin are regulated by adrenal status and corticosterone in the rat. Endocrinology. 133: 1192-1196.

[89] Tamura M, (1995) Improvement of hypothyroidism after glucocorticoid replacement adrenocorticotropin deficiency. Intern. Med. 34: 559-563.

[90] Nagai Y, Ieki Y, Ohsawa K, Kobayashi K (1997) Simultaneouslly found transient hypothyroidism due to Hashimoto's thyroiditis, autoimmune hepatitis and isolated ACTH deficiency after cessation of glucocorticoid administration. Endocr. J. 44: 453-458.

[91] Yue L, Wang F, Li G (1998) Changes of peripheral tissue thyroid hormone metabolism in rats fed with selenium- and vitamin E-deficient artificial semisynthetic diet. Clin Med. J. 111: 854-857.

[92] Haraguchi K, Onaya T (1991) Autoimmune thyroid dysfunction after treatment for Cushing's syndrome. N. Engl. J. Med. 325: 1708-1712.

[93] Mastorakos G, Ilias I (2000) Maternal hypothalamic–pituitary–adrenal axis in pregnancy and the postpartum period: postpartum–related disorders Ann. N.Y. Acad. Sci. 900: 95-106.

[94] Wick G, Hu Y, Schwarz S, Kroemer G (1993) Immunoendocrine communication via the hypothalamo–pituitary–adrenal axis in autoimmune diseases. Endocr. Rev. 14: 539-563.

Chapter 12

Novel Aspects of Glucocorticoids Actions on Energy Homeostasis and Hydromineral Balance

Silvia Graciela Ruginsk, Rodrigo Cesar Rorato,
Beatriz de Carvalho Borges, Ernane Torres Uchoa,
Lucila Leico Kagohara Elias and Jose Antunes-Rodrigues

Additional information is available at the end of the chapter

1. Introduction

Glucocorticoids can readily diffuse into the cells due to their lipophilic nature and bind to glucocorticoid (GR) and mineralocorticoid (MR) receptors, which, in the inactive form, are associated with other proteins in the cytosol. MR was shown to bind most of the glucocorticoids under basal conditions. However, after an increase in the circulating levels of glucocorticoids (i.e. caused by exposure to stress or during the circadian and ultradian peaks of glucocorticoid secretion) GRs are predominantly activated (de Kloet et al., 2005). The activated receptor undergoes conformational changes followed by the translocation of the ligand-bound complex to the nucleus. Within this subcellular compartment, this complex can form homo or heterodimers and bind to responsive elements (GREs) in the promoter region of target genes, a mechanism known as transactivation, or interact with transcription factors as monomers to modulate the transcription of responsive genes, a mechanism known as transrepression. The main transcriptional factors involved in these responses are the nuclear factor kappa B (NFκB) and the AP-1 protein family.

More recently, it has been suggested that nontranscriptional actions may account for the very rapid effects observed with acute glucocorticoid treatment (Limbourg & Liao, 2003). These actions differ from the classic genomic responses by the targets, type of interaction and period of action, being detected within few minutes after hormone secretion (Mikics et al., 2004; Sandi et al., 1996). The administration of high doses of dexamethasone was shown to protect the myocardial tissue from infarction and stroke through the prompt activation of endothelial nitric oxide (NO) system (Hafezi-Moghadam et al., 2002). During the 1990's, NO has been identified as a potent vasodilatatory gas. Its properties in decreasing blood pressure are still clinically explored by the use of NO donors as anti-hypertensive drugs.

More recently, NO has also been implicated in neuromodulation, exerting its actions in an autocrine or paracrine manner in the central nervous system (CNS).

In general, these rapid effects mediated by glucocorticoids seem to modulate signaling (through actions on ion channels, neuromodulators, neurotransmitters and other receptors systems), being very distinctive depending on the brain areas involved. It is generally accepted that glucocorticoids increase the excitability in some areas, like hippocampus and amygdala, and potentially decrease neuronal activity in others, such as the hypothalamus. Since the expression of glucocorticoid receptors vary considerably in the CNS, glucocorticoids are likely to modulate not only the activity of the hypothalamic-pituitary-adrenal (HPA) axis, but also indirectly modify the inputs to hypothalamic neurons, projecting from the limbic system and cerebral cortex.

The classic glucocorticoid receptors GR and MR have already been identified in neuronal and non-neuronal cellular membranes, although their involvement in these nongenomic responses is still controversial (Gametchu et al., 1993; Lipositis & Bohn, 1993). In pituitary-derived cells, the use of a GR antagonist prevented the dexamethasone-induced translocation of annexin-1, which was implicated in the rapid inhibition of adrenocorticotrophic hormone (ACTH) release (Buckingham et al., 2003; Solito et al., 2003; Tierney et al., 2003). Nevertheless, a GR-independent pathway has been also reported in the fast feedback mechanism at the pituitary level *in vivo* (Hinz & Hirschelmann, 2000).

Another line of evidence suggests that most of nongenomic responses are mediated by the glucocorticoid binding to G-coupled protein receptors (Liu & Chen, 1995; Orchinik et al., 1991). In tumor-derived cells, a receptor coupled to an inhibitory G-protein (Gi) has been implicated in the glucocorticoid-induced inhibition of ACTH release (Iwasaki et al., 1997). In the hypothalamus, however, the production and release of neuromodulators (endocannabinoids and NO) seem to be driven by the activation of a membrane receptor associated with a stimulatory G-protein (Gs) (Di et al., 2009). Endocannabinoids were shown to mediate most of the nongenomic actions of the glucocorticoids, including the rapid negative feedback on the HPA axis (Evanson et al., 2010). Accordingly, several signaling pathways have been implicated in the responses induced by glucocorticoids downstream from the putative membrane receptors, mainly including protein kinase A (PKA)- and protein kinase C (PKC)-derived mechanisms (Han et al., 2002, 2005; Lou & Chen, 1998; Qiu et al, 1998, 2003).

2. Glucocorticoids and energy balance

2.1. The control of food intake by glucocorticoids: novel aspects

The motivated behaviour of eating comprises one of the most primordial responses in all species. It is regulated by several factors, including adiposity (leptin and insulin) and satiety signals (such as mechanical and chemical stimulation of stomach and small intestine), as well as hormones [such as cholecystokinin (CCK)] (Schwartz et al., 2000). The adiposity factors are involved in the long-term control of energy balance and act primarily in hypothalamic neurons expressing orexigenic or anorexigenic neuropeptides (Schwartz et al., 2000). Neuropeptide Y (NPY) and agouti related protein (AgRP) in the arcuate nucleus of the hypothalamus (ARC), and orexins and melanin-concentrating hormone (MCH) in the lateral hypothalamic area (LHA), represent the main hypothalamic orexigenic neuropeptides (Gehlert, 1999; Smith & Ferguson, 2008; Valassi et al., 2008). In contrast, proopiomelanocortin (POMC) and cocaine and amphetamine-regulated transcript (CART) in the ARC, and corticotrophin-releasing factor (CRF) and oxytocin (OT) in the paraventricular nucleus of the hypothalamus (PVN) are the main mediators involved in the inhibition of food intake (Schwartz et al., 2000; Valassi et al., 2008). The localization of the above mentioned neuropeptides in hypothalamic nuclei is summarized in Table 1. The satiety signals, in turn, are implicated in the short-term control of food intake and have their actions mediated by brainstem areas, primarily by the nucleus of the solitary tract (NTS), which is implicated in the control of meal size (Havel, 2001). It is well established that the hypothalamic nuclei involved in the control of food intake have reciprocal connections with the brainstem (Sawchenko & Swanson, 1982; Swanson & Kuypers, 1980). This evidence provides the neuroanatomical basis for the hypothesis that adiposity signals may modulate satiety (Matson & Ritter, 1999; Wang et al., 2000).

Neuropeptides	Localization in the hypothalamus
NPY	ARC
AgRP	ARC
Orexins	LHA and PFA
MCH	LHA
POMC	ARC
CART	ARC, PVN and SON
CRF	PVN
OT	PVN and SON

Table 1. Hypothalamic localization of the neuropeptides involved in the control of food intake. NPY, neuropeptide Y; ARC, arcuate nucleus of the hypothalamus; AgRP, agouti related protein; LHA, lateral hypothalamic area; PFA, perifornical area MCH, melanin-concentrating hormone; POMC, proopiomelanocortin; CART, cocaine and amphetamine-regulated transcript; PVN, paraventricular nucleus of the hypothalamus; SON, supraoptic nucleus of the hypothalamus; CRF, corticotrophin-releasing factor; OT, oxytocin.

Glucocorticoids play an important role in the control of energy balance (La Fleur, 2006). It is well established that a peak in the concentration of glucocorticoids occurs immediately before or at the onset of the activity period, with a progressive decrease in the HPA axis activity being detected over the remaining period within 24 hours, resulting in the classic circadian rhythm (Moreira & Leal, 1997). In addition, this rhythm occurs due to glucocorticoids release from the adrenal gland in discrete pulses, which results in an ultradian rhythm. Changes in the amplitude of these pulses, and to a lesser extent in their frequency, determine the pattern of the circadian rhythm (Lightman et al., 2008). In fact, it has been also demonstrated that feeding is a major synchronizer of the HPA axis rhythmicity (Leal & Moreira, 1997), being the size of the meal directly related to glucocorticoid secretion (Honma et al., 1983). At the same time, increased food intake and body weight gain have been observed in humans following glucocorticoid treatment (Tataranni et al., 1996). Stress conditions, characterized by elevated circulating glucocorticoids levels, are also associated with increased food intake, body weight gain and obesity (Dallman et al., 2003; La Fleur, 2006; Spencer & Tilbrook, 2011).

Consistent with the importance of glucocorticoids on energy homeostasis are two very prevalent clinical conditions: 1) Cushing's syndrome, which is characterized by clinical findings that include abnormalities in the HPA axis rhythmicity, insulin resistance and hyperglycaemia secondary to hypercortisolism. The most common cause of Cushing's syndrome is the administration of pharmacological doses of oral, parenteral and, rarely, by topical glucocorticoids. Endogenous glucocorticoid excess may arise from ACTH–secreting pituitary tumors, ectopic (nonpituitary) ACTH production, or adrenal tumors. Hypercortisolaemia is associated with increased glucose production, decreased glucose transport and utilization, decreased protein synthesis, increased protein degradation in muscle and body weight gain (Nieuwenhuizen & Rutters, 2008; Shibli-Rahhal et al., 2006); (2) Addison's disease or primary adrenal insufficiency, first described by Addison in 1855, is characterized by an inability of the adrenal cortex to synthesize and secrete glucocorticoids and mineralocorticoids. Chronically, the main clinical findings observed in patients with Addison's disease include malaise, fatigue, anorexia, weight loss, darkening of the skin, hyponatraemia, hypoglycaemia and hyperkalaemia (Nieman and Chanco Turner, 2006).

It has been shown that the effects of glucocorticoids on food intake can vary according to their concentration in the circulation (Devenport et al., 1989). Low doses of corticosterone administered to adrenalectomized (ADX) rats activate MR and induce a stimulatory effect on fat intake, body weight gain and fat depot, being these effects prevalent at the late phase of the feeding period, the same period in which HPA axis activity is reduced during the circadian variation (Tempel & Leibowitz, 1994, 1989; Tempel et al., 1991). In contrast, GRs are activated by higher doses of circulating corticosterone, being this effect observed just before or at the first hours after the beginning of the feeding period, mimicking the peak of glucocorticoids secretion within the 24 hours of circadian rhythm. Such high levels of circulating glucocorticoids produce an increase in carbohydrate ingestion and metabolism (Goldstein et al., 1993; Kumar & Leibowitz, 1988; Kumar et al., 1988; Tempel & Leibowitz, 1994, 1989; Tempel et al., 1993). In addition, extremely high corticosterone plasma concentrations, such as those observed in response to stress or food restriction, stimulate fat and protein catabolism (mainly from muscular source) and, consequently, body weight loss, which increases the availability of gluconeogenesis substrates and enhances glucose plasma concentrations (Tempel & Leibowitz, 1994; Tomas et al., 1979).

Historically, the brain has been considered the main regulator of hunger and satiety. However, the existence of a unique hypothalamic satiety or hunger center, as proposed a few decades ago, is no longer acceptable. It has been demonstrated that dexamethasone injection into the lateral ventricle not only stimulates food intake but also enhances body weight gain in rats, being these effects accompanied by hyperleptinaemia and hyperinsulinaemia (Cusin et al., 2001; Zakrzewska et al., 1999). These central effects of glucocorticoids seem to be mediated by their interaction with neurons co-expressing glucocorticoid receptors and neuropeptides involved in the control of energy homeostasis (Aronsson et al., 1988; Hisano et al., 1988). This hypothesis has been evaluated by Zakrzewska and co-workers (1999), who demonstrated that the hypothalamic levels of NPY and CRF were, respectively, increased and decreased in response to the intracerebroventricular administration of dexamethasone. In addition, circulating glucocorticoids were shown to be required for the feeding-induced decrease in the expression of orexigenic neuropeptides in the ARC, as well as for the increased expression of the anorexigenic neuropeptide POMC in the same nucleus (Uchoa et al., 2012). It has been hypothesized by these authors that these effects would occur either by a direct effect of glucocorticoids on ARC neurons or indirectly by the feeding-induced secretion of leptin and insulin.

The removal of endogenous glucocorticoids induced by bilateral ADX surgery is one of the most used experimental models for replicating the human Addison's disease. The food intake and body weight gain are reduced in ADX animals, being these effects reversed by glucocorticoid replacement (Freedman et al., 1985; Uchoa et al., 2009a, 2009b, 2010). Furthermore, ADX is effective in diminishing hyperphagia and obesity under diverse experimental conditions (Bruce et al., 1982; Dubuc and Wilden, 1986; Yukimura et al., 1978). The ADX-induced hypophagia has been associated with a decrease of hypothalamic NPY and AgRP mRNA expression (Strack et al., 1995; Uchoa et al., 2012). Conversely, ADX induces an increase in the expression of CRF and OT in PVN (Uchoa et al., 2009b and 2010). The actions on these two peptides in the control of food intake were confirmed by the central administration of OT and CRF-2 receptor antagonists, which were able to reverse the ADX-induced hypophagic effect (Uchoa et al., 2009b and 2010).

It has been hypothesized that the stimulatory action of glucocorticoids on food intake may involve an increased drive for eating. Accordingly, it is believed that the ADX-induced hypophagia is caused, at least in part, by a reduction of this motivated behaviour. However, there are few evidences concerning the role of glucocorticoids on the satiety-related responses. Recent studies have demonstrated that the hypophagic response induced by ADX is associated with increased activation of satiety-related responses mediated by brainstem and hypothalamic circuits (Uchoa et al., 2009a, 2009b). Accordingly, the activation of NTS neurons, assessed by the increased number of cells expressing the nuclear c-Fos protein, is increased in ADX animals after feeding, indicating that this nucleus may be involved in the increased satiety responses following glucocorticoid deficiency (Uchoa et al., 2009a). Interestingly, the activation of CRF and OT neurons was also enhanced in the PVN of fed ADX rats, indicating that, besides the brainstem, the hypothalamus may be also involved in these satiety-related responses. Furthermore, this increased activation of satiety-related responses in the NTS following ADX is reversed by CRF$_2$ receptor antagonist, indicating that CRF also plays an important functional neuromodulatory role in the brainstem (Uchoa et al., 2010).

In addition to the reduced drive to eat and the increased satiety observed in ADX animals, a change in both the concentration as well as in the sensitivity to peripheral factors seems to underlie the hypophagic effect of glucocorticoid deficiency. Accordingly, ADX reduces plasma leptin levels in *ad libitum* rats (Germano et al., 2007; Savontaus et al., 2002), as well as the meal-induced insulin secretion (Germano et al., 2008; Uchoa et al., 2012), whereas glucocorticoid treatment increases leptin secretion and leptin expression in adipocytes (Jahng et al., 2008; Slieker et al., 1996; Zakrzewska et al., 1999). Furthermore, the sensitivity to insulin and leptin seems to be enhanced after ADX (Chavez et al., 1997; Zakrzewska et al., 1997), although CCK administration did not significantly alter food intake in ADX rats (Uchoa et al, 2009a). Another hormone that arises as a candidate for the modulation by glucocorticoids is ghrelin, although the effects of this hormone on food intake may also be produced independently of glucocorticoid action.

The physiological instinct of obtaining energy through food intake is parallel to the equally important development of satiation signals, which may terminate the ingestive behaviour as soon as the organism is replenished. Glucocorticoids have a well established role in both processes, contributing to the enhanced drive to eat as well as to the reduction of satiety-related responses. However, it is believed that, particularly in humans, the initiation of a meal often starts in the absence of any depletion signal, which means that it is possible for other brain areas such as the cortex and the limbic system to overcome the inputs coming from the hypothalamus and the brainstem, turning the organism into an ingestive mode, which actually exceeds its needs. Accordingly, both real and potential challenges that activate the HPA axis and, consequently, alter the secretion of glucocorticoids, may also disrupt this balance.

2.2. Glucocorticoids in the interface of immune challenges and food intake

Under acute immune challenges, the body produces a strong inflammatory response to the pathogens. This generalized reaction, triggered by the organism in order to safeguard the host homeostasis, comprises physiological and behavioural changes (Langhans, 2000). However, in a severe condition in which the overwhelming infection leads to life-threatening low blood pressure and decreased tissue perfusion, a medical emergency known as septic shock may contribute to organ damage and death. Microbial products such as lipopolisaccharides (LPS) from the outer lipid bilayer of gram-negative bacteria cell walls are commonly used to model acute illness, leading to the development of sepsis or endotoxaemia, depending on the dose of the endotoxin (Borges et al., 2007; 2011; Giusti-Paiva et al., 2002).

Hypophagia is part of the acute-phase response to illness. During endotoxaemia, food intake is limited and there is an impairment of energy expenditure. Experimental models have demonstrated that LPS dramatically reduces food consumption (Gautron et al., 2005; Sachot et al., 2004), being this hypophagic effect mainly elicited by the production of proinflammatory cytokines (Johnson, 1998; Wise et al., 2006). Consistent with the contribution of proinflammatory cytokines to this illness-induced hypophagia are the studies showing that their peripheral or central administration restrains eating, and that the acute antagonism of their actions attenuates this anorexic response (Asarian & Langhans, 2010).

The systemic administration of LPS triggers the synthesis and release of interleukin (IL)-1β, IL-6 and tumor necrosis factor (TNF)-α by monocytes and macrophages. In turn, these cytokines can exert local actions as signaling molecules to activate the immune system and the HPA axis (Turnbull and Rivier, 1999; Turnbull et al., 1998). Accordingly, it has been demonstrated that cytokines induce intense nuclear c-Fos immunoreactivity in CRF parvocellular neurons of the PVN (Matsunaga et al., 2000). Endotoxin also increases CRF synthesis and secretion, stimulating ACTH release from the pituitary corticotrophs and, consequently, the secretion of glucocorticoids from the adrenal cortex (Borges et al., 2007; Turnbull & Rivier, 1999). In turn, glucocorticoids inhibit the induction of proinflammatory cytokines, mostly by interacting with the intracellular GR, which culminates with the activation of NFκB and AP-1 (Conat et al., 1990; Munoz et al., 1996). After glucocorticoid binding to the cytosolic GR, the activated complex is translocated to the cell nucleus, where it interacts with the specific transcription factors AP-1 and NF-κB and prevents the transcription of targeted genes, in a process called transrepression. Glucocorticoids are able to prevent the transcription of many inflammation-associated genes, such as those ones encoding cytokines, including interleukins IL-1B, IL-4, IL-5 and IL-8, chemokines, arachidonic acid metabolites and adhesion molecules. The immunosuppressant action exerted by glucocorticoids may be also evidenced by the increased hypothalamic messenger RNA (mRNA) expression of cytokines and IL-1β plasma levels observed in response to LPS administration to ADX rats (Goujon et al., 1996).

Within this context, glucocorticoids appear as crucial hormones involved in the mobilization of stored peripheral energy, directing the metabolism to the production of key substrates utilized by the liver to sustain gluconeogenesis. Studies performed in rats show that the search and consumption of palatable foods are stimulated by corticosterone in a dose-related fashion (Dallman et al., 2007). Accordingly, these authors have also demonstrated that ADX rats exhibit poor weight gain, low fat content and increased sympathetic and HPA axis outflow, effects that are, in general, reversed by replacement with corticosterone. The removal of the negative feedback exerted by glucocorticoids in ADX animals has been also implicated in the increased expression of CRF mRNA in the PVN (Herman & Morrison, 1996; Rorato et al., 2008). In addition to its essential function in the control of HPA axis activity, CRF also has a physiological role in the control of food intake, as evidenced by the anorexigenic response induced by central administration of CRF and CRF-related peptides to experimental animals (Kalra et al., 1999; Richard et al., 2002), as previously discussed in this chapter. Furthermore, the use of a CRF receptor antagonist partially reverses the reduction in food intake induced by different stress paradigms (Hotta et al., 1999; Krahn et al., 1986). Accordingly, Borges and coworkers (2007) observed that increased CRF mRNA expression in the PVN precedes LPS-induced anorexia. Hence, an interchange between feeding control and HPA axis activity is conceivable to operate in basal conditions as well as following an immune challenge.

Recently, Saito and Watanabe (2008) have described that dexamethasone treatment attenuates the production of multiple proinflammatory cytokines by the brain and liver, suggesting a potential preventive effect of glucocorticoids on the LPS-induced hypophagia.

Furthermore, Rorato and coworkers (2008) reported that the anorexigenic effect induced by LPS is amplified in ADX rats and that the ADX-induced glucocorticoid deficiency promotes an increased activation of hypothalamic CRF and POMC neurons. It has been already demonstrated that the activation of POMC neurons promotes the release of α-melanocyte stimulating hormone (α-MSH), which, in turn, activates melanocortin 4 receptor (MC4R) (Cone, 2005). Melanocortin has been also implicated in the LPS-induced hypophagia, since the administration of exogenous α-MSH intensified, whereas the antagonism of MC4R attenuated the inhibitory effect of LPS on food intake (Fan et al., 1997; Huang et al., 1999). Within this context, glucocorticoids appear as negative regulators of melanocortin signaling, since ADX was shown not only to reduce AgRP expression in the hypothalamus of wild type mice, but also to reverse obese phenotype and restore hypothalamic melanocortin tone to control levels in leptin-deficient *ob/ob* mice (Makimura et al., 2000).

A growing body of evidence has recently linked obesity to a chronic low-grade inflammatory state (Paternain et al., 2011; Trayhurn & Wood, 2005). In fact, inflammation may contribute to a range of metabolic disturbances related to obesity, such as diabetes mellitus and cardiovascular diseases (Oren et al., 2007). Rats fed with high-fat diet express high levels of TNF-α, IL-6 and IL-1β in the hypothalamus, which is consistent with the development of an inflammatory process (Milanski et al., 2009). Cani and coworkers (2007) have demonstrated that endotoxaemia dysregulates the inflammatory tone and induces body weight gain and diabetes in mice, showing that a 4-week high-fat diet induced a two to three-fold increase in plasma LPS concentrations. The bacterial endotoxin is normally present in the human intestinal tract (Kelly et al., 2012). Accordingly, LPS is detectable in the circulation of both healthy and obese individuals, but it may transiently raises following energy-rich meals. It has also been shown that the intake of fat-rich diet acts as an inducer of chronic stress, elevating basal glucocorticoid levels and enhancing HPA axis responses to stress (Tannenbaum et al., 1997), suggesting that glucocorticoids are likely to participate in the pathogenesis of metabolic syndrome and obesity (Milagro et al., 2007; Paternain et al., 2011), even though obese individuals and patients with metabolic syndrome do not necessarily show elevated systemic glucocorticoid concentrations (Pereira et al., 2012).

In face of these findings, efforts are now being turned to clarify the significance of glucocorticoids in counteracting the pathophysiology of illness-induced hypophagia. The better understanding of these processes may place glucocorticoids as important pharmacological targets to deal with obesity and metabolic syndrome, in which inflammatory modulators seem to play a key role.

3. Endocannabinoids as potential intermediates of glucocorticoids actions

3.1. Endocannabinoids: general aspects

The pharmacological properties of the plant *Cannabis sativa* are knwon since ancient times. The first cannabinoid receptor (CB1R) was characterized in 1988 and its predominant distribution through the CNS initially suggested a relationship with the control of cognitive function. However, over the past few years, the number of studies investigating the participation of CB1R in several areas has increased dramatically. Pioneer studies revealed that the exogenous administration of "cannabis-like" compounds inhibits the activity of diverse neuroendocrine functions (Lomax, 1970; Rettori et al., 1990; Tyrey, 1978). Accordingly, it has been demonstrated that the mRNA for the CB1R is expressed in the hypothalamus and in the external layer of the median eminence of rodents (Herkenham et al., 1991; Wittmann et al., 2007), as well as in both the anterior and intermediate lobes of the human pituitary gland (Pagotto et al., 2001). The evidence of the local production of endocannabinoids provided by this later group further suggested a role for these substances on the direct control of pituitary function.

In this context, the CB1R has been implicated in most, if not all, the actions of endogenously produced cannabinoids in neurotransmission. It has been also demonstrated that hippocampal astrocytes functionally express the CB1R and respond with elevations in intracellular calcium concentrations to the stimulation by neurotransmitters released locally from neuronal sources (Navarrete & Araque, 2008). This evidence suggests that non-neuronal populations can also contribute to the complexity of the responses elicited by endocannabinoids within the CNS. Differently from CB1R, the second cannabinoid receptor (CB2R) was identified in immune cells, being predominantly distributed in the peripheral organs, but not restricted to them. Most of the actions of the endocannabinoid system are mediated by the interaction of endogenous ligands with CB1R or CB2R, although the precise actions of orphan receptors, such as GPR55, still remain to be elucidated.

The identification of this receptor system, as well as the description of well-known effects induced by the consumption or administration of "cannabis-like" substances in humans, suggested the existence of endogenous ligands to be discovered. Anandamide (AEA) was the first one, followed by 2-araquidonoilglicerol (2-AG), the main endocannabinoids studied so far. AEA binds to CB1R with high affinity and regulates the signaling cascade as a partial agonist (Bouaboula et al., 1995). On the other hand, 2-AG, besides being the most abundant endocannabinoid produced by the CNS, has a lower affinity for CB1R when compared to AEA but stimulates the intracellular signaling pathway as a full agonist (Mechoulam et al., 1995). Both AEA and 2-AG are synthesized on demand from membrane phospholipids after the activation of membrane-associated glucocorticoid receptors. AEA and 2-AG are also metabolized by independent enzymatic pathways (Freund et al., 2003). Indeed, AEA acts as a very promiscuous ligand, since it can also bind to type 1 vanilloid (TRPV1) receptors with high affinity (Tóth et al., 2005). Accordingly, some of the effects induced by AEA cannot be mimicked by the administration of the synthetic cannabinoid agonist WIN55,212-2 (Al-Hayani et al., 2001) and the well-known AEA-induced antinociception is still preserved in experimental animals lacking the CB1R gene (Di Marzo et al., 2000).

3.2. Endocannabinoids and the ingestive behaviour

3.2.1. Food intake

It has been demonstrated that glucocorticoids increase endocannabinoid levels in hypothalamic PVN slices, supporting the hypothesis that at least part of the effects induced by glucocorticoids on food intake are mediated by these lipid-derived mediators (Malcher-Lopes et al., 2006). In this study, Malcher-Lopes and colleagues also demonstrated that the glucocorticoid-mediated activation of a membrane receptor coupled to a Gαs–cAMP–PKA signaling cascade leads to an increase in endocannabinoid synthesis. Accordingly, increased hypothalamic levels of endocannabinoids have been also observed *in vivo* following glucocorticoid treatment (Hill et al., 2010).

Both endocannabinoids and glucocorticoids injected into hypothalamic areas induce similar effects on eating behaviour, increasing food consumption (Jamshidi & Taylor, 2001; Tempel et al., 1992). The synthesis of endocannabinoids in the hypothalamus and the expression of both endocannabinoids and glucocorticoid receptors in synapses and in hypothalamic neurons that synthesize peptides with a key role in food consumption reinforce this assumption (Castelli et al., 2007; Cota et al., 2003; Deli et al. 2009; Di Marzo et al., 2001; Malcher-Lopes et al., 2006). In fact, the neuropeptides CRF, OT and TRH, which have well described anorexigenic properties (Arletti et al., 1989, 1990; Morley et al., 1983; Steward et al., 2003), appear as potential targets for endocannabinoid-mediated actions induced by glucocorticoids. Therefore, the glucocorticoid-mediated blockade of excitatory glutamatergic synapses induced by endocannabinoids via CB1R has been already described in CRF, OT and TRH hypothalamic neurons (Di et al., 2003).

Although feeding is one of the main synchronizers of the HPA axis activity and both the endocannabinoid system and glucocorticoids seem to drive the organism into an increased ingestive behaviour under physiological conditions, several studies reported both stimulatory and inhibitory roles for endocannabinoids in the control of stress responses. In the experiments conducted by Patel and co-workers (2004), mice pretreated with a CB1R antagonist exhibited a robust increase in the restraint-induced glucocorticoid release and c-Fos immunolabeling in the PVN. In addition, the administration of a CB1R agonist, an inhibitor of endocannabinoid transport or a FAAH inhibitor attenuated the restraint-induced increase in glucocorticoid secretion. Although these authors hypothesized that the activation of endogenous CB1R may negatively modulate the HPA axis activity, they also demonstrated that the hypothalamic contents of 2-AG were, respectively, decreased and enhanced after acute and sustained stress. This finding is not consistent with an endocannabinoid-mediated inhibition of the HPA axis activity, but rather indicates that glucocorticoids may centrally inhibit the production of endocannabinoids. Similar results were obtained by Borges and colleagues (2011), who reported decreased hypothalamic 2-AG contents after acute LPS administration. Additionally, increased CRF mRNA expression, glucocorticoid plasma concentrations and hypophagia were found by this group in experimental animals submitted to a single LPS injection, being all these responses completely restored to basal levels following repeated LPS administration.

Conversely, an increase in hypothalamic 2-AG levels after acute restraint stress has also been recently reported (Evanson et al., 2010). According to these findings, these authors proposed that the CB1R-mediated signaling is required for glucocorticoid negative feedback, but not for the initial HPA axis response to restraint. In addition, a down-regulation of CB1R and an impaired glucocorticoid-mediated inhibition of excitatory inputs to parvocellular PVN neurons were observed in hypothalamic slices from rats submitted to repeated immobilization stress (Wamsteeker et al., 2010). Interestingly, application of a CB1R agonist to the bath did not suppress the excitatory inputs onto PVN neurons, suggesting that the CB1R-mediated signaling may be disrupted after prolonged exposure to stress. It has been recently reported by our group that the pharmacological blockade of the CB1R-mediated signaling during LPS-induced endotoxaemia produces a remarkable increase in the activation of CRF neurons in the parvocellular subdivision of the PVN, which is associated with a pronounced hypophagia (Rorato et al., 2011). Although further studies are needed to clarify the precise actions of endocannabinoids on stress responses, the majority of studies suggest that the endocannabinoid system may mediate the fast negative feedback exerted by glucocorticoids at both hypothalamic and pituitary levels, avoiding the overloading of this system and making it continuously responsive to other potential challenges.

It has been also observed that the peripheral nutrition-related hormone leptin reverses the increases in PVN endocannabinoid levels induced by glucocorticoids, indicating a central crosstalk between glucocorticoids and this satiety signal (Malcher-Lopes et al., 2006). In fact, Obese Zucker rats, which do not express leptin receptors, are hyperphagic and exhibit elevated glucocorticoid plasma levels (Ahima, 2000; Freedman et al., 1985) and increased hypothalamic levels of endocannabinoids (Di Marzo et al., 2001; Kirkham et al., 2002). Within this context, the study of the CB1R-mediated signaling has a great clinical relevance and expectation, since obesity is emerging as a very concerning heath problem worldwide, either considered alone or in association with other chronic degenerative diseases. Accordingly, an increasing number of recent studies have focused on the glucocorticoid-related effects mediated by CB1R, such as the central control of food consumption (Di Marzo et al., 2001) and satiety (Matias & Di Marzo, 2007), as well as the peripheral control of adiposity, a predictor of several chronic metabolic disorders (Westerink & Visseren, 2011).

Although the endocannabinoid system has been implicated in several physiological and pathological functions related to the control of food intake and body weight by glucocorticoids (Ameri, 1999; Bisogno et al., 2005; Di Marzo & Matias, 2005; Marco et al., 2011), it has been also demonstrated that these lipid-derived mediators can act independently of the glucocorticoid-mediated signalling (Jamshidi & Taylor, 2001; Kirkham & Williams, 2001; Williams & Kirkham, 1999; Williams et al. 1998). Most of these effects are also mediated by the activation of the CB1R, since the administration of the CB1R antagonist rimonabant reverses the cannabinoid-induced increase in food intake (Jamshidi & Taylor, 2001; Williams & Kirkham, 2002). Consistent with the CB1R-mediated orexigenic effects of endocannabinoids, transgenic mice that lack this receptor subtype or experimental animals treated with the CB1R antagonist exhibit decreased food consumption (Colombo et al. 1998; Di Marzo et al. 2001; Pertwee, 2005).

This rimonabant-induced decrease in food intake is, at least in part, mediated by changes in endocannabinoid signalling within the hypothalamus (Cota et al., 2003; Mailleux & Vanderhaeghen, 1992; Marsicano & Lutz, 1999). It has been already reported that the CB1R is co-expressed with several anorexigenic peptides such as CART and CRF (Asakawa et al.,

2001; Cota et al., 2003; Füzesi et al., 2008; Morley et al., 1983; Vrang et al., 2000). Accordingly, CB1R knockout mice exhibit increased CRF mRNA expression in the PVN (Cota et al., 2003). It has been also demonstrated that acute rimonabant treatment induces an increase in the co-localization of c-Fos with CART in the PVN and ARC and with POMC in the ARC, as well as promotes a decrease in both the protein and the mRNA for NPY in the ARC (Verty et al., 2009a). Conversely, no changes in NPY or POMC mRNA expression were found in the ARC of lean rats treated with rimonabant (Doyon et al., 2006), although the administration of AM251, a selective CB1R antagonist, blocked NPY release from hypothalamic explants (Gamber et al., 2005) and the POMC-expressing neurons were shown to release endocannabinoids under basal conditions (Hentges et al. 2005).

In the brainstem, the CB1R and the enzyme that metabolizes AEA, fatty acid amide hydrolase (FAAH), are expressed in the dorsal vagal complex, which includes the NTS (Van Sickle et al., 2001). In addition, peripheral vagal afferents expressing CB1R and the local production of AEA by the gastrointestinal tract are important food-stimulated signals involved with the control of food intake and meal size (Burdyga et al., 2004, 2010; Gómez et al., 2002; Jelsing et al., 2009a,b). Accordingly, our group has recently demonstrated that the previous CB1R blockade potentiates LPS-induced increase in the number of TH-expressing neurons of the NTS co-localizing c-Fos, suggesting that endocannabinoids may modulate satiety during an immune challenge.

Endocannabinoids can also modulate the hedonistic component of food intake. It has been demonstrated that the cannabinoid agonist THC increases the motivation to eat palatable food (Gallate et al., 1999), whereas the CB1R antagonism reduces this response (Simiand et al., 1998). Changes in content of endocannabinoids in the limbic forebrain regions were shown to be correlated with the nutritional status in experimental animals (Kirkham et al., 2002). Furthermore, the expression of the CB1R in the accumbens shell nucleus (NAcS), a key structure involved with motivation and reward, reinforce this hypothesis (Di Marzo et al., 2009). It is already known that dopamine release within NAcS is associated with rewarding associated with the addictive properties of abuse drugs (Volkow et al., 2007). Interestingly, it was observed that the administration of a CB1R antagonist attenuates the increases in dopamine release within this nucleus induced by a novel high palatable food (Melis et al., 2007), indicating that endocannabinoids may account for the integrated control of feeding-associated motivated behaviour.

In addition to their central effects on the control of hunger and satiety, the endocannabinoid signalling has been also implicated in the peripheral control of body weight through changes in energy storage and expenditure (Silvestri et al., 2011). Interestingly, SV40 immortalised murine white and brown adipocytes treated with rimonabant show increased uncoupling protein 1 (UCP1) expression (Perwitz et al., 2010), which is associated with the preferential production of heat. Furthermore, Quarta and colleagues (2010) have demonstrated that mice lacking CB1R exhibit a lean phenotype due to an increased lipid oxidation and thermogenesis. Accordingly, prolonged rimonabant administration was shown to increase lipolysis and decrease fat storage in white adipose tissue of mice with diet-induced obesity (Jbilo et al., 2005). A recent report from Verty and co-workers (2009b) has proposed that this response may be mediated by the autonomic nervous system, since the denervation of the sympathetic afferents blocked the effect of rimonabant on body weight.

3.2.2. Fluid intake

Although the endocannabinoid system has a great impact on the regulation of energy homeostasis, its participation in the control of fluid intake remains elusive. A pioneer study has demonstrated that the exogenous administration of compounds derived from the plant *Cannabis sativa* inhibits water intake (Sofia & Knobloch, 1976). On the other hand, the CB1R blockade significantly reduced water intake in the experiments conducted by Gardner & Mallet (2006). Recent studies have also reported that endocannabinoids increase the preference for palatable solutions such as sucrose (Higgs et al., 2003; Jarrett et al., 2005), without altering the drinking of salty solutions or distilled water induced by fluid deprivation (Yoshida et al., 2010). However, these conflicting results could be explained, at least in part, by the parallel effects of the endocannabinoid system in the control of locomotor activity, which could directly interfere with the search for eating and drinking.

The specific appetite for sodium and water is a very important adaptative response recruited to restore body fluid homeostasis. However, the excessive intake of sodium in industrialized food has a great impact in modern society, since it may be directly associated with the impairment of cardiovascular and renal functions. The neuropeptide OT appears as an important negative modulator of salt appetite in rats, being particularly relevant in osmolality- but not in the sodium-dependent inhibition of this ingestive behaviour (Blackburn et al., 1993). Furthermore, OT has been implicated in the central inhibition of water intake induced by water deprivation, hypertonic saline administration and angiotensin II injection (Arletti et al., 1990). More recently, studies developed by Verty and co-workers (2004) revealed that these effects of OT on water intake may be partially mediated by CB1R.

An empirical and very interesting observation is that animals that undergo periods of restricted or no access to water also reduce their food consumption, being this anorexic state as long as the water restriction persists. It is believed that this reduction in food intake is a compensatory mechanism, since a slight change in the osmolality of the gastrointestinal tract circulation may be detected after the beginning of the digestive process. This would contribute to a further increase in the already enhanced plasma osmolality, constituting a very life-threatening situation. Although some studies suggest the participation of central increases in CRF in this anorexic response induced by chronic exposure to osmotic stress (Koob et al., 1993; Krahn et al., 1986; Morley, 1987), it is clear that this decreased food intake occurs earlier than the activation of the HPA axis. Accordingly, no changes in c-Fos/CRF immunoreactivity or CRF mRNA expression were found in the hypothalamus of animals submitted to 24 hours (h) water restriction, despite the fact that the anorexigenic response, as well as the decrease in body weight, had already been observed after this short period (Ruginsk et al., 2011).

Furthermore, it has been also demonstrated by Ruginsk and coworkers (2011) that the number of CART neurons activated to produce c-Fos is increased in the hypothalamus of 24h water-deprived rats. Since CART is a well-known anorexigenic peptide, these results suggest a possible intersection between pathways controlling food and fluid intake. These results further propose the existence of an osmolality-related mechanism in this interface, since the immunoreactivity for c-Fos/CART and the CART mRNA expression in the PVN and supraoptic (SON) nuclei of the hypothalamus were increased after hypertonic but not isotonic extracellular volume expansion (Ruginsk et al., 2011).

4. Endocannabinoids and the control of hydromineral homeostasis

The magnocellular neurosecretory system consists of a group of neurons whose cell bodies are located at the PVN and SON in the hypothalamus and whose terminals, located at the neurohypophysis, release vasopressin (AVP) and OT in response to depolarization. Both neuropeptides act in the kidneys to control the excretion of water and electrolytes. AVP is mostly known for its antidiuretic and vasoconstrictor effects, while OT, together with atrial natriuretic peptide (ANP) produced by the heart, are the two major circulating hormones stimulating natriuresis and diuresis.

Immunohistochemical studies have revealed that GR and MR are co-localized in the parvocellular subdivision of the PVN, but not in magnocellular neurons, which predominantly express MR (Han et al., 2005). Accordingly, it has been demonstrated that high doses of dexamethasone can inhibit OT but not AVP secretion in response to hypertonic extracellular volume expansion (Durlo et al., 2004; Ruginsk et al., 2007) and central cholinergic, angiotensinergic and osmotic stimulation (Lauand et al., 2007). These effects were also correlated with immunohistochemical data, showing that the magnocellular neurons of the PVN and SON are inhibited by dexamethasone administration (Ruginsk et al., 2007).

More recently, the activation of membrane-associated glucocorticoid receptors has been proposed using hypothalamic slice preparations. It has been demonstrated that glucocorticoids could activate at least two divergent intracellular pathways mediated by $G_{\alpha}s$ and $G_{\beta\gamma}$ subunits. The local production of endocannabinoids and NO would then result in two synapse-specific mechanisms, respectively: 1) suppression of excitatory (glutamatergic) synaptic inputs and 2) facilitation of inhibitory (GABAergic) synaptic inputs to the hypothalamic magnocellular neurosecretory system (Di et al., 2003, 2005, 2009), consequently decreasing AVP and OT release from neurohypophyseal terminals. These actions on glutamatergic neurotransmission would be dependent on the activation of the CB1R, located mainly at presynaptic terminals. Accordingly, it has been recently demonstrated that the administration of rimonabant potentiates AVP and OT release as well as the number of c-Fos/AVP and c-Fos/OT double immunoreactive neurons in the PVN and SON of experimental animals submitted to hypertonic extracellular volume expansion (Ruginsk et al., 2010). Furthermore, the participation of the CB1R in the glucocorticoid-induced inhibition of the magnocellular neurosecretory system was clearly demonstrated by the same group, since the previous administration of rimonabant reversed the inhibitory effects of dexamethasone on hormone release (Ruginsk et al., 2012).

Although many brain regions seem to share similar cellular mechanisms triggered by endocannabinoids, their central actions can vary widely within the CNS. Several studies suggest that the endocannabinoid system can mediate not only the central effects of glucocorticoids but also independently modulate the excitability of postsynaptic terminals after the dendritic-mediated release of neuropeptides like OT (Hirasawa et al., 2004; McDonald et al., 2008; Oliet et al., 2007). This mechanism is likely to be implicated in the intra-hypothalamic feedback on hormone release and neuroplasticity (de Kock et al., 2003). The CB1R is also expressed in the NTS (Tsou et al., 1998), a key structure involved in the control of cardiovascular function that projects to the hypothalamus. Accordingly, the central administration of CB1R agonists was shown to reduce blood pressure and heart rate (Lake et al., 1997), while the microinjection of a CB1R antagonist into the NTS resulted in prolonged hypotension after activation of the baroreflex in experimental animals (Rademacher et al., 2003).

Besides participating in the central control of cardiovascular function, recent reports also suggest a role for peripherally-synthesized cannabinoids in the control of blood pressure. This hypothesis is supported by the evidence that the CB1R is expressed by human, rat and guinea-pig atria (Bonz et al., 2003; Kurz et al., 2008; Sterin-Borda et al., 2005). Within the heart, the activation of the CB1R induces a negative inotropic response on muscular fibers, thus reducing blood pressure. This is of particular interest for the study of the integrated cardiovascular and neuroendocrine responses to an increase in the circulating volume, since the distension of cardiac chambers (especially the right atria) in response to such experimental condition is the main stimulus for ANP secretion. Indeed, a role for the CB1R in ANP release has been recently proposed (Ruginsk et al., 2012), although further studies are needed to support this hypothesis.

5. Conclusions and perspectives

Besides the well-known effects on energy homeostasis and metabolism, the ability of glucocorticoids to suppress inflammatory responses has been extensively explored in therapeutics during the last fifty years. However, the clinical potential of glucocorticoids has not been fully achieved because of the severe dose-limiting side effects as well as the development of glucocorticoid resistance. More recently, a lot of expectation was put on characterization of non-steroidal dissociated GR agonists and modulators, which try to uncouple the desired and adverse effects of glucocorticoid administration based on the type of GR interaction with the DNA (transactivation and trasnrepression). However, the difficulty to transpose the effects to *in vivo* set-ups and their still unproved long-term safety have limited the use of these drugs in clinical practice so far.

In this context, different approaches to improve the benefit/risk ratio of glucocorticoids also include the development of drugs that selectively target the activation of membrane-associated GRs and its downstream nongenomic events, without evoking adverse effects, primarily attributed to the activation of genomic pathways. Therefore, the study of the nongenomic actions of glucocorticoids has introduced a novel player in the complexity of the circuitries regulated by the HPA axis and the integrated control of homeostasis. The endocannabinoid system appears as an important mediator of both central and peripheral effects of glucocorticoids, constituting a possible target by which several aspects of stress-mediated responses and energy acquisition/expenditure could be manipulated under diverse physiological and pathological conditions.

Author details

Silvia Graciela Ruginsk, Rodrigo Cesar Rorato, Beatriz de Carvalho Borges,
Ernane Torres Uchoa, Lucila Leico Kagohara Elias and Jose Antunes-Rodrigues
Department of Physiology, School of Medicine of Ribeirao Preto, University of Sao Paulo, Brazil

6. References

Al-Hayani, A., Wease, K.N., Ross, R.A., Pertwee, R.G., Davies, S.N. (2001). The endogenous cannabinoid anandamide activates vanilloid receptors in the rat hippocampal slice. *Neuropharmacology* Vol.41, No.8, pp. 1000-1005, ISSN 0028-3908

Ahima, R.S. (2000). Leptin and the neuroendocrinology of fasting. *Frontiers of Hormone Research* Vol.26, pp. 42-56, ISSN 0301-3073

Ameri, A. (1999). The effects of cannabinoids on the brain. *Progress in Neurobiology* Vol.58, No.4, pp.315-348, ISSN 0301-0082

Arletti, R., Benelli, A. & Bertolini, A. (1989). Influence of oxytocin on feeding behavior in the rat. *Peptides* Vol.10, No.1, pp. 89-93, ISSN 0196-9781

Arletti, R., Benelli, A.& Bertolini, A. (1990). Oxytocin inhibits food and fluid intake in rats. *Physiology and Behavior* Vol.48, No.6, pp. 825-830, ISSN 0031-9384

Aronsson, M., Fuxe, K., Dong, Y., Agnati, L.F., Okret, S., Gustafsson, J.A. (1988). Localization of glucocorticoid receptor mRNA in the male rat brain by in situ hybridization. *Proceedings of the National Academy of Sciences of the United States of America* Vol. 85, No. 23, pp. 9331-9335, ISSN 1091-6490

Asakawa, A., Inui, A., Yuzuriha, H., Nagata, T., Kaga, T., Ueno, N., Fujino, M.A., Kasuga, M. (2001). Cocaine-amphetamine-regulated transcript influences energy metabolism, anxiety and gastric emptying in mice. *Hormone and Metabolic Research* Vol.33, No.9, pp. 554–558, ISSN 1439-4286

Asarian, L., Langhans, W. (2010). A new look on brain mechanisms of acute illness anorexia. *Physiology and Behavior* Vol.100, No.5, pp. 464-471, ISSN: 0031-9384

Bisogno, T., Ligresti, A. & Di Marzo, V. (2005). The endocannabinoid signalling system: biochemical aspects. *Pharmacology, Biochemistry and Behavior* Vol.81, No.2, pp. 224-238, ISSN 0091-3057

Blackburn, R.E., Samson, W.K., Fulton, R.J., Stricker, E.M., Verbalis, J.G. (1993). Central oxytocin inhibition of salt appetite in rats: evidence for differential sensing of plasma sodium and osmolality. *Proceedings of the National Academy of Sciences of the United States of America* Vol.90, No.21, pp. 10380-10384, ISSN 0027-8424

Bonz, A., Laser, M., Küllmer, S., Kniesch, S., Babin-Ebell, J., Popp, V., Ertl. G., Wagner, J.A. (2003). Cannabinoids acting on CB1 receptors decrease contractile performance in human atrial muscle. *Journal of Cardiovascular Pharmacology* Vol.41, No.4, pp. 657-664, ISSN 1533-4023

Borges, B.C., Antunes-Rodrigues, J., Castro, M., Bittencourt, J.C., Elias, C.F., Elias, L.L. (2007). Expression of hypothalamic neuropeptides and the desensitization of pituitary-adrenal axis and hypophagia in the endotoxin tolerance. *Hormones and Behavior* Vol.52, No.4, pp. 508-519, ISSN: 0018-506X

Borges, B.C., Rorato, R., Avraham, Y., da Silva, L.E., Castro, M., Vorobiav, L., Berry, E., Antunes-Rodrigues, J, Elias, L.L. (2011). Leptin resistance and desensitization of hypophagia during prolonged inflammatory challenge. *American Journal of Physiology. Endocrinology and Metabolism* Vol.300, No.5, pp. E858-869, ISSN 1522-1555

Bouaboula, M., Poinot-Chazel, C., Bourrié, B., Canat, X., Calandra, B., Rinaldi-Carmona, M., Le Fur, G., Casellas, P. (1995). Activation of mitogen-activated protein kinases by stimulation of the central cannabinoid receptor CB1. *Biochemical Journal* Vol.312, No. 2, pp. 637-641, ISSN 0264-6021

Bruce, B.K., King, B.M., Phelps, G.R., Veitia, M.C. (1982). Effects of adrenalectomy and corticosterone administration on hypothalamic obesity in rats. *American Journal of Physiology* Vol. 243, No. 2, pp. E152-157, ISSN 0002-9513

Buckingham, J.C., Solito, E., John, C., Tierney, T., Taylor, A., Flower, R., Christian, H., Morris, J. (2003). Annexin 1: a paracrine/juxtacrine mediator of glucocorticoid action in the neuroendocrine system. *Cell Biochemistry and Function* Vol.21, pp. 217–221, ISSN 1099-0844

Burdyga, G., Lal, S., Varro, A., Dimaline, R., Thompson, D.G., Dockray, G.J. (2004). Expression of cannabinoid CB1 receptors by vagal afferent neurons is inhibited by cholecystokinin. *The Journal of Neuroscience* 2004 Vol.24, No.11, pp. 2708-2715, ISSN 0270-6474

Burdyga, G., Varro, A., Dimaline, R., Thompson, D.G., Dockray, G.J. (2010). Expression of cannabinoid CB1 receptors by vagal afferent neurons: kinetics, and role in influencing neurochemical phenotype. *American Journal of Physiology. Gastrointestinal and Liver Physiology* Vol.299, No.1, pp. G63-G69, ISSN 1522-1547

Cani, P.D., Amar, J., Iglesias, M.A., Poggi, M., Knauf, C., Bastelica, D., Neyrinck, A.M., Fava, F., Tuohy, K.M., Chabo, C., Waget, A., Delmée, E., Cousin, B., Sulpice, T., Chamontin, B., Ferrières, J., Tanti, J.F., Gibson, G.R., Casteilla, L., Delzenne, N.M., Alessi, M.C., Burcelin, R. (2007). Metabolic endotoxemia initiates obesity and insulin resistance. *Diabetes* Vol.56, No.7, pp. 1761-1772, ISSN: 1939-327X

Castelli, M.P., Piras, A.P., Melis, T., Succu, S., Sanna, F., Melis, M.R., Collu, S., Ennas, M.G., Diaz, G., Mackie, K., Argiolas, A. (2007). Cannabinoid CB1 receptors in the paraventricular nucleus and central control of penile erection: immunocytochemistry, autoradiography and behavioral studies. *Neuroscience* Vol.147, No.1, pp. 197-206, ISSN 0306-4522

Chavez, M., Seeley, R.J., Green, P.K., Wilkinson, C.W., Schwartz, M.W., Woods, S.C. (1997). Adrenalectomy increases sensitivity to central insulin. *Physiology and Behavior* Vol. 62, No. 3, pp. 631-634, ISSN 1873-507X

Colombo, G., Agabio, R., Diaz, G., Lobina, C., Reali, R., Gessa, G.L. (1998). Appetite suppression and weight loss after the cannabinoid antagonist SR 141716. *Life Sciences* Vol.63, No.8, pp. PL113–PL117, ISSN 0024-3205

Cone, D.R. (2005). Anatomy and regulation of the central melanocortin system. *Nature Neuroscience* Vol.8, No.5, pp. 571-578, ISSN: 1546-1726

Cota, D., Marsicano, G., Tschöp, M., Grübler, Y., Flachskamm, C., Schubert, M., Auer, D., Yassouridis, A., Thöne-Reineke, C., Ortmann, S., Tomassoni, F., Cervino, C., Nisoli, E., Linthorst, A.C., Pasquali, R., Lutz, B., Stalla, G.K., Pagotto, U. (2003). The endogenous cannabinoid system affects energy balance via central orexigenic drive and peripheral lipogenesis. *The Journal of Clinical Investigation* Vol.112, No.3, pp. 423-431, ISSN 0021-9738

Cusin, I., Rouru, J., Rohner-Jeanrenaud, F. (2001). Intracerebroventricular glucocorticoid infusion in normal rats: induction of parasympathetic-mediated obesity and insulin resistance. *Obesity Research* Vol. 9, No. 7, pp. 401-406, ISSN 1550-8528

Dallman, M.F., Pecoraro, N., Akana, S.F., La Fleur, S.E., Gomez, F., Houshyar, H., Bell, M.E., Bhatnagar, S., Laugero, K.D., Manalo, S. (2003). Chronic stress and obesity: a new view of "comfort food". *Proceedings of the National Academy of Sciences of the United States of America* Vol. 100, No. 20, pp. 11696-11701, ISSN 1091-6490

Dallman, M.F., Akana, S.F., Pecoraro, N.C., Warne, J.P., La Fleur, S.E., Foster, M.T. (2007). Glucocorticoids, the etiology of obesity and the metabolic syndrome. *Current Alzheimer Research* Vol.4, No.2, pp. 199-204, ISSN: 1875-5828

De Kloet, E.R., Joëls & M., Holsboer, F. (2005). Stress and the brain: from adaptation to disease. *Nature Reviews Neuroscience* Vol.6, No.6, pp. 463-475, ISSN 1471-003X

De Kock, C.P., Wierda, K.D., Bosman, L.W., Min, R., Koksma, J.J., Mansvelder, H.D., Verhage, M., Brussaard, A.B. (2003). Somatodendritic secretion in oxytocin neurons is upregulated during the female reproductive cycle. *The Journal of Neuroscience* Vol.23, No.7, pp. 2726-2734, ISSN 0270-6474

Deli, L., Wittmann, G., Kalló, I., Lechan, R.M., Watanabe, M., Liposits, Z., Fekete, C. (2009). Type 1 cannabinoid receptor-containing axons innervate hypophysiotropic thyrotropin-releasing hormone-synthesizing neurons. *Endocrinology* Vol.150, No.1, pp. 98-103, ISSN 1945-7170

Devenport, L., Knehans, A., Sundstrom, A., Thomas, T. (1989). Corticosterone's dual metabolic actions. *Life Science* Vol. 45, No. 15, pp. 1389-1396, ISSN 1879-0631

Di, S., Malcher-Lopes, R., Halmos, K.C., Tasker, J. (2003). Nongenomic glucocorticoid inhibition via endocannabinoid release in the hypothalamus: a fast feedback mechanism. *The Journal of Neuroscience* Vol.23, No.12, pp. 4850-4857, ISSN 0270-6474

Di, S., Malcher-Lopes, R., Marcheselli, V.L., Bazan, N.G., Tasker, J.G. (2005). Rapid glucocorticoid-mediated endocannabinoid release and opposing regulation of glutamate and γ-aminobutiric acid inputs to hypothalamic magnocellular neurons. *Endocrinology* Vol.145, No.10, pp. 4292-4301, ISSN 1945-7170

Di, S., Maxson, M.M., Franco, A., Tasker, J.G. (2009). Glucocorticoids regulate glutamate and GABA synapse-specific retrograde transmission via divergent nongenomic signaling pathways. *The Journal of Neuroscience* Vol.29, No.2, pp. 393-401, ISSN 0270-6474

Di Marzo, V., Breivogel, C.S., Tao, Q., Bridgen, D.T., Razdan, R.K., Zimmer, A.M., Zimmer, A., Martin, B.R. (2000). Levels, metabolism, and pharmacological activity of anandamide in CB(1) cannabinoid receptor knockout mice: evidence for non-CB(1), non-CB(2)receptor-mediated actions of anandamide in mouse brain. *Journal of Neurochemistry* Vol.75, No.6, pp. 2434-2444, ISSN 1471-4159

Di Marzo, V., Goparaju, S.K., Wang, L., Liu, J., Batkai, S., Jarai, Z., Fezza, F., Miura, G.I., Palmiter, R.D., Sugiura, T., Kunos, G. (2001). Leptin-regulated endocannabinoids are involved in maintaining food intake. *Nature* Vol.410, pp. 822-825, ISSN 0028-0836

Di Marzo, V. & Matias, I. (2005). Endocannabinoid control of food intake and energy balance. *Nature Neuroscience* Vol.8, No.5, pp. 585-589, ISSN 1546-1726

Di Marzo, V., Ligresti, A. & Cristino, L. (2009). The endocannabinoid system as a link between homoeostatic and hedonic pathways involved in energy balance regulation. *International Journal of Obesity* Vol.33, No.2, pp. S18-S24, ISSN 1476-5497

Doyon, C., Denis, R.G., Baraboi, E.D., Samson, P., Lalonde, J., Deshaies, Y., Richard, D. (2006). Effects of rimonabant (SR141716) on fasting-induced hypothalamic-pituitary-adrenal axis and neuronal activation in lean and obese Zucker rats. *Diabetes* Vol.55, No.12, pp. 3403-3410, ISSN 1939-327X

Dubuc, P.U., Wilden, N.J (1986). Adrenalectomy reduces but does not reverse obesity in ob/ob mice. *International Journal of Obesity* Vol. 10, No. 2, pp. 91-98, ISSN 0307-0565

Durlo, F.V., Castro, M., Elias, L.L.K., Antunes-Rodrigues, J. (2004). Interaction of prolactin, ANPergic, oxytocinergic and adrenal systems in response to extracellular volume expansion in rats. *Experimental Physiology* Vol.89, No.5, pp. 541-548, ISSN 1469-445X

Evanson, N.K., Tasker, J.G., Hill, M.N., Hillard, C.J., Herman, J.P. (2010). Fast feedback inhibition of the HPA axis by glucocorticoids is mediated by endocannabinoid signaling. *Endocrinology* Vol.151, No.10, pp. 4811-4819, ISSN 1945-7170

Fan,W., Boston, B.A., Kesterson, R.A., Hruby,W.J., Cone, R.D. (1997). Role of melanocortinergic neurons in feeding and the agouti obesity syndrome. *Nature* Vol.385, No.6612, pp. 165–168, ISSN: 1476-4687

Freedman, M.R., Castonguay, T.W. & Stern, J.S. (1985). Effect of adrenalectomy and corticosterone replacement on meal patterns of Zucker rats. *The American Journal of Physiology* Vol.249, R584-R594, ISSN 0002-9513

Freund, T.F., Katona, I. & Piomelli, D. (2003). Role of endogenous cannabinoids in synaptic signaling (review). *Physiological Reviews* Vol.83, pp. 1017-1066, ISSN 1522-1210

Füzesi, T., Sánchez, E., Wittmann, G., Singru, P.S., Fekete, C., Lechan, R.M. (2008). Regulation of cocaine- and amphetamine-regulated transcript-synthesising neurons of the hypothalamic paraventricular nucleus by endotoxin; implications for lipopolysaccharide-induced regulation of energy homeostasis. *Journal of Neuroendocrinology* Vol.20, No.9, pp. 1058-1066, ISSN 1365-2826

Gallate, J.E., Saharov, T., Mallet, P.E., McGregor, I.S. (1999). Increased motivation for beer in rats following administration of a cannabinoid CB1 receptor agonist. *European Journal of Pharmacology* Vol.370, No.3, pp. 233-240, ISSN 0014-2999

Gamber, K.M., Macarthur, H. & Westfall, T.C. (2005). Cannabinoids augment the release of neuropeptide Y in the rat hypothalamus. *Neuropharmacology* Vol.49, No.5, pp. 646-652, ISSN 0028-3908

Gametchu, B., Watson, C.S. & Wu, S. (1993). Use of receptor antibodies to demonstrate membrane glucocorticoid receptor in cells from human leukemic patients. *The FASEB Journal* Vol.7, No.13, pp. 1283-1292, ISSN 1530-6860.

Gardner, A. & Mallet, P.E. (2006). Supression of feeding, drinking, and locomotion by a putative cannabinoid receptor 'silent antagonist'. *European Journal of Pharmacology* Vol.530, pp. 103-106, ISSN 0014-2999

Gautron, L., Mingam, R., Moranis, A., Combe, C., Laye, S. (2005). Influence of feeding status on neuronal activity in the hypothalamus during lipopolysaccharide-induced anorexia in rats. *Neuroscience* Vol.134, No.3, pp. 933-946, ISSN: 0306-4522

Gehlert, D.R. (1999). Role of hypothalamic neuropeptide Y in feeding and obesity. *Neuropeptides* Vol. 33, No. 5, pp. 329-338, ISSN 0143-4179

Germano, C.M., Castro, M., Rorato, R., Laguna, M.T., Antunes-Rodrigues, J., Elias, C.F., Elias, L.L. (2007). Time course effects of adrenalectomy and food intake on cocaine- and amphetamine-regulated transcript expression in the hypothalamus. *Brain Research* Vol. 1166, pp. 55-64, ISSN 1872-6240

Germano, C.M., Castro, M., Rorato, R., Costa, D.B., Antunes-Rodrigues, J., Elias, C.F., Elias, L.L. (2008). Downregulation of melanocortin-4 receptor during refeeding and its modulation by adrenalectomy in rats. *Hormone and Metabolic Research* Vol. 40, No. 12, pp. 842-847, ISSN 1439-4286

Giusti-Paiva, A., De Castro, M., Antunes-Rodrigues, J., Carnio, E.C. (2002). Inducible nitric oxide synthase pathway in the central nervous system and vasopressin release during experimental septic shock. *Critical Care Medicine* Vol.30, No.6, pp. 1306–1310, ISSN: 1530-0293

Goldstein, R.E., Wasserman, D.H., McGuinness, O.P., Lacy, D.B., Cherrington, A.D., Abumrad, N.N. (1993). Effects of chronic elevation in plasma cortisol on hepatic carbohydrate metabolism. *American Journal of Physiology* Vol. 264, No. 1 Pt 1, pp. E119-E127, ISSN 0002-9513

Gómez, R., Navarro, M., Ferrer, B., Trigo, J.M., Bilbao, A., Del Arco, I., Cippitelli, A., Nava, F., Piomelli, D., Rodríguez de Fonseca, F. (2002). A peripheral mechanism for CB1 cannabinoid receptor-dependent modulation of feeding. *The Journal of Neuroscience* Vol.22, No.21, pp. 9612-9617, ISSN 0270-6474

Goujon, E., Parnet, P., Laye, S., Combe, C., Dantzer, R. (1996). Adrenalectomy enhances pro-inflammatory cytokines gene expression, in the spleen, pituitary and brain of mice in response to lipopolysaccharide. *Brain Research* Vol.36, No.1, pp. 53–62, ISSN: 0006-8993

Hafezi-Moghadam, A., Simoncini, T., Yang, Z., Limbourg, F.P., Plumier, J.C., Rebsamen, M.C., Hsieh, C.M., Chui, D.S., Thomas, K.L., Prorock, A.J., Laubach, V.E., Moskowitz, M.A., French, B.A., Ley, K., Liao, J.K. (2002). Acute cardiovascular protective effects of corticosteroids are mediated by non-transcriptional activation of endothelial nitric oxide synthase. *Nature Medicine* Vol.8, No.5, pp. 473-479, ISSN 1078-8956

Han, J.Z., Lin, W., Lou, S.J., Qiu, J., Chen, Y.Z. (2002). A rapid, nongenomic action of glucocorticoids in rat B103 neuroblastoma cells. *Biochimica et Biophysica Acta* Vol.1591, pp. 21–27, ISSN 0006-3002

Han, J.Z., Lin,W. & Chen, Y.Z. (2005). Inhibition of ATP-induced calcium influx in HT4 cells by glucocorticoids: involvement of protein kinase A. *Acta Pharmacologica Sinica* Vol.26, pp. 199–204, ISSN 1745-7254

Han F, Ozawa H, Matsuda K, Nishi M, Kawata M. (2005). Colocalization of mineralocorticoid receptor and glucocorticoid receptor in the hippocampus and hypothalamus. *Neuroscience Research* Vol.51, No.4, pp. 371-381, ISSN 0168-0102

Havel, P.J (2001). Peripheral signals conveying metabolic information to the brain: short-term and long-term regulation of food intake and energy homeostasis. *Experimental Biology and Medicine* Vol. 226, No. 11, pp. 963-977, ISSN 1535-3699

Hentges, S.T., Low, M.J. & Williams, J.T. (2005). Differential regulation of synaptic inputs by constitutively released endocannabinoids and exogenous cannabinoids. *The Journal of Neuroscience* Vol.25, No.42, pp. 9746-9751, ISSN 0270-6474

Herkenham, M., Lynn, A.B., Johnson, M.R., Melvin, L.S., de Costa, B.R., Rice, K.C. (1991). Characterization and localization of cannabinoid receptors in rat brain: a quantitative in vitro autoradiographic study. *The Journal of Neuroscience* Vol.11, No.2, pp. 563-83, ISSN 0270-6474

Herman, J.P., Morrison, D.G. (1996). Immunoautoradiographic and in situ hybridization analysis of corticotropin-releasing hormone biosynthesis in the hypothalamic paraventricular nucleus. *Journal of Chemical Neuroanatomy* Vol.11, No.1, pp. 49–56, ISSN: 0891-0618

Higgs, S., Williams, C.M. & Kirkham, T.C. (2003). Cannabinoid influences on palatability: Microstructural analysis of sucrose drinking after delta(9)-tetrahydrocannabinol, anandamide, 2-arachidonoyl glycerol and SR141716. *Psychopharmacology (Berlin)* Vol.165, pp. 370–377, ISSN 0033-3158

Hill, M.N., Karatsoreos, I.N., Hillard, C.J., McEwen, B.S. (2010). Rapid elevations in limbic endocannabinoid content by glucocorticoid hormones in vivo. *Psychoneuroendocrinology* Vol.35, No.9, pp. 1333-1338, ISSN 0306-4530

Hinz, B., Hirschelmann, R. (2000). Rapid non-genomic feedback effects of glucocorticoids on CRF-induced ACTH secretion in rats. *Pharmaceutical Research* Vol.17, No.10, pp. 1273-1277, ISSN 1573-904X

Hirasawa, M., Schwab, Y., Natah, S., Hillard, C.J., Mackie, K., Sharkey, K.A., Pittman, Q.J. (2004). Dendritically released transmitters cooperate via autocrine and retrograde actions to inhibit afferent excitation in rat brain. *The Journal of Physiology* Vol.559, No.2, pp. 611-624, ISSN 1469-7793

Hisano, S., Kagotani, Y., Tsuruo, Y., Daikoku, S., Chihara, K., Whitnall, M.H. (1988). Localization of glucocorticoid receptor in neuropeptide Y-containing neurons in the arcuate nucleus of the rat hypothalamus. *Neuroscience Letters* Vol. 95, No. 1-3, pp.13-18, ISSN 1872-7972

Honma, K.I., Honma, S., Hiroshige, T. (1983). Critical role of food amount for prefeeding corticosterone peak in rats. *American Journal of Physiology* Vol. 245, No. 3, pp. R339-R344, ISSN 0002-9513

Hotta, M., Shibasaki, T., Arai, K., Demura, H. (1999). Corticotropin-releasing factor receptor type 1 mediates emotional stress-induced inhibition of food intake and behavioral changes in rats. *Brain Research* Vol.823, No. 1-2, pp. 221–225, ISSN: 0006-8993

Huang, Q.H., Hruby, V.J., Tatro, J.B. (1999). Role of central melanocortins in endotoxin-induced anorexia. *American Journal of Physiology – Regulatory, Integrative and Comparative Physiology* Vol.276, No.3, pp. 864–871, ISSN: 1522-1490

Iwasaki, Y., Aoki, Y., Katahira, M., Oiso, Y., Saito, H. (1997). Non-genomic mechanisms of glucocorticoid inhibition of adrenocorticotropin secretion: possible involvement of GTP-binding protein. *Biochemical and Biophysical Research Communications* Vol.235, pp. 295–299, ISSN 0006-291X

Jahng, J.W., Kim, N.Y., Ryu, V., Yoo, S.B., Kim, B.T., Kang, D.W., Lee, J.H. (2008). Dexamethasone reduces food intake, weight gain and the hypothalamic 5-HT concentration and increases plasma leptin in rats. *European Journal of Pharmacology* Vol. 581, No. 1-2, pp. 64-70, ISSN 1879-0712

Jamshidi, N. & Taylor, D.A. (2001). Anandamide administration into the ventromedial hypothalamus stimulates appetite in rats. *British Journal of Pharmacology* Vol.134, No.6, pp. 1151-1154, ISSN 1476-5381

Jbilo, O., Ravinet-Trillou, C., Arnone, M., Buisson, I., Bribes, E., Péleraux, A., Pénarier, G., Soubrié, P., Le Fur, G., Galiègue, S., Casellas, P. (2005). The CB1 receptor antagonist rimonabant reverses the diet-induced obesity phenotype through the regulation of lipolysis and energy balance. *FASEB Journal* Vol.19, No.11, pp. 1567-1569, ISSN 1530-6860

Jarrett, M.M., Limebeer, C.L. & Parker, L.A. (2005). Effect of Delta9-tetrahydrocannabinol on sucrose palatability as measured by the taste reactivity test. *Physiology and Behavior* Vol.86, pp. 475–479, ISSN 0031-9384

Jelsing, J., Galzin, A.M., Guillot, E., Pruniaux, M.P., Larsen, P.J., Vrang, N. (2009a). Localization and phenotypic characterization of brainstem neurons activated by rimonabant and WIN55,212-2. *Brain Research Bulletin* Vol.78, No.4-5, pp. 202-210, ISSN 0361-9230

Jelsing, J., Larsen, P.J., Vrang, N. (2009b). The effect of leptin receptor deficiency and fasting on cannabinoid receptor 1 mRNA expression in the rat hypothalamus, brainstem and nodose ganglion. *Neuroscience Letters* Vol.463, No.2, pp. 125-129, ISSN 0304-3940

Johnson, R.W. (1998). Immune and endocrine regulation of food intake in sick animals. *Domestic Animal Endocrinology* Vol.15, No.5, pp. 309-319, ISSN: 0739-7240

Jonat, C., Rahmsdorf, H.J., Park, K.K., Cato, A.C.B., Gebel, S.,Ponta, H., Herrlich, P. (1990). Antitumor promotion and antiinflammation: down-modulation of AP-1 (Fos/Jun) activity by glucocorticoid hormone. *Cell* Vol.62, No.6, pp. 1189–1204, ISSN: 0092-8674

Kalra, S.P., Dube, M.G., Pu, S., Xu, B., Horvath, T.L., Kalra, P.S. (1999). Interacting appetite-regulating pathways in the hypothalamic regulation of body weight. *Endocrine Reviews* Vol.20, No.1, pp. 68–100, ISSN: 1945-7189

Kelly, C.J., Colgan, S.P., Frank, D.N. (2012). Of Microbes and Meals: The Health Consequences of Dietary Endotoxemia. *Nutrition in Clinical Practice* [Epub ahead of print], ISSN: 1941-2452

Kirkham, T.C. & Williams, C.M. (2001). Endogenous cannabinoids and appetite. *Nutrition Research Reviews* Vol.14, No.1, pp. 65-86, ISSN 1475-2700

Kirkham, T.C., Williams, C.M., Fezza, F., Di Marzo, V. (2002). Endocannabinoid levels in rat limbic forebrain and hypothalamus in relation to fasting, feeding and satiation: stimulation of eating by 2-arachidonoyl glycerol. *British Journal of Pharmacology* Vol.136, No.4, pp. 550-557, ISSN 1476-5381

Koob, G.F., Heinrichs, S.C., Merlo Pich, E., Menzaghi, F., Baldwin, H., Miczek, K., Britton, K.T. (1993). The role of corticotropin releasing factor in behavioural responses to stress. In: *Corticotropin Releasing Factor*, Ciba Foundation Symposium, Wiley, Chichester, UK, pp. 277-295.

Krahn, D.D., Gosnell, B.A., Grace, M., Levine, A.S. (1986). CRF antagonist partially reverses CRF- and stress-induced effects on feeding. *Brain Research Bulletin* Vol.17, pp. 285-289, ISSN 0361-9230

Kumar, B.A., Leibowitz, S.F. (1988). Impact of acute corticosterone administration on feeding and macronutrient self-selection patterns. *American Journal of Physiology* Vol. 254, No. 2 Pt 2, pp. R222-R228, ISSN 0002-9513

Kumar, B.A., Papamichael, M., Leibowitz, S.F. (1988). Feeding and macronutrient selection patterns in rats: adrenalectomy and chronic corticosterone replacement. *Physiology and Behavior* Vol. 42, No. 6, pp. 581-589, ISSN 1873-507X

Kurz, C.M., Gottschalk, C., Schlicker, E., Kathmann, M. (2008). Identification of a presynaptic cannabinoid CB1 receptor in the guinea-pig atrium and sequencing of the guinea-pig CB1 receptor. *Journal of Physiology and Pharmacology* Vol.59, No.1, pp. 3-15, ISSN 0867-5910

La Fleur, S.E., (2006). The effects of glucocorticoids on feeding behavior in rats. *Physiology and Behavior* Vol. 89, No. 1, pp.110-114, ISSN 1873-507X

Lake, K.D., Compton, D.R., Varga, K., Martin, B.R., Kunos, G. (1997). Cannabinoid-induced hypotension and bradycardia in rats mediated by CB1-like cannabinoid receptors.

Journal of Pharmacology and Experimental Therapeutics Vol.281, No.3, pp. 1030-1037, ISSN 1521-0103

Langhans, W. (2000). Anorexia of infection: current prospects. *Nutrition* Vol.16, No.10, pp. 996-1005, ISSN: 0899-9007

Lauand, F., Ruginsk, S.G., Rodrigues, H.L., Reis, W.L., De Castro, M., Elias, L.L., Antunes-Rodrigues, J., 2007. Glucocorticoid modulation of atrial natriuretic peptide, oxytocin, vasopressin and Fos expression in response to osmotic, angiotensinergic and cholinergic stimulation. *Neuroscience* Vol.147, No.1, pp. 247-257, ISSN 0306-4522

Leal, A.M., Moreira, A.C. (1997). Food and the circadian activity of the hypothalamic-pituitary-adrenal axis. *Braz. J. Med. Biol. Res.*, Vol. 30, No. 12, pp. 1391-1405, ISSN 1414-431X Limbourg, F.P. & Liao, J.K. (2003). Nontranscriptional actions of the glucocorticoid receptor. *Journal of Molecular Medicine (Berlin)* Vol.81, No.3, pp. 168-174, ISSN 1432-1440

Lightman, S.L., Wiles, C.C., Atkinson, H.C., Henley, D.E., Russell, G.M., Leendertz, J.A., McKenna, M.A., Spiga, F., Wood, S.A., Conway-Campbell, B.L. (2008). The significance of glucocorticoid pulsatility. *European Journal of Pharmacology* Vol.583, No.2-3, pp. 255-262, ISSN 1879-0712

Liposits, Z. & Bohn, M.C. (1993). Association of glucocorticoid receptor immunoreactivity with cell membrane and transport vesicles in hippocampal and hypothalamic neurons of the rat. *Journal of Neuroscience Research* Vol.35, No.1, pp. 14-19, ISSN 1097-4547

Liu, X. & Chen, Y.Z. (1995). Membrane mediated inhibition of corticosterone on the release of arginine vasopressin from rat hypothalamic slices. *Brain Research* Vol.704, No.1, pp. 19-22, ISSN 0006-8993

Lomax, P., 1970. The effect of marihuana on pituitary-thyroid activity in the rat. *Agents and Actions* Vol.1, No.5, pp. 252-257, ISSN 0065-4299

Lou, S.J. & Chen, Y.Z. (1998). The rapid inhibitory effect of glucocorticoid on cytosolic free Ca^{2+} increment induced by high extracellular K and its underlying mechanism in PC12 cells. *Biochemical and Biophysical Research Communications* Vol.244, pp. 403–407, ISSN 0006-291X

Mailleux, P. & Vanderhaeghen, J.J. (1992). Distribution of neuronal cannabinoid receptor in the adult rat brain: a comparative receptor binding radioautography and in situ hybridization histochemistry. *Neuroscience* Vol.48, No.3, pp. 655–668, ISSN 0306-4522

Makimura, H., Mizuno, T.M., Roberts, J., Silverstein, J., Beasley, J., Mobbs, C.V. (2000). Adrenalectomy reverses obese phenotype and restores hypothalamic melanocortin tone in leptin-deficient ob/ob mice. *Diabetes* Vol.49,No.11, pp. 1917–1923, ISSN: 1939-327X

Malcher-Lopes, R., Di, S., Marcheselli, V.S., Weng, F.J., Stuart, C.T., Bazan, N.G., Tasker, J.G. (2006). Opposing crosstalk between leptin and glucocorticoids rapidly modulates synaptic excitation via endocannabinoid release. *The Journal of Neuroscience* Vol.26, No.24, PP. 6643-6650, ISSN 0270-6474

Marco, E.M., García-Gutiérrez, M.S., Bermúdez-Silva, F.J., Moreira, F.A., Guimarães, F., Manzanares, J., Viveros, M.P. (2011). Endocannabinoid system and psychiatry: in search of a neurobiological basis for detrimental and potential therapeutic effects. *Frontiers in Behavioral Neuroscience* [Epub ahead of print], ISSN 1662-5153

Marsicano, G. & Lutz, B. (1999). Expression of the cannabinoid receptor CB1 in distinct neuronal subpopulations in the adult mouse forebrain. *The European Journal of Neuroscience* Vol.11, No.12, pp. 4213-4225, ISSN 1460-9568

Matias, I. & Di Marzo, V. (2007). Endocannabinoids and the control of energy balance. *Trends in Endocrinology and Metabolism* Vol.18, No.1, pp. 27-37, ISSN 1043-2760

Matias, I., Cristinol, L. & Di Marzo, V. (2008). Endocannabinoids: Some like it fat (and sweet too). *Journal of Neuroendocrinology* Vol.20, No.1, pp. 100-109, ISSN 1365-2826

Matson, C.A., Ritter, R.C., (1999). Long-term CCK-leptin synergy suggests a role for CCK in the regulation of body weight. *American Journal of Physiology* Vol. 276, No. 4 Pt 2, pp. R1038-R1045, ISSN 0002-9513

Mechoulam, R., Ben-Shabat, S., Hanus, L., Ligumsky, M., Kaminski, N.E., Schatz, A.R., Gopher, A., Almog, S., Martin, B.R., Compton, D.R., et al., 1995. Identification of an endogenous 2-monoglyceride, present in canine gut, that binds to cannabinoid receptors. *Biochemical Pharmacology* Vol.50, No.1, pp. 83-90, ISSN 0006-2952

Melis, T., Succu, S., Sanna, F., Boi, A., Argiolas, A., Melis, M.R. (2007). The cannabinoid antagonist SR 141716A (Rimonabant) reduces the increase of extra-cellular dopamine release in the rat nucleus accumbens induced by a novel high palatable food. *Neuroscience Letters* Vol.419, No.3, pp. 231–235, ISSN 0304-3940

Mikics, E., Kruk, M.R. & Haller, J. (2004). Genomic and non-genomic effects of glucocorticoids on aggressive behavior in male rats. *Psychoneuroendocrinology* Vol.29, No.5, pp. 618-635, ISSN 0306-4530

Milagro, F.I., Campion, J., Martinez, J.A. (2007). 11-Beta hydroxysteroid dehydrogenase type 2 expression in white adipose tissue is strongly correlated with adiposity. *The Journal of Steroid Biochemistry and Molecular Biology* Vol.104, No.1–2, pp. 81–84, ISSN: 0960-0760

Milanski, M., Degasperi, G., Coope, A., Morari, J., Denis, R., Cintra, D.E., Tsukumo, D.M., Anhe, G., Amaral, M.E., Takahashi, H.K., Curi, R., Oliveira, H.C., Carvalheira, J.B., Bordin, S., Saad, M.J., Velloso, L.A. (2009). Saturated fatty acids produce an inflammatory response predominantly through the activation of TLR4 signaling in hypothalamus: implications for the pathogenesis of obesity. *The Journal of Neuroscience* Vol.29, No.2, pp. 359-370, ISSN: 1529-2401

Morley, J.E., Levine, A.S. & Rowland, N.E. (1983). Minireview: stress-induced eating. *Life Sciences* Vol.32, No.19, pp. 2169–2182, ISSN 0024-3205

Morley, J.E. (1987). Neuropeptide regulation of appetite and weight. *Endocrine Reviews* Vol.8, pp. 256-287, ISSN 1945-7189

Munoz, C., Pascual-Salcedo, D., Castellanos, M.C., Alfranca,A., Aragones, J., Vara, A., Redondo, J.M., de Landázuri, M.O. (1996). Pyrrolidine dithiocarbamate inhibits the production of interleukin-6, interleukin-8, and granulocyte-macrophage colony-stimulating factor by human endothelial cells in response to inflammatory mediators: modulation of NF-κB and AP-1 transcription factors activity. *Blood* Vol.88, No.9, pp. 3482–3490, ISSN: 1528-0020

Navarrete, M., Araque, A., 2008. Endocannabinoids mediate neuron-astrocyte communication. *Neuron* Vol.57, No.6, pp. 883-893, ISSN 0896-6273

Nieman, L.K., Chanco Turner, M.L. (2006). Addison's disease. *Clinics in Dermatology* Vol. 24, No. 4, pp. 276-280, ISSN 1879-1131

Nieuwenhuizen, A.G., Rutters, F. (2008). The hypothalamic-pituitary-adrenal-axis in the regulation of energy balance. *Physiol. Behav.*, Vol. 94, No.2, pp.169-177, ISSN 1873-507X

Oliet, S.H., Baimoukhametova, D.V., Piet, R., Bains, J.S., 2007. Retrograde regulation of GABA transmission by the tonic release of oxytocin and endocannabinoids governs postsynaptic firing. *The Journal of Neuroscience* Vol. 27, No.6, pp. 1325-1333, ISSN 0270-6474

Orchinik, M., Murray, T.F. & Moore, F.L. (1991). A corticosteroid receptor in neuronal membranes. *Science* Vol.252, No.5014, pp. 1848-1851, ISSN 1095-9203

Oren, H., Erbay,A.R., Balci, M., Cehreli, S.(2007). Role of novel biomarkers of inflammation in patients with stable coronary heart disease. *Angiology* Vol.58, No.2, pp. 148–155, ISSN: 0003-3197

Pagotto, U., Marsicano, G., Fezza, F., Theodoropoulou, M., Grübler, Y., Stalla, J., Arzberger, T., Milone, A., Losa, M., Di Marzo, V., Lutz, B., Stalla, G.K. (2001). Normal human pituitary gland and pituitary adenomas express cannabinoid receptor type 1 and synthesize endogenous cannabinoids: first evidence for a direct role of cannabinoids on hormone modulation at the human pituitary level. *The Journal of Clinical Endocrinology and Metabolism* Vol.86, No.6, pp. 2687-2696, ISSN 0021-972X

Patel, S., Roelke, C.T., Rademacher, D.J., Cullinan, W.E., Hillard, C.J. (2004). Endocannabinoid signaling negatively modulates stress-induced activation of the hypothalamic-pituitary-adrenal axis. *Endocrinology* Vol.145, No.12, pp. 5431-5438, ISSN 1945-7170

Paternain, L., García-Diaz, D.F., Milagro, F.I., González-Muniesa, P., Martinez, J.A., Campión, J. (2011). Regulation by chronic-mild stress of glucocorticoids, monocyte chemoattractant protein-1 and adiposity in rats fed on a high-fat diet. *Physiology and Behavior* Vol.103, No.2, pp. 173-180, ISSN: 0031-9384

Pereira, C.D., Azevedo, I., Monteiro, R., Martins, M.J. (2012). 11β-Hydroxysteroid dehydrogenase type 1: relevance of its modulation in the pathophysiology of obesity, the metabolic syndrome and type two diabetes mellitus. *Diabetes, Obesity and Metabolism* [Epub ahead of print], ISSN: 1463-1326

Pertwee, R.G. (2005). Inverse agonism and neutral antagonism at cannabinoid CB1 receptors. *Life Sciences* Vol.76, No.12, pp. 1307-1324, ISSN 0024-3205

Perwitz, N., Wenzel, J., Wagner, I., Büning, J., Drenckhan, M., Zarse, K., Ristow, M., Lilienthal, W., Lehnert, H., Klein, J. (2010). Cannabinoid type 1 receptor blockade induces transdifferentiation towards a brown fat phenotype in white adipocytes. *Diabetes, Obesity and Metabolism* Vol.12, No., pp. 158-166, ISSN 1463-1326

Qiu, J., Lou, L.G., Huang, X.Y., Lou, S.J., Pei, G., Chen, Y.Z. (1998). Nongenomic mechanisms of glucocorticoid inhibition of nicotine-induced calcium influx in PC12 cells: involvement of protein kinase C. *Endocrinology* Vol.139, pp. 5103–5108, ISSN 1945-7170

Qiu, J., Wang, C.G., Huang, X.Y., Chen, Y.Z. (2003). Nongenomic mechanism of glucocorticoid inhibition of bradykinin-induced calcium influx in PC12 cells: possible involvement of protein kinase C. *Life Science* Vol.72, pp. 2533–2542, ISSN 0024-3205

Quarta, C., Bellocchio, L., Mancini, G., Mazza, R., Cervino, C., Braulke, L.J., Fekete, C., Latorre, R., Nanni, C., Bucci, M., Clemens, L.E., Heldmaier, G., Watanabe, M., Leste-Lassere, T., Maitre, M., Tedesco, L., Fanelli, F., Reuss, S., Klaus, S., Srivastava, R.K., Monory, K., Valerio, A., Grandis, A., De Giorgio, R., Pasquali, R., Nisoli, E., Cota, D., Lutz, B., Marsicano, G., Pagotto, U. (2010). CB(1) signaling in forebrain and sympathetic neurons is a key determinant of endocannabinoid actions on energy balance. *Cell Metabolism* Vol.11, No.4, pp. 273-285, ISSN 1550-4131

Rademacher, D.J., Patel, S., Hopp, F.A., Dean, C., Hillard, C.J., Seagard, J.L. (2003). Microinjection of a cannabinoid receptor antagonist into the NTS increases baroreflex duration in dogs. *American Journal of Physiology - Heart and Circulatory Physiology* Vol.284, pp. H1570–H1576, ISSN 1522-1539

Rettori, V., Aguila, M.C., Gimeno, M.F., Franchi, A.M., McCann, S.M., 1990. In vitro effect of delta 9-tetrahydrocannabinol to stimulate somatostatin release and block that of luteinizing hormone-releasing hormone by suppression of the release of prostaglandin E2. *Proceedings of the National Academy of Sciences of the United States of America* Vol.87, No.24, pp. 10063-10066, ISSN 0027-8424

Richard, D., Lin, Q., Timofeeva, E. (2002). The corticotropin-releasing factor family of peptides and CRF receptors: their roles in the regulation of energy balance. *European Journal of Pharmacology* Vol.440, No.2-3, pp. 189–197, ISSN: 0014-2999

Rorato, R., Castro, M., Borges, B.C., Benedetti, M., Germano, C.M., Antunes-Rodrigues, J., Elias, L.L. (2008). Adrenalectomy enhances endotoxemia-induced hypophagia: higher activation of corticotrophin-releasing-factor and proopiomelanocortin hypothalamic neurons. *Hormomes and Behavior* Vol.54, No.1, pp. 134-142, ISSN: 0018-506X

Rorato, R., Reis, W.L., Carvalho Borges, B.D., Antunes-Rodrigues, J., Kagohara Elias, L.L. (2011). Cannabinoid CB(1) receptor restrains accentuated activity of hypothalamic corticotropin-releasing factor and brainstem tyrosine hydroxylase neurons in endotoxemia-induced hypophagia in rats. *Neuropharmacology* [Epub ahead of print], ISSN 0028-3908

Ruginsk, S.G., Oliveira, F.R.T., Margatho, L.O., Vivas, L., Elias, L.L.K., Antunes-Rodrigues, J., 2007. Glucocorticoid modulation of neuronal activation and hormone secretion induced by blood volume expansion. *Experimental Neurology* Vol.206, No.2, pp. 192-200, ISSN 0014-4886

Ruginsk, S.G., Uchoa, E.T., Elias, L.L., Antunes-Rodrigues, J. (2010). CB(1) modulation of hormone secretion, neuronal activation and mRNA expression following extracellular volume expansion. *Experimental Neurology* Vol.224, No.1, pp. 114-122, ISSN 0014-4886

Ruginsk, S.G., Uchoa, E.T., Elias, L.L., Antunes-Rodrigues, J., Llewellyn-Smith, I.J. (2011). Hypothalamic cocaine- and amphetamine-regulated transcript and corticotrophin releasing factor neurons are stimulated by extracellular volume and osmotic changes. *Neuroscience* Vol.186, pp. 57-64, ISSN 0306-4522

Ruginsk, S.G., Uchoa, E.T., Elias, L.L.K., Antunes-Rodrigues, J. (2012). Cannabinoid CB(1) receptor mediates glucocorticoid effects on hormone secretion induced by volume and osmotic changes. *Clinical and Experimental Pharmacology and Physiology* Vol.39, No.2, pp. 151-154, ISSN 1440-1681

Sachot, C., Poole, S., Luheshi, G.N. (2004). Circulating leptin mediates lipopolysaccharide-induced anorexia and fever in rats. *The Journal of Physiology* Vol.15, No.561 , pp. 263-272, ISSN: 1469-7793

Saito, M., Watanabe, S. (2008). Differential modulation of lipopolysaccharide- and zymosan-induced hypophagia by dexamethasone treatment. *Pharmacology, Biochemistry and Behavior* Vol.90, No.3, pp. 428-433, ISSN: 0091-3057

Sandi, C., Venero, C. & Guaza, C. (1996). Novelty-related rapid locomotor effects of corticosterone in rats. *European Journal of Neuroscience* Vol.8, No.4, pp. 794-800, ISSN 1460-9568

Savontaus, E., Conwell, I.M., Wardlaw, S.L. (2002). Effects of adrenalectomy on AGRP, POMC, NPY and CART gene expression in the basal hypothalamus of fed and fasted rats. *Brain Research* Vol. 958, No. 1, pp. 130-138, ISSN 1872-6240

Sawchenko, P.E., Swanson, L.W. (1982). The organization of noradrenergic pathways from the brainstem to the paraventricular and supraoptic nuclei in the rat. *Brain Research* Vol. 257, No. 3, pp. 275-325, ISSN 1872-6240

Schwartz, M.W., Woods, S.C., Porte Jr., D., Seeley, R.J., Baskin, D.G. (2000). Central nervous system control of food intake. *Nature* Vol.404, pp. 661–671, ISSN 1476-4687

Silvestri, C., Ligresti, A. & Di Marzo, V. (2011). Peripheral effects of the endocannabinoids system in energy homeostasis: Adipose tissue, liver and skeletal muscle. *Reviews in Endocrine and Metabolic Disorders* Vol.12, No.3, pp. 153-162, ISSN 1573-2606

Simiand, J., Keane, M., Keane, P.E., Soubrié, P. (1998). SR 141716, a CB1 cannabinoid receptor antagonist, selectively reduces sweet food intake in marmoset. *Behavioural Pharmacology* Vol.9, No.2, pp. 179-181, ISSN 1473-5849

Shibli-Rahhal, A., Van Beek, M., Schlechte, J.A. (2006). Cushing's syndrome. *Clinics in Dermatology* Vol. 24, No. 4, pp.260-265, ISSN 1879-1131

Slieker, L.J., Sloop, K.W., Surface, P.L., Kriauciunas, A., LaQuier, F., Manetta, J., Bue-Valleskey, J., Stephens, T.W. (1996). Regulation of expression of ob mRNA and protein by glucocorticoids and cAMP. *The Journal of Biological Chemistry* Vol. 271, No. 10, pp. 5301-5304, ISSN 1083-351X

Smith, P.M., Ferguson, A.V. (2008). Neurophysiology of hunger and satiety. *Developmental Disabilities Research Reviews* Vol.14, No. 2, pp. 96-104, ISSN 1940-5529

Sofia, R.D. & Knobloch, L.C. (1976). Comparative effects of various naturally occurring cannabinoids on food, sucrose and water consumption by rats. *Pharmacology Biochemistry and Behavior* Vol.4, pp. 591-599, ISSN 0091-3057

Solito, E., Mulla, A., Morris, J.F., Christian, H.C., Flower, R.J., Buckingham, J.C. (2003). Dexamethasone induces rapid serine-phosphorylation and membrane translocation of annexin 1 in a human folliculostellate cell line via a novel nongenomic mechanism involving the glucocorticoid receptor, protein kinase C, phosphatidylinositol 3-kinase, and mitogen-activated protein kinase. *Endocrinology* Vol.144, pp. 1164–1174, ISSN 1945-7170

Spencer, S.J., Tilbrook, A. (2011). The glucocorticoid contribution to obesity. *Stress* Vol. 14, No. 3, pp. 233-246, ISSN 1607-8883

Sterin-Borda, L., Del Zar, C.F. & Borda, E. (2005). Differential CB1 and CB2 cannabinoid receptor-inotropic response of rat isolated atria: endogenous signal transduction pathways. *Biochemical Pharmacology* Vol.69, No.12, pp. 1705-1713, ISSN 0006-2952

Steward, C.A., Horan, T.L., Schuhler, S., Bennett, G.W., Ebling, F.J. (2003). Central administration of thyrotropin releasing hormone (TRH) and related peptides inhibits feeding behavior in the Siberian hamster. *Neuroreport* Vol.14, No.5, pp. 687-691, ISSN 1473-558X

Strack, A.M., Sebastian, R.J., Schwartz, M.W., Dallman, M.F. (1995). Glucocorticoids and insulin: reciprocal signals for energy balance. *American Journal of Physiology* Vol. 268, No. 1 Pt 2, pp. R142-R149, ISSN 0002-9513

Swanson, L.W., Kuypers, H.G. (1980). The paraventricular nucleus of the hypothalamus: cytoarchitectonic subdivisions and organization of projections to the pituitary, dorsal vagal complex, and spinal cord as demonstrated by retrograde fluorescence double-labeling methods. *The Journal of Comparative Neurology* Vol. 194, No. 3, pp. 555-570, ISSN 1096-9861

Tannenbaum, B.M., Brindley, D.N., Tannenbaum, G.S., Dallman, M.F., McArthur, M.D., Meaney, M.J. (1997). High-fat feeding alters both basal and stress-induced hypothalamic–pituitary–adrenal activity in the rat. *American Journal of Physiology, Endocrinology and Metabolism* Vol.273, No.6, pp. 1168–1177, ISSN: 1522-1555

Tataranni, P.A., Larson, D.E., Snitker, S., Young, J.B., Flatt, J.P., Ravussin, E. (1996). Effects of glucocorticoids on energy metabolism and food intake in humans. *American Journal of Physiology* Vol. 271, No. 2 Pt 1, pp. E317-E325, ISSN 0002-9513

Tempel, D.L., Leibowitz, S.F. (1989). PVN steroid implants: effect on feeding patterns and macronutrient selection. *Brain Research Bulletin* Vol. 23, No. 6, pp. 553-560, ISSN 1873-2747

Tempel, D.L., McEwen, B.S. & Leibowitz, S.F. (1992). Effects of adrenal steroid agonists on food intake and macronutrient selection. *Physiology and Behavior* Vol.52, No.6, pp. 1161-1166, ISSN 0031-9384

Tempel, D.L., McEwen, B.S., Leibowitz, S.F. (1993). Adrenal steroid receptors in the PVN: studies with steroid antagonists in relation to macronutrient intake. *Neuroendocrinology* Vol. 57, No. 6, pp. 1106-1113, ISSN 1423-0194

Tempel, D.L, Leibowitz, S.F. (1994). Adrenal steroid receptors: interactions with brain neuropeptide systems in relation to nutrient intake and metabolism. *Journal of Neuroendocrinology* Vol. 6, No. 5, pp. 479-501, ISSN 1365-2826

Tierney, T., Christian, H.C., Morris, J.F., Solito, E., Buckingham, J.C. (2003). Evidence from studies on co-cultures of TtT/GF and AtT20 cells that Annexin 1 acts as a paracrine or juxtacrine mediator of the early inhibitory effects of glucocorticoids on ACTH release. *Journal of Neuroendocrinology* Vol.15, pp. 1134–1143, ISSN 1365-2826

Tomas, F.M., Munro, H.N., Young, V.R. (1979). Effect of glucocorticoid administration on the rate of muscle protein breakdown in vivo in rats, as measured by urinary excretion of N tau-methylhistidine. *Biochemistry Journal* Vol. 178, No. 1, pp. 139-146, ISSN 1470-8728

Tóth, A., Boczán, J., Kedei, N., Lizanecz, E., Bagi, Z., Papp, Z., Edes, I., Csiba, L., Blumberg, P.M., 2005. Expression and distribution of vanilloid receptor 1 (TRPV1) in the adult rat brain. *Brain research. Molecular brain research* Vol.135, No.1-2, pp. 162-168, ISSN 0169-328X

Trayhurn, P., Wood, I.S. (2005). Signalling role of adipose tissue: adipokines and inflammation in obesity. *Biochemical Society Transactions* Vol.33, No.5, pp. 1078-1081, ISSN: 0300-5127

Tsou, K., Brown, S., Sanudo-Pena, M., Mackie, K., Walker, J. (1998). Immunohistochemical distribution of cannabinoid CB1 receptors in the rat central nervous system. *Neuroscience* Vol.83, No.2, pp. 393-411, ISSN 0014-4886

Turnbull, A.V., Lee, S., Rivier, C. (1998). Mechanisms of hypothalamic-pituitary-adrenal axis stimulation by immune signals in the adult rat. *Annals of the New York Academy of Sciences* Vol.840, pp. 434-443, ISSN: 1749-6632

Turnbull, A.V., Rivier, C.L. (1999). Regulation of the hypothalamic-pituitary-adrenal axis by cytokines: actions and mechanisms of action. *Physiology Reviews* Vol.79, No.1, pp. 1–71. ISSN: 1522-1210

Tyrey, L., 1978. Delta-9-Tetrahydrocannabinol suppression of episodic luteinizing hormone secretion in the ovariectomized rat. *Endocrinology* Vol.102, No.6, pp. 1808-1814, ISSN 1945-7170

Uchoa, E.T., Sabino, H.A., Ruginsk, S.G., Antunes-Rodrigues, J., Elias, L.L. (2009a). Hypophagia induced by glucocorticoid deficiency is associated with an increased activation of satiety-related responses. *Journal of Applied Physiology* Vol. 106, No. 2, pp. 596-604, ISSN 1522-1601

Uchoa, E.T., Silva, L.E., de Castro, M., Antunes-Rodrigues, J., Elias, L.L. (2009b). Hypothalamic oxytocin neurons modulate hypophagic effect induced by adrenalectomy. *Hormones and Behavior* Vol. 56, No. 5, pp. 532-538, ISSN 1095-6867

Uchoa, E.T., Silva, L.E., de Castro, M., Antunes-Rodrigues, J., Elias, L.L. (2010). Corticotrophin-releasing factor mediates hypophagia after adrenalectomy, increasing meal-related satiety responses. *Hormones and Behavior* Vol. 58, No. 5, pp. 714-719, ISSN 1095-6867

Uchoa, E.T., Silva, L.E., de Castro, M., Antunes-Rodrigues, J., Elias, L.L. (2012). Glucocorticoids are required for meal-induced changes in the expression of hypothalamic neuropeptides. *Neuropeptides* Vol.46, No.3, pp. 119-124, ISSN 1532-2785

Valassi, E., Scacchi, M., Cavagnini, F. (2008). Neuroendocrine control of food intake. *Nutrition, Metabolism and Cardiovascular Diseases* Vol. 18, No. 2, pp. 158-168, ISSN 1590-3729

Van Sickle, M.D., Oland, L.D., Ho, W., Hillard, C.J., Mackie, K., Davison, J.S., Sharkey, K.A. (2001). Cannabinoids inhibit emesis through CB1 receptors in the brainstem of the ferret. *Gastroenterology* Vol.121, No.4, pp. 767-774, ISSN 0016-5085

Verty, A.N., McFarlane, J.R., McGregor, I.S., Mallet, P.E. (2004). Evidence for an interaction between CB1 cannabinoid and oxytocin receptors in food and water intake. *Neuropharmacology* Vol.47, No.4, pp. 593-603, ISSN 0028-3908

Verty, A.N., Boon, W.M., Mallet, P.E., McGregor, I.S., Oldfield, B.J. (2009a). Involvement of hypothalamic peptides in the anorectic action of the CB receptor antagonist rimonabant (SR 141716). *The European Journal of Neuroscience* Vol.29, No.11, pp. 2207-2016, ISSN 1460-9568

Verty, A.N., Allen, A.M. & Oldfield, B.J. (2009b). The effects of rimonabant on brown adipose tissue in rat: implications for energy expenditure. *Obesity* Vol.17, No.2, pp. 254-261, ISSN 1930-739X

Volkow, N.D., Fowler, J.S., Wang, G.J., Swanson, J.M. (2004). Dopamine in drug abuse and addiction: results from imaging studies and treatment implications. *Molecular Psychiatry* Vol.9, No.6, pp. 557-569, ISSN 1359-4184

Vrang, N., Larsen, P.J., Kristensen, P., Tang-Christensen, M. (2000). Central administration of cocaine-amphetamine-regulated transcript activates hypothalamic neuroendocrine neurons in the rat. *Endocrinology* Vol.141, No.2, pp. 794-801, ISSN 1945-7170

Wamsteeker, J.I., Kuzmiski, J.B. & Bains, J.S. (2010). Repeated stress impairs endocannabinoid signaling in the paraventricular nucleus of the hypothalamus. *The Journal of Neuroscience* Vol.30, No 33, pp. 11188-11196, ISSN 0270-6474

Wang, L., Barachina, M.D., Martínez. V., Wei, J.Y., Taché, Y. (2000). Synergistic interaction between CCK and leptin to regulate food intake. *Regulatory Peptides* Vol. 92, No. 1-3, pp. 79-85, ISSN 1873-1686

Westerink, J. & Visseren, F.L. (2011). Pharmacological and non-pharmacological interventions to influence adipose tissue function. *Cardiovascular Diabetology* Vol.10, No.1, pp. 13, ISSN 1475-2840

Williams, C.M., Rogers, P.J. & Kirkham, T.C. (1998). Hyperphagia in pre-fed rats following oral delta9-THC. *Physiology and Behavior* Vol.65, No.2, pp. 343-346, ISSN 0031-9384

Williams, C.M. & Kirkham, T.C. (1999). Anandamide induces overeating: mediation by central cannabinoid (CB1) receptors. *Psychopharmacology* Vol.143, No.3, pp. 315-317, ISSN 1432-2072

Williams, C.M. & Kirkham, T.C. (2002). Reversal of delta 9-THC hyperphagia by SR141716 and naloxone but not dexfenfluramine. *Pharmacology, Biochemistry and Behavior* Vol.71, No.1-2, pp. 333-340, ISSN 0091-3057

Wisse, B.E., Ogimoto, K., Schwartz, M.W. (2006). Role of hypothalamic interleukin-1beta (IL-1beta) in regulation of energy homeostasis by melanocortins. *Peptides* Vol.27, No.2, p. 265-273, ISSN: 0196-9781

Wittmann, G., Deli, L., Kalló, I., Hrabovszky, E., Watanabe, M., Liposits, Z., Fekete, C. (2007). Distribution of type 1 cannabinoid receptor (CB1)-immunoreactive axons in the mouse hypothalamus. *The Journal of Comparative Neurolology* Vol.503, No.2, pp. 270-9, ISSN 1096-9861

Yoshida, R., Ohkuri, T., Jyotaki, M., Yasuo, T., Horio, N., Yasumatsu, K., Sanematsu, K., Shigemura, N., Yamamoto, T., Margolskee, R.F., Ninomiya, Y. (2010). Endocannabinoids selectively enhance sweet taste. *Proceedings of the National Academy of Sciences of the United States of America* Vol.107, No.2, pp. 935-939, ISSN 0027-8424

Yukimura, Y., Bray, G.A., Wolfsen, A.R. (1978). Some effects of adrenalectomy in the fatty rat. *Endocrinology* Vol. 103, No.5, pp. 1924-1928, ISSN 1945-7170

Zakrzewska, K.E., Cusin, I., Sainsbury, A., Rohner-Jeanrenaud, F., Jeanrenaud, B. (1997). Glucocorticoids as counterregulatory hormones of leptin: toward an understanding of leptin resistance. *Diabetes* Vol. 46, No. 4, pp. 717-719, ISSN 1939-327X

Zakrzewska, K.E., Cusin, I., Stricker-Krongrad, A., Boss, O., Ricquier, D., Jeanrenaud, B., Rohner-Jeanrenaud, F. (1999). Induction of obesity and hyperleptinemia by central glucocorticoid infusion in the rat. *Diabetes* Vol. 48, No. 2, pp. 365-370, ISSN 1939-327X

Permissions

The contributors of this book come from diverse backgrounds, making this book a truly international effort. This book will bring forth new frontiers with its revolutionizing research information and detailed analysis of the nascent developments around the world.

We would like to thank Dr. Xiaoxiao Qian, for lending her expertise to make the book truly unique. She has played a crucial role in the development of this book. Without her invaluable contribution this book wouldn't have been possible. She has made vital efforts to compile up to date information on the varied aspects of this subject to make this book a valuable addition to the collection of many professionals and students.

This book was conceptualized with the vision of imparting up-to-date information and advanced data in this field. To ensure the same, a matchless editorial board was set up. Every individual on the board went through rigorous rounds of assessment to prove their worth. After which they invested a large part of their time researching and compiling the most relevant data for our readers. Conferences and sessions were held from time to time between the editorial board and the contributing authors to present the data in the most comprehensible form. The editorial team has worked tirelessly to provide valuable and valid information to help people across the globe.

Every chapter published in this book has been scrutinized by our experts. Their significance has been extensively debated. The topics covered herein carry significant findings which will fuel the growth of the discipline. They may even be implemented as practical applications or may be referred to as a beginning point for another development. Chapters in this book were first published by InTech; hereby published with permission under the Creative Commons Attribution License or equivalent.

The editorial board has been involved in producing this book since its inception. They have spent rigorous hours researching and exploring the diverse topics which have resulted in the successful publishing of this book. They have passed on their knowledge of decades through this book. To expedite this challenging task, the publisher supported the team at every step. A small team of assistant editors was also appointed to further simplify the editing procedure and attain best results for the readers.

Our editorial team has been hand-picked from every corner of the world. Their multi-ethnicity adds dynamic inputs to the discussions which result in innovative outcomes. These outcomes are then further discussed with the researchers and contributors who give their valuable feedback and opinion regarding the same. The feedback is then collaborated with the researches and they are edited in a comprehensive manner to aid the understanding of the subject.

Apart from the editorial board, the designing team has also invested a significant amount of their time in understanding the subject and creating the most relevant covers. They scrutinized every image to scout for the most suitable representation of the subject and create an appropriate cover for the book.

The publishing team has been involved in this book since its early stages. They were actively engaged in every process, be it collecting the data, connecting with the contributors or procuring relevant information. The team has been an ardent support to the editorial, designing and production team. Their endless efforts to recruit the best for this project, has resulted in the accomplishment of this book. They are a veteran in the field of academics and their pool of knowledge is as vast as their experience in printing. Their expertise and guidance has proved useful at every step. Their uncompromising quality standards have made this book an exceptional effort. Their encouragement from time to time has been an inspiration for everyone.

The publisher and the editorial board hope that this book will prove to be a valuable piece of knowledge for researchers, students, practitioners and scholars across the globe.

List of Contributors

Rosalie M. Uht
Institute for Aging and Alzheimer's Disease Research and Department of Pharmacology and Neuroscience University of North Texas Health Science Center, USA

Xing-Ming Shi
Institute of Molecular Medicine and Genetics, Department of Pathology, Georgia Health Sciences University, Augusta, GA, USA

Norman Chutkan
Department of Orthopaedic Surgery, Georgia Health Sciences University, Augusta, GA, USA

Mark W. Hamrick
Departments of Cellular Biology & Anatomy and Orthopaedic Surgery, Georgia Health Sciences University, Augusta, GA, USA

Carlos M. Isales
Institute of Molecular Medicine and Genetics, Departments of Orthopaedic Surgery and Medicine, Georgia Health Sciences University, Augusta, GA, USA

Mingxi Tang
Department of Pathology, Luzhou Medical College, Sichuan, P. R. China

Anu Joseph, Qian Chen, Jianwei Jiao and Ya-Ping Tang
Department of Cell Biology and Anatomy, Louisiana State University Health Sciences Center, New Orleans, LA, USA

Anna-Mart Engelbrecht and Benjamin Loos
Dept of Physiological Sciences, Stellenbosch University, Stellenbosch, South Africa

Hümeyra Ünsal and Muharrem Balkaya
Adnan Menderes University, Faculty of Veterinary Medicine, Department of Physiology, Işikli, Aydin, Turkey

Feodora I. Kostadinova and Thomas Brunner
Division of Biochemical Pharmacology, Department of Biology, University of Konstanz, Germany

Nina Hostettler and Pamela Bianchi
Division of Experimental Pathology, Institute of Pathology, University of Bern, Switzerland

Ilhem Berrou, Marija Krstic-Demonacos, Constantinos Demonacos
University of Manchester, School of Pharmacy and Faculty of Life Sciences, Manchester, UK

Huapeng Fan and Eric F. Morand
Centre for Inflammatory Diseases, Monash University, Australia

Carine Smith
Stellenbosch University, South Africa

Fhionna R. Moore
School of Psychology, College of Art and Social Science, University of Dundee, UK

Liliya Nadolnik
Department of Bioregulators, Institute of Bioorganic Chemistry National Academy of Sciences of Belarus, Belarus

Silvia Graciela Ruginsk, Rodrigo Cesar Rorato, Beatriz de Carvalho Borges, Ernane Torres Uchoa, Lucila Leico Kagohara Elias and Jose Antunes-Rodrigues
Department of Physiology, School of Medicine of Ribeirao Preto, University of Sao Paulo, Brazil